Practical Surgery
Short Clinical Cases

Practical Surgery
Short Clinical Cases
(Diagnosis, Viva Voce and Discussion)

Third Edition

TC Goel

MBBS MS (Surgery)
Professor (Retd), Department of Surgery
King George's Medical University
Professor Emeritus, Career Institute Dental Sciences
Chief Consultant Surgeon, Mayo Medical Centre, Gomti Nagar
Consulting Surgeon, Satyashiv Hospital, Mahanagar Extension, Lucknow, Uttar Pradesh, India

Apul Goel

MBBS MS (Surgery) MCh (Urology)
Professor, Department of Urology
King George's Medical University, Lucknow, Uttar Pradesh, India

Foreword

Rama Kant

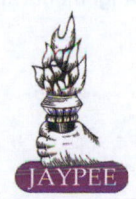

The Health Sciences Publisher

New Delhi | London | Philadelphia | Panama

Jaypee Brothers Medical Publishers (P) Ltd

Headquarters

Jaypee Brothers Medical Publishers (P) Ltd
4838/24, Ansari Road, Daryaganj
New Delhi 110 002, India
Phone: +91-11-43574357
Fax: +91-11-43574314
Email: jaypee@jaypeebrothers.com

Overseas Offices

J.P. Medical Ltd
83, Victoria Street, London
SW1H 0HW (UK)
Phone: +44-20 3170 8910
Fax: +44(0)20 3008 6180
Email: info@jpmedpub.com

Jaypee-Highlights Medical Publishers Inc
City of Knowledge, Bld. 237, Clayton
Panama City, Panama
Phone: +1 507-301-0496
Fax: +1 507-301-0499
Email: cservice@jphmedical.com

Jaypee Medical Inc
The Bourse
111 South Independence Mall East
Suite 835, Philadelphia, PA 19106, USA
Phone: +1 267-519-9789
Email: jpmed.us@gmail.com

Jaypee Brothers Medical Publishers (P) Ltd
17/1-B Babar Road, Block-B, Shaymali
Mohammadpur, Dhaka-1207
Bangladesh
Mobile: +08801912003485
Email: jaypeedhaka@gmail.com

Jaypee Brothers Medical Publishers (P) Ltd
Bhotahity, Kathmandu
Nepal
Phone: +977-9741283608
Email: kathmandu@jaypeebrothers.com

Website: www.jaypeebrothers.com
Website: www.jaypeedigital.com

Practical Surgery: Short Clinical Cases (Diagnosis, Viva Voce and Discussion)

First Edition: 1996

Second Edition: 1999

Third Edition: **2015**

ISBN 978-93-5152-678-0

Printed at Replika Press Pvt. Ltd.

Foreword

It is an honor and pleasure to write foreword for the book *Practical Surgery: Short Clinical Cases, (Diagnosis, Viva Voce and Discussion)* authored by Professor TC Goel and Professor Apul Goel. The book actually fulfills the void befitting exactly the need of students appearing in the final year or postgraduate examinations in surgery. This is based on their decades of experience as expert clinicians and both undergraduate and postgraduate examiners. Thus, with excellent format of discussion and photographs, I feel confident that examination may remain no more a scare and students will be greatly benefited by this excellent book.

With best regards.

Rama Kant MS FICS FLCS
Professor and Head (Retd)
Department of Surgery (General)
King George's Medical University,
Lucknow, Uttar Pradesh, India

Preface to the Third Edition

The response to previous two editions of *Practical Surgery: Short Clinical Cases* has been good. We thank the readers.

The whole book has been updated. Many chapters have been rewritten, and necessary corrections have been made.

The most important feature of this edition is addition of clinical photographs of patients, investigative pictures and line diagrams. The previous two editions have none of them.

Some more short cases have been added with clinical diagnosis, viva voce and discussion.

One new chapter on non-clinical practical examination is also added. It will guide the candidates through the non-clinical examination.

With best wishes.

TC Goel
Apul Goel

Preface to the First Edition

A short case constitutes an important part of the practical examination in surgery. Usually, three short cases are allotted to each candidate who has to make a clinical diagnosis, give reasons for making the diagnosis, tell about the investigations and treatment, and answer a few viva voce questions about the disease in question—everything in brief and in a limited time, as one does in surgical outpatient department of the hospital.

This book is prepared according to the requirements of the practical examination on short cases in surgery. The common cases that are seen frequently are described, as one requires to know for replying in the practical examination.

All the textbooks of surgery describe the details of all the diseases one sees or gets in the examination. Many times it becomes very difficult to give an exact or calculated answer to the questions asked by the examiners based on the knowledge obtained from these books. This book is an effort in that direction and prepares the candidate for giving accurate and to-the-point answers.

To appear in any examination is an art (apart from science and knowledge) and a medical student should master this art as he/she would face examinations and interviews more or less throughout life.

We hope this book will be helpful to the candidates who are appearing in various surgical practical examinations. We will welcome suggestions for improvement.

With best wishes.

TC Goel
Apul Goel

Acknowledgments

We remember with gratitude and great respect late Shri MK Garg who encouraged us and provided the basic facility to do medical writing work.

We are thankful to our friends and colleagues of King George's Medical University who have helped us by providing clinical pictures and investigation-records of various problems described in this book—Professor Sandeep Kumar, Professor D Dalela, Professor Ashish Wakhlu, Professor Rajiv Agarwal, Professor SP Agarwal, Professor KD Varma, Professor MN Mathur, Professor RK Tandon, Professor Divya Mehrotra, and Professor Sandeep Tewari.

These colleagues of Mayo Medical Centre, Gomti Nagar, Lucknow, Uttar Pradesh, have helped us—Dr PR Gupta, Dr Sunil Bisen, Dr Divya Narain, Dr Ajay Kr Chaudhary, Dr MK Srivastava, Dr Sushil Upadhyaya, Dr Uttam Garg, and Dr MK Srivastava (Oncology). We are grateful and thankful to them.

We also thank Professor RK Agrawal (Retd) and Professor AK Khare of Rabindranath Tagore Medical College, Udaipur, Rajasthan, who sent many interesting pictures of clinical problems. We are grateful to Dr GP Kaushal and Dr Suresh Talwar for help.

Dr SS Sarkar of Sarkar Diagnostic Institute sent us many interesting and investigative pictures. We gratefully acknowledge his help and thank him. We thank Sarkar Foundation for help.

We also acknowledge the encouragement and facilitation given by the Research Cell, King George's Medical University, Lucknow, Uttar Pradesh.

Mrs Aruna Goel (senior author's wife) did a lot of work with proofs. We thank her. Ms Alpana also helped in some computer work.

Mr Jai Prakash is our trusted and sincere computer associate who has done all the computer work. We are very thankful to him.

Mr Laxman, our office helper has kept us in constant contact with Mr Jai Prakash and many of our friends and helpers. We thank him.

We thank M/s Jaypee Brothers Medical Publishers (P) Ltd, New Delhi, for bringing this work to light.

Contents

A Short Case

A short case is one where the details of the history and the physical examination are not required for making a clinical diagnosis. Here, the diagnosis can be arrived on the basis of the patient's complaints and relevant and brief local examination.

Many times the diagnosis is made just by a look at the patient and a look at the lesion. It is called 'spot diagnosis'. It is the usual practice of making a clinical diagnosis in surgical outpatients in most of the hospitals.

In most of the clinical examination settings, 3 to 5 minutes per patient are allotted to a candidate for making a diagnosis, and for writing on the reply sheet—the diagnosis, the reasons for making it and the treatment in a few lines. For following this time-discipline the students should do this drill repeatedly during their clinical posting in surgical outdoor clinics.

Sample Reply Sheet

Diagnosis: Phimosis

Reasons: Prepuce cannot be retracted to expose the glans penis

Treatment: Circumcision

Usually the examiners do not see the reply sheet; they are more interested in taking the viva voce of the candidate. The 'Sheet' goes in the records of the examination office.

Cases given to us in practical examination

Senior author:

MBBS: Carcinoma of penis, umbilical hernia, leukoplakia of cheek

MS: Carcinoma of lip, femoral hernia, anal fissure

Junior author:

MBBS: Scrotal hydrocele, branchial cyst, osteomyelitic sinus

MS: Right oblique inguinal hernia, phimosis, sebaceous cyst

MCh: Stricture of urethra, pelviureteric junction obstruction, bladder tumor

Verbal Examination: The Viva Voce

Four questions are likely to be asked from a candidate on a short case:
1. What is your diagnosis?
2. What are the reasons for making this diagnosis?
3. Do you need any investigations? If yes, what are the investigations?
4. How will you treat this case?

Primary questions:

The four questions mentioned above are the primary questions as they are asked on every case from every candidate. Hence one must prepare and set the answers to these questions before the viva starts, so that one can give correct and to-the-point replies to these questions. Most of the time, the success in the practical clinical examination is determined by the replies given in response to these questions. Also, subsequently in the practical life as a doctor, one has to deal with or solve these four quaries throughout the clinical carrier.

Secondary questions:

These questions arise from the answers given in response to the primary questions. They are not asked from every candidate. If the primary questions are answered well then lesser number of secondary questions are asked. The examples of secondary questions are:

- From the answer to question no. 1.
  - What is this disease (name of the disease)?
  - How will you differentiate it from (some resembling disease)?
- From the answer to question no. 2.
  - What is the cause of (symptom or sign)?
  - How will you examine the patient to elicit this sign?
- From the answer to question no. 3.
  - What will you find on examination of blood?
  - What will you find on radiological investigations?
  - What are the endoscopic features of this disease?
- From the answer to question no. 4: The treatment of most of the surgical diseases is usually some surgical procedure. Hence, the examinee tells the name of the operation in response to this question. The secondary questions to this response are:
  - What is done in this operation?
  - What are the indications for this operation?
  - What will be the nature of anesthesia?
  - What are the complications of this operation?
  - What are the results of treatment?
  - Is there any non-operative or medical treatment?

It is not necessary that all of the secondary questions given above are asked from every candidate. The number of questions depends on the availability of time. The viva on short cases usually finishes with secondary questions.

There can be tertiary questions also which may arise from the answers given to secondary questions. They are rarely asked on a short case. They may be asked in a long case. Further, they may be asked from a candidate who is being considered for a position of merit.

If a candidate organizes himself/herself as suggested above and answers to the questions as described in the pages of this book, he/she is likely to come out of the practical clinical examination with a brilliant success.

With best wishes and best of luck.

Tumor or Tumor-like Swellings

CASE 1: LIPOMA

CLINICAL DIAGNOSIS

1. The patient presents with a painless, slow growing swelling anywhere where there is fat, especially head and neck area, abdominal wall and thigh (Fig. 1).
2. The surface is lobulated or smooth.
3. It is soft and may give a false sense of fluctuation (pseudo-fluctuation).
4. The edge is well defined and slips under the examining finger (slipping sign).
5. The overlying skin is free and cutaneous dimples appear on the surface when the swelling is pushed away.
6. It is not translucent.

VIVA VOCE

1. **What is a lipoma?**
   It is a benign tumor of fat composed of fat cells of adult type.
2. **What is the cause of dimples on the overlying skin when the swelling is pushed away?**
   It is because of the pull of fibrous strands which traverse the lipoma and are attached to overlying skin.
3. **What is a universal tumor?**
   A lipoma is called a 'universal tumor' because it can occur anywhere in the body where there is fat.
4. **What are the sites where it does not occur?**
   It does not occur inside the brain as there is no fat there.
5. **What are the anatomical types?**
   Anatomically, a lipoma can be of following types (Fig. 2):

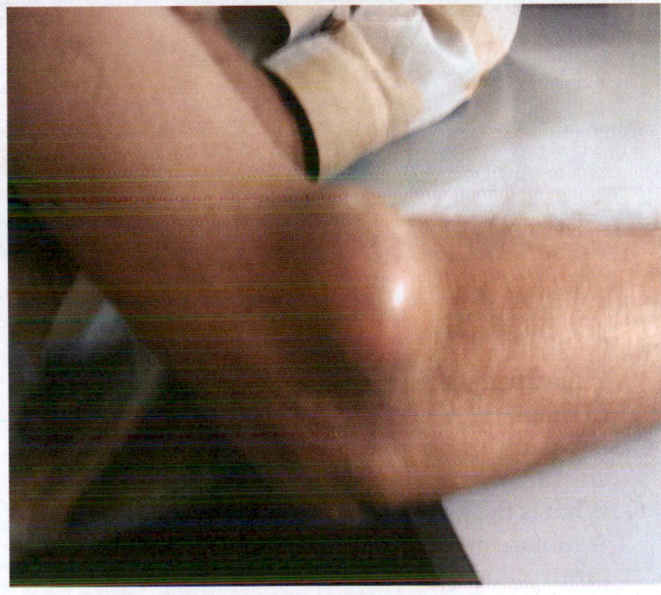

Fig. 1: Lipoma of the elbow region
(*Courtesy:* Dr MK Srivastava)

- Subcutaneous
- Subaponeurotic or subfascial
- Subserous
- Retroperitoneal
- Extradural
- Parosteal
- Intra-articular
- Intermuscular
- Intraglandular
- Intraosseous.

6. **What is lipoma arborescens?**
   It is a subcutaneous lipoma that is pedunculated.

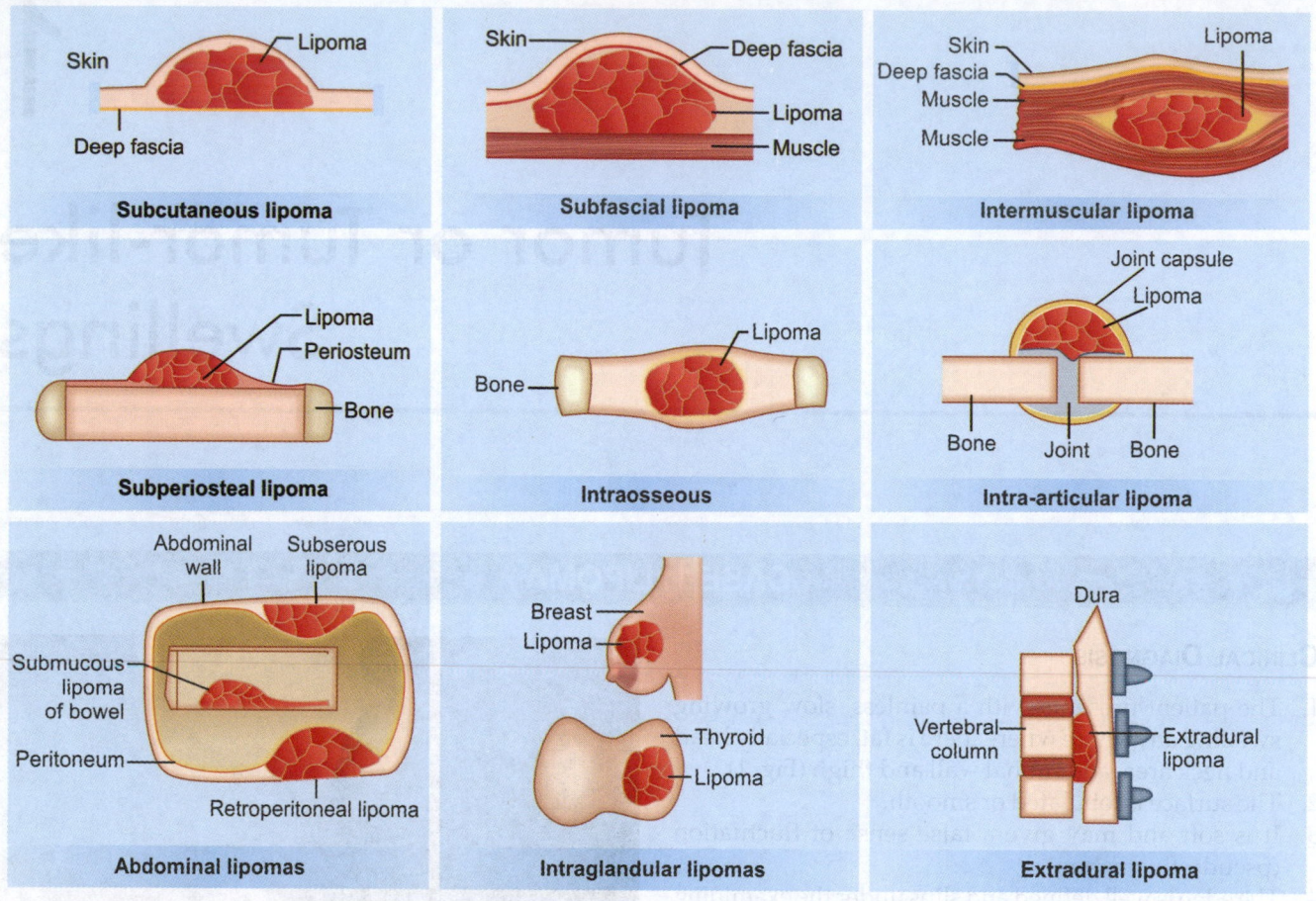

Fig. 2: Anatomical types of lipoma

7. **What are the sites of occurrence of a subaponeurotic lipoma?**
   It occurs under the palmar or plantar fascia or epicranial aponeurosis.

8. **What is the peculiarity of this type?**
   A subfascial lipoma, because of tough fascia, tends to ramify and go in between the tissue planes. A subepicranial lipoma may indent the underlying skull.

9. **Where does a submucous lipoma occur?**
   It occurs under the mucosa of respiratory or alimentary tract.

10. **How does a submucous lipoma of intestine present?**
    It is usually present with signs of intussusception.

11. **What is the site of occurrence of an extradural lipoma?**
    Spinal extradural space.

12. **Can the presence of a lipoma indicate the presence of a congenital abnormality?**
    Yes, a lipoma may be present over the site of spina bifida occulta.

13. **Does a lipoma have a capsule?**
    A localized lipoma is usually encapsulated, while a diffuse one does not have a capsule.

14. **What is a fibrolipoma?**
    It has a mixture of fibrous and fatty tissues.

15. **What are the clinical signs of a nevolipoma?**
    This lipoma has a mixture of hemangiomatous and fatty tissues.

16. **What are the clinical signs of a nevolipoma?**
    The clinical signs are:
    - Bluish discoloration of overlying skin
    - It blanches on pressure
    - It is partially compressible.

17. **What is a neurolipoma?**
    It contains a mixture of nerve and adipose tissue.

18. **What is Dercum's disease?**
    It is associated with multiple, painful and diffuse or nodular deposits of fat (neurolipomatosis).

19. **What is a hibernoma?**
    A variant of lipoma presenting as benign solitary swelling on the back of children or adults and

comprising of brown fat cells similar to those found in hibernating animals.

20. What is a pedunculated lipoma?

Some lipomas, especially those of gluteal region or thigh develop a peduncle with passage of time when the lipoma hangs like a tomato on its pedicle. It is called pedunculated lipoma (Fig. 3).

21. What are the complications?

A lipoma can have many complications:
- Malignant transformation into a liposarcoma
- Myxomatous degeneration
- Saponification
- Calcification
- Ulceration.

22. Are these complications common?

No, they occur only occasionally.

23. Which lipomas are likely to undergo malignant change?

The lipomas that may undergo malignant change are:
- Retroperitoneal lipoma
- Lipoma of thigh, especially the intermuscular type
- Lipoma of shoulder region.

24. What are the investigations?

The diagnosis can be confirmed by FNAC. Deep-seated lipomas can be seen by imaging methods, e.g. a retroperitoneal lipoma by CT scan (Fig. 4), a large lipoma may cast a soft tissue shadow on radiography (Fig. 5).

25. How do you treat a lipoma?

It is treated by excision (Fig. 6).

26. Do all lipomas require surgical excision?

No, surgical excision is particularly indicated if the lipoma is large, unsightly or troublesome.

27. What are the complications of excision?

The complications are:
- Hematoma, seroma (commonest)
- Wound infection
- Flap necrosis.

28. Do you know of any recent development in the treatment?

Yes, recently lipomas have been removed by suction lipolysis through a small incision.

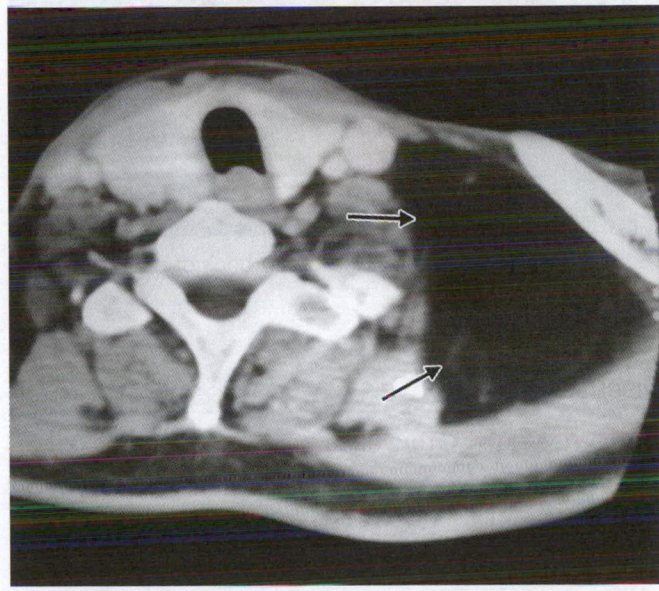

Fig. 4: CT scan showing a supraclavicular lipoma extending into the chest. Fat looks hypodense on CT scan

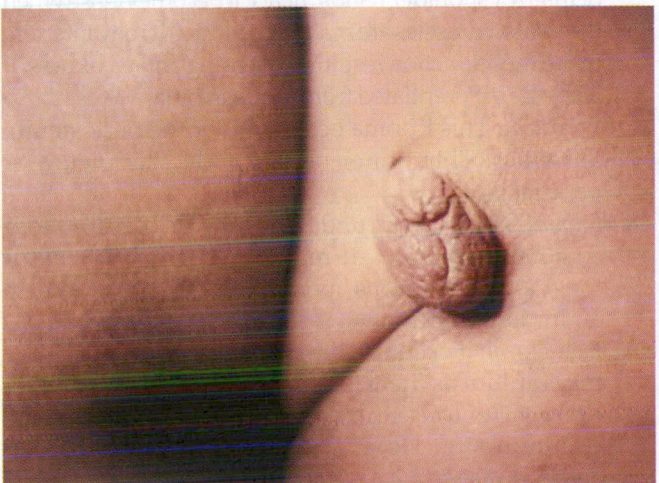

Fig. 3: Pedunculated lipoma of gluteal region

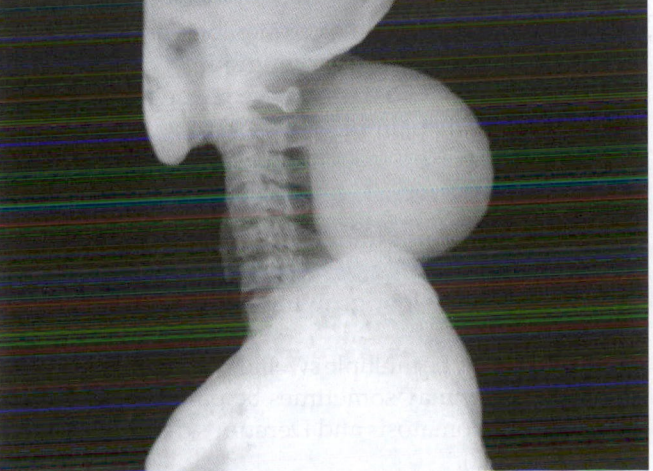

Fig. 5: Radiograph of the neck, lateral view showing a large, round soft tissue shadow at nape of neck. The cervical spine has lost its normal anterior convexity. Lipoma of nape of neck

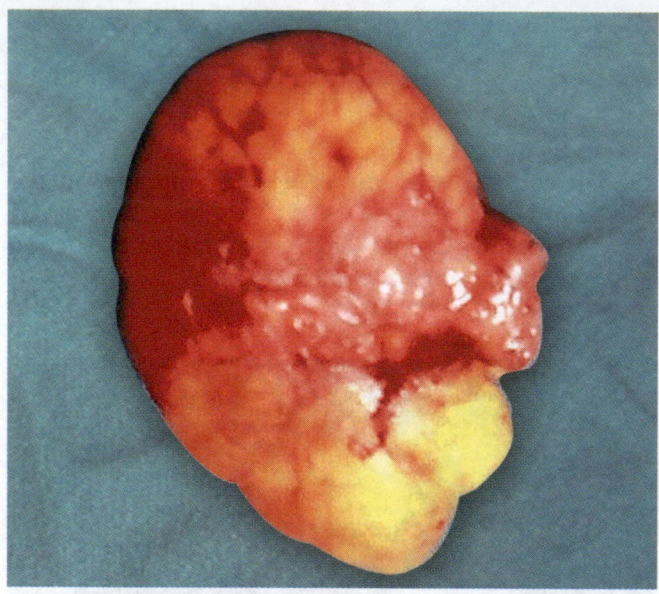

Fig. 6: Lipoma (excised from back of chest)

DISCUSSION

Lipoma is a slowly growing tumor composed of fat cells of adult type.

Etiology: Not known.

Pathology: It contains normal fat that is arranged in lobules separated by fibrous septa enclosed in a delicate capsule. From the capsule, fibrous bands pass to the overlying skin. This is the reason for dimpling of the skin when the tumor is moved. Other histological types of lipoma are:

1. Fibrolipoma: It contains excessive amount of fibrous tissue.
2. Nevolipoma: It contains considerable vascularity often with telangiectasis of overlying skin.
3. Neurolipoma: It contains nerve tissue in addition to fat. It is usually painful.

Clinical Features

- **Age and sex:** This tumor can affect anybody.
- **Symptoms**
  1. A painless slow growing swelling of insidious onset.
  2. There may be multiple swelling of small or moderate size; they may sometimes be painful as occurs in neurolipomatosis and Dercum's disease (adiposis dolorosa).

- **Signs**
  1. It can occur anywhere in the body where fat is found (universal or ubiquitous tumor), especially head and neck area, abdominal wall and thigh.
  2. The size is variable.
  3. The surface is usually lobulated but may be smooth.
  4. It is soft and a sense of fluctuation (pseudofluctuation) may be obtained.
  5. It has a definite edge that slips under the finger.

Anatomical Types

1. *Subcutaneous:* It is the commonest type and can occur anywhere in the body especially in the shoulder region or back. It is commonly present over the site of spina bifida occulta. It is usually hemispherical and sessile. It may occasionally become pedunculated when it is called as lipoma arborescens.
2. *Subfascial:* This type of lipoma occurs under the palmar or plantar fascia or epicranial aponeurosis. In the hand or foot, it may be mistaken for tuberculous tenosynovitis as the tough fascia covering it masks the lobulation and edge of the tumor. Further, because of tough fascia, the tumor tends to ramify and go in various tissue planes. A lipoma of areolar layer under the epicranial aponeurosis may erode the underlying bone producing a depression in the skull.
3. *Intra-articular:* It occurs inside a joint and is extremely rare.
4. *Subsynovial:* It occurs under the synovial membrane in the fat pad. It is usually seen in the knee joint where it can be confused with Morrant Baker's cyst or bursitis.
5. *Intermuscular:* This tumor occurs in between the muscles of thigh or shoulder region, hence it becomes tense when the related muscles are made to contract. It may interfere in the muscle action resulting in aching and weakness. It has to be differentiated from fibrosarcoma.
6. *Parosteal:* This lipoma occurs under the periosteum.
7. *Subserous:* This tumor occurs under the pleura or peritoneum.
8. *Submucous:* It occurs under the mucosa of respiratory or alimentary tract. It may occur in the larynx or tongue. A submucous lipoma of intestine may initiate an intussusception.
9. *Extradural:* It occurs in the spinal space but not inside the cranium as there is no fat there.
10. *Retroperitoneal:* Retroperitoneum is one of the common site. Here, a lipoma can grow into an enormous size.

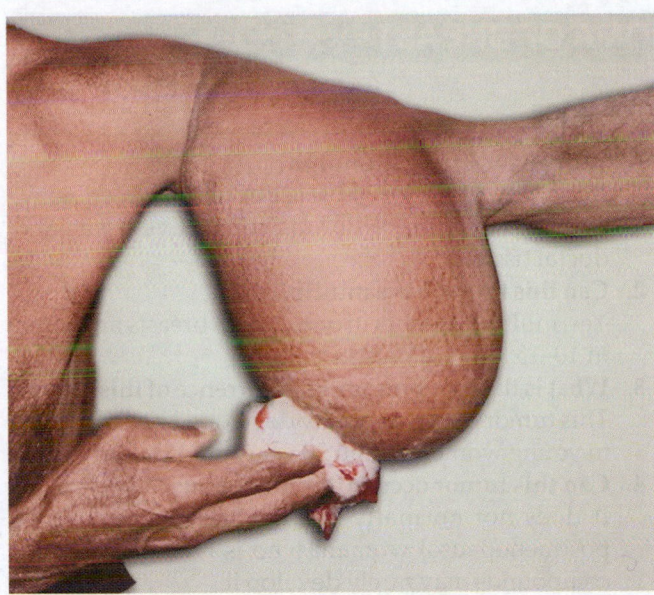

Fig. 7: Liposarcoma of left upper arm. This patient has a lipoma for 11 years which is growing rapidly in size for one year. It has ulcerated

11. *Intraglandular:* A lipoma can rarely occur in pancreas, kidney (subcapsular) or breast.

Compliactions

1. *Sarcomatous change:* It occurs occasionally in large lipomas of thigh, shoulder region and retroperitoneum (Fig. 7).
2. Myxomatous degeneration.
3. Saponification.
4. Calcification.

Treatment

- If it is causing symptoms or some troubles, it should be excised. It confirms the diagnosis and restores normal skin contour.
- It can also be removed by suction lipolysis that is a minimally invasive technique.

CASE 2: FIBROADENOMA OF BREAST

CLINICAL DIAGNOSIS

1. The patient is usually a young girl or woman 15 to 25 years of age who presents with a painless and slow growing swelling of the breast of insidious onset.
2. It is discrete, nontender, firm or hard and often almond shaped (Figs 8 and 9).
3. It is freely mobile and may be lost in the breast from time to time (breast mouse), if the breast is large.
4. The regional lymph nodes are normal.

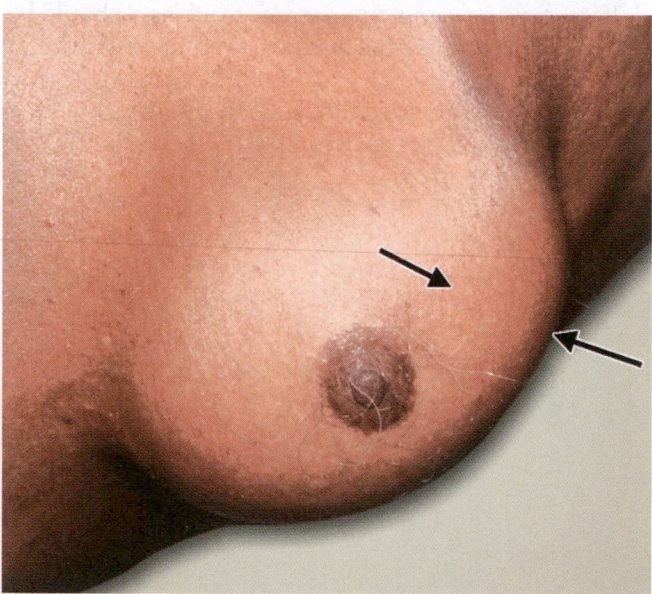

Fig. 8: Fibroadenoma of upper and outer quadrant of the breast where the breast is somewhat more prominent. This tumor is usually not visible but palpable, because of its small size in proportion to the size of breast

VIVA VOCE

1. **What is a fibroadenoma?**
   It is a benign tumor of breast of unknown etiology, having a mixture of fibrous connective tissue and ductal tissue.
2. **Can this tumor have multiplicity?**
   Yes, multiple tumors in one or both breasts are found in 10–15% of patients.
3. **What is the common age of occurrence of this tumor?**
   This tumor occurs in a fully developed breast mostly in young women within 20 years after puberty.
4. **Can this tumor occur after menopause?**
   It does not normally occur after menopause. A postmenopausal woman, who is taking estrogenic compounds may rarely develop it.
5. **What investigations will you do in this tumor?**
   Apart from routine investigations no other specific investigation is required. FNAC may be done as it confirms the diagnosis. The tumor and its extent can be seen by mammography (Fig. 10).
6. **Will you like to biopsy the tumor?**
   It is usually not required; if required FNAC may be done. After excision of this tumor, the whole specimen is sent for histopathological examination.
7. **What are the complications of this disease?**
   Usually, there are no complications.
8. **Will it not undergo malignant change?**
   Malignant change is very rare.

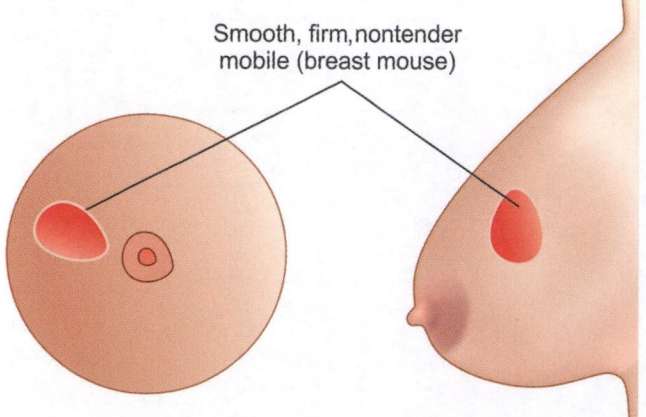

Smooth, firm, nontender mobile (breast mouse)

Fig. 9: Fibroadenoma of breast

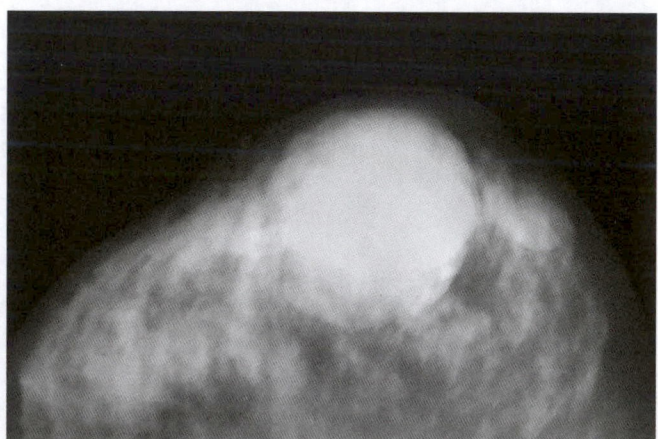

Fig. 10: Mammogram showing a large fibroadenoma of left breast

9. **How do you treat a fibroadenoma?**
   A small fibroadenoma need not be treated. A large fibroadenoma is excised through a cosmetically appropriate incision.

10. **What are the complications of this operation?**
    The complications are:
    - Hematoma
    - Seroma
    - Wound infection
    - Gaping of the wound.

11. **What is cystosarcoma phylloides?**
    It is a type of fibroadenoma with cellular stroma that tends to grow rapidly and attain a large size. It is usually a benign tumor and rarely malignant. It occurs in women over 40 years of age (Fig. 11).

12. **Why is this name?**
    It is now called phylloid tumor as it is rarely cystic and usually not malignant (sarcoma). It is a type of fibroadenoma with cellular stroma that tends to grow rapidly.

13. **What are the clinical signs of a phylloid tumor?**
    The patient has a massive swelling of the breast which has an unevenly bosselated surface with prominent veins. It is firm, nontender and mobile on the chest wall (Fig. 11).

14. **How do you treat this tumor?**
    It is treated by local excision of the mass with a margin of surrounding breast tissue.

15. **What will happen if it is excised inadequately?**
    There will be local recurrence.

16. **Which histological component of a malignant phylloid tumor is malignant?**

The stromal component is malignant (sarcoma) and not the epithelial one.

17. **How do you treat a malignant phylloid tumor?**
    It is treated by complete excision with a rim of normal tissue around. Sometime, simple mastectomy is required.

DISCUSSION

Fibroadenoma of breast is a benign local tumor of unknown etiology having glandular and mesenchymal elements. It has a relationship to estrogen sensitivity. It arises from hyperplasia of a single lobule and usually grows up to 2 to 3 cm in size.

Pathology

Gross: It is characteristic with sharp circumscription and smooth boundaries. The cut surface is glistening white. If epithelial elements are excessive, they may appear as light brown areas. This tumor is surrounded by a well defined capsule from which it can be enucleated (Fig. 12).

Microscopic: Fibrous tissue composes most of the lesion; the stroma may surround rounded and easily definable duct-like epithelial structures or epithelium may be skewed into a curvilinear arrangement (Fig. 13).

Clinical Features

1. The patient is usually in second or third decade of life and presents with a painless and slow growing lump in the breast of insidious onset.

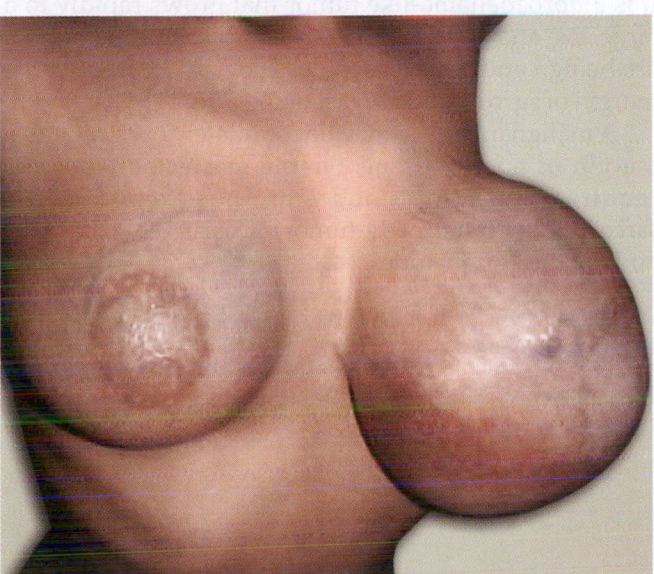

Fig. 11: Phylloid tumor of left breast
(*Courtesy:* Professor Sandeep Kumar)

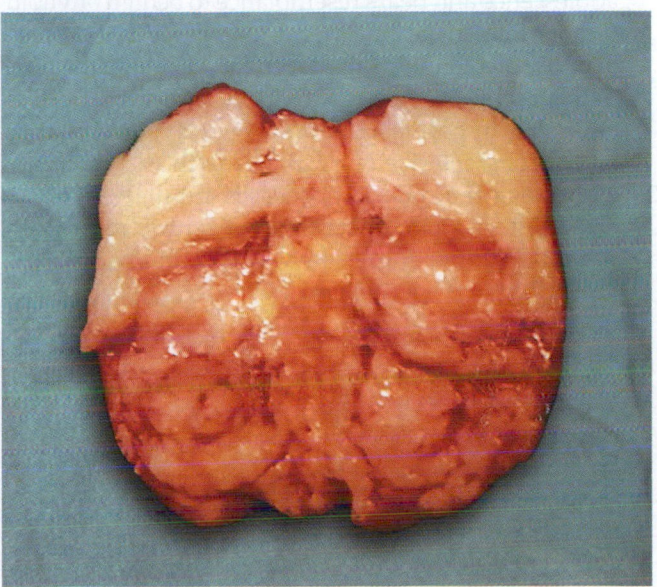

Fig. 12: Opened-up fibroadenoma of breast

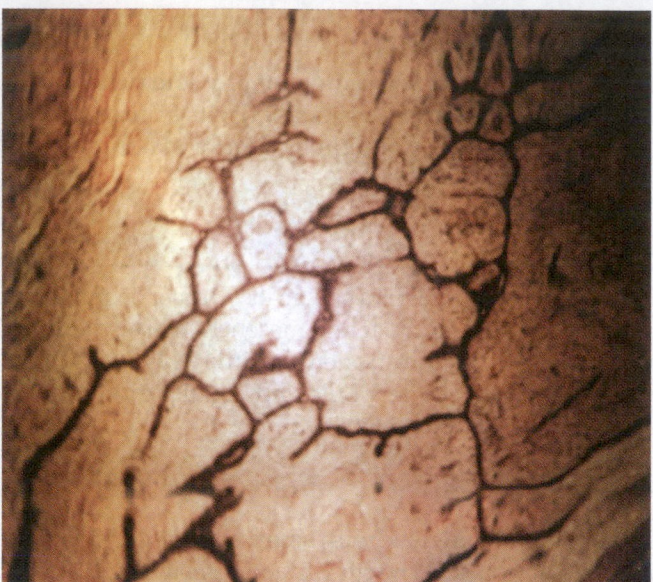

Fig. 13: Microscopic appearance of a fibroadenoma of breast
(*Courtesy:* Professor PK Agarwal)

2. It is discrete, nontender, firm or hard and often almond shaped.
3. It is freely mobile and may be lost in the breast tissue from time to time.
4. The regional lymph nodes are normal.

Variants

1. **Adolescent cellular fibroadenoma:** It has increased cellularity of stroma and/or epithelium, occurs in adolescence and bears resemblance to benign phylloid tumors, thus suggesting a term 'juvenile adenofibroma'. 5 to 10% of adenofibromas occur at and about the time of menarche; they frequently have a ductal pattern of epithelial hyperplasia and stromal hypercellularity and are characterized by rapid growth.
2. **Tubular adenoma:** It possesses tubular elements arranged in a circumscribed concentric mass with minimal supporting stroma. It has fine nodularity, uniform tubular structures and the absence of lobular anatomy.

The lactating adenoma is analogous to tubular adenoma and represents the physiologic response to pregnancy.

Investigations

1. Mammography: It is usually not required as the diagnosis is obvious clinically (Fig. 10).
2. FNAC or needle biopsy confirms the diagnosis.

Complications

It may evolve into a phylloid tumor but does not undergo malignant change.

Treatment

- A small tumor may be left as such
- The indications for excision are: suspicious cytology, very large tumor or if the patient wants the tumor to be removed.

  The tumor is excised through a cosmetically appropriate incision
- Newer methods of treatment:
  1. Vacuum-assisted core needle removal with pathological examination of specimen.
  2. Cryoablation or freezing: It is not appropriate for large fibroadenomas or if the diagnosis is not certain.

Phylloid Tumor

It is a fibroadenoma-like tumor that grows rapidly to a large size and has a cellular stroma. Most of the tumors are benign and have a capsule. They are excised with a margin of surrounding breast tissue (Fig. 11).

A malignant tumor may be completely excised with a margin of normal tissue. Simple mastectomy may be required, but lymph nodes are not excised as the sarcomatous portion of the tumor metastasizes to the lungs and not the lymph nodes.

CASE 3: KELOID

CLINICAL DIAGNOSIS

1. The patient presents with painless and progressive enlargement of a scar usually associated with itching.
2. It may be the scar of burn, cut, prick or operation.
3. It can occur anywhere but commonly seen in front of the sternum, face, ear lobule and neck (Figs 14 and 15).
4. It is pink and smooth with fine capillaries at the edge of the swelling.
5. It is firm and irregular with claw-like processes invading into healthy skin.

VIVA VOCE

1. **What is a keloid?**
   Keloid is a tumor-like swelling arising from connective tissue elements of the dermis and growing beyond the margins of the original injury or scar.
2. **What is the cause of this problem?**
   It is not exactly known. Probably, it is due to inhibition of maturation and stabilization of collagen fibrils.
3. **What are the predisposing factors?**
   The predisposing factors are:
   - Site of scar, vertical scar in the neck and ear lobule are common sites
   - Nature: Vaccination scars and scar of burns are more prone for keloid formation
   - Race: Negroes are commonly affected.
   - Tuberculous diathesis: It is common in patients of tuberculosis
   - Pregnancy: Sometimes keloids occur on the scars of the wounds inflicted during pregnancy.
4. **How do you differentiate a keloid from a hypertrophied scar?**
   The differences are as follows:

Differentiating feature	Keloid	Hypertrophied scar
Growth	Continues to grow beyond the scar into normal tissues	Does not grow after sometime (6 months) and never beyond the limits of scar
Vascularity	More vascular	Less vascular
Itching	Usually present	Usually absent
Tenderness	Margins may be tender	Nontender
Histology	Contains thick collagen and increased levels of epidermal hyaluronic acid	Nodular microscopic structure with fine collagen bundles and increased levels of α-actin

5. **What is the microscopic picture?**
   Microscopically, it contains thick collagen with a higher than usual proportion of type III collagen, immature fibroblasts and immature blood vessels.

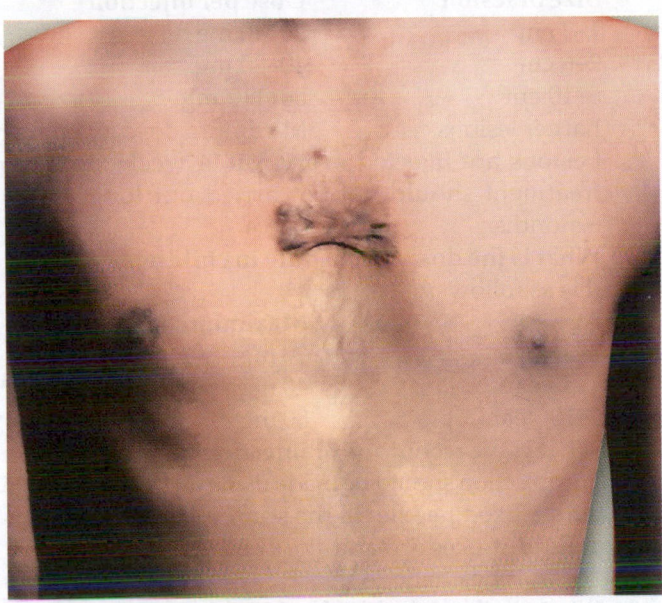

Fig. 14: Keloid of presternal region

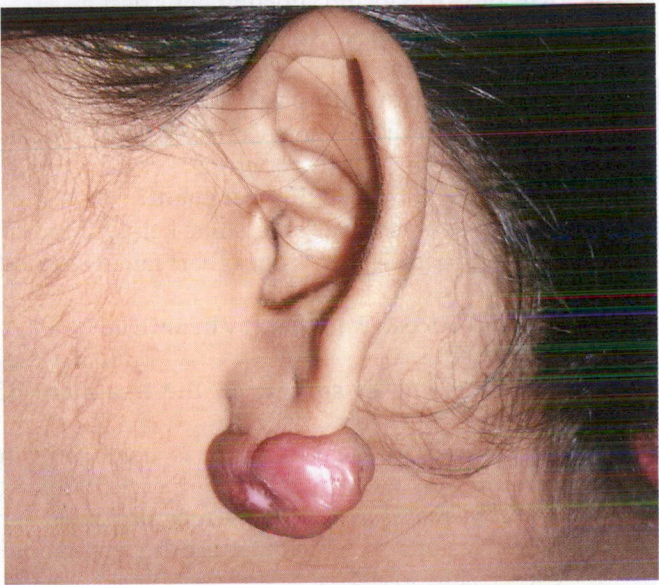

Fig. 15: Keloid of lobule of external ear
(*Courtesy:* Professor Rajiv Agarwal)

6. **How do you treat a keloid?**
A keloid is treated by a variety of methods including intrakeloidal injection of triamcinolone acetonide, surgical excision and radiotherapy, the treatment of choice being the first one.

7. **What is the dosage schedule of steroid injection?**
The following is the dosage schedule:

Size of lesion	Dose per injection
1–2 cm²	20–40 mg
2–6 cm²	40–80 mg
6–10 cm²	80–110 mg
Larger lesions	Maximum dose 120 mg

Lesions are injected every 3 to 4 weeks, and the treatment should not be carried out longer than 6 months.

8. **What is the dosage schedule in children?**
It is as follows:

Age	Maximum dose
1–2 years	20 mg
3–5 years	40 mg
6–10 years	80 mg

9. **What is the technique of injection?**
The injection should be made using an insulin syringe with a fixed needle till the scar becomes white. It is painful procedure and the children may require a general anesthetic.

10. **What are the risks involved in this treatment?**
The complications of this procedure are:
- Atrophy of skin and subcutaneous tissue
- Depigmentation
- Telangiectasia.

11. **What is the cause of atrophy?**
It happens if the drug is given too frequently or in too high a dose or into the hypodermis.

12. **What is the response to this treatment?**
The response is very variable, some keloids become flat after 2 to 3 injections, while others fail to respond at all.

13. **Is topical corticosteroid therapy beneficial?**
It is of no value.

14. **What is the role of surgery in the treatment of keloids?**
- At present surgical excision is used only in conjunction with intralesional corticosteroid therapy. Excision is usually recommended for larger lesions in which steroid therapy would exceed safe dosages
- When surgical excision is being done, care should be taken so as not to extend into the normal skin around the keloid as the growth of a new keloid may occur in new scars (intralesional excision).

15. **What is the schedule of corticosteroid therapy with surgical excision?**
The wound is injected at the time of excision and subsequently postoperatively in the schedule already described.

16. **What is the role of radiation therapy?**
Radiotherapy is also effective. Hence, can be used in intractable keloids. It may cause radiation injury, especially in young patients. It may be given after excision to reduce the recurrence rate.

17. **How will you treat a keloid of ear lobule?**
These keloids are usually of such a size as to require surgical excision. Postoperatively, prompt application of pressure clip on ear rings may be effective in preventing recurrence.

18. **How will you treat keloids of the sternal region?**
Butterfly presternal keloids (Fig. 14) may be treated by shaving the scar to its base and application of split skin graft. It should be followed by the use of a properly fitting pressure garment.
If the keloid is small, it may be left as such or given intralesional corticosteroids.

19. **How do you prevent keloid formation in a keloid-prone person?**
Prompt application of pressure on a scar is the most effective prophylactic measure. It requires the use of properly fitting elastic pressure garment that may need to be worn continuously for up to 1-year.

20. **How does the pressure help?**
It helps by increasing collagenase activity and decreasing collagen synthesis.

21. **What is the role of silicon dressing or oil?**
It is better for a hypertrophic scar than a keloid. It probably works through an immune mechanism.

DISCUSSION

Keloid is a hypertrophic scar arising from the connective tissue elements of the dermis and growing beyond the margins of original scar.

Etiology

- They may develop months or years after injury, often apparently in response to hormonal stimuli at puberty or during pregnancy
- *Skin type:* Dark-skinned people, especially of African genetic origin are 15 times more likely to have them. They have never occurred in albino skin.
- *Familial occurrence:* Both autosomal recessive and dominant inheritance is seen. They may occur in Ehlers-Danlos syndrome and scleroderma

- *Site and lie of the scar:* Scars of cuts across the Langer's lines, e.g. a vertical scar in the neck, are more prone to this lesion
- *Nature of scar:* Vaccination scars and scars of burns are more likely to become keloidal.

Pathology

- A keloid is associated with abnormal collagen metabolism resulting in a higher than usual proportion of type III collagen
- A keloid is more likely to develop in wounds that undergo inflammation without resolution for over 3 weeks and associated with tissue hypoxia and sustained levels of transforming growth factor (TGF) β_1 and β_2 (rather than TGF β_3) within the wound
- Histologically, it contains thick collagen and has increased levels of epidermal hyaluronic acid. There occurs proliferation of immature fibroblasts and also immature blood vessels.

Clinical Features

This disease is frequently a familial condition and occurs more commonly in females. The patient presents with painless and progressive enlargement of a scar of burn, cut, prick or operation. It can occur anywhere but commonly seen in front of sternum, face and neck (Fig. 15).

It is pink and smooth with fine capillaries at the edge of the swelling. It is firm, may be tender, and irregular with claw-like processes invading into healthy skin.

Complications

1. Recurrence: The most characteristic feature of a keloid is recurrence after excision.

2. It never undergoes malignant change.

Treatment

Keloid is a difficult condition to treat.

1. Pressure from massage or compressive dressings: It is the simplest treatment. It helps by increasing collagenase activity and decreasing collagen synthesis. It can be used as a preventive measure in patients who are prone for keloid formation.
2. Silicon dressing or oil: It has a better effect on a hypertrophic scar than on a keloid. It probably helps via an immune mechanism.
3. Intralesional injection of triamcinolone results in atrophy of the keloid. One should be careful not to inject into the hypodermis for fear of hypodermal fat atrophy. It may be combined with cryotherapy to improve the effectivity.
4. Radiotherapy is also effective. It may be considered for intractable keloids. But one must be careful in using it in young patients as they are likely to live long enough to develop the long-term sequel of radiation injury.
5. Surgical excision: The keloids can be excised but the wound should be closed without tension using a local flap. It has a 50 to 80 percent recurrence rate. To reduce the recurrence rate, excision may be combined with intralesional steroid injection preoperatively and post-operatively or with radiation treatment. Local pressure may also be applied following excision for at least 2 months.

Intralesional excision: It is excision of keloid leaving the rim of the original scar behind. It has a lower recurrence rate and suboptimal cosmesis. It may be just fooling the scar into not knowing that it has been mostly excised.

CASE 4: PLEOMORPHIC ADENOMA OF PAROTID

CLINICAL DIAGNOSIS

1. The patient is usually a middle-aged person, commonly a male, who presents with a painless and slow growing swelling in the parotid region (Figs 16 and 17).

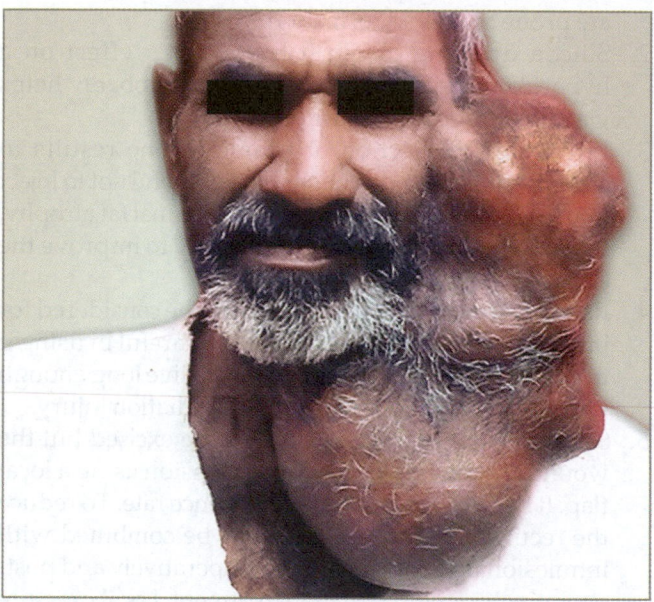

Fig. 16: A large pleomorphic adenoma of left parotid. Facial nerve intact, mobile, firm, lobulated swelling, no lymphadenopathy

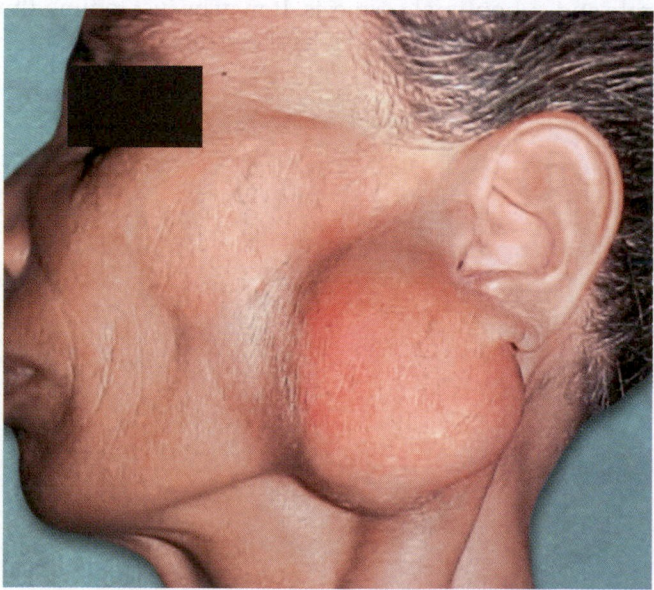

Fig. 17: Pleomorphic adenoma of left parotid gland (*Courtesy:* Professor Sandeep Kumar)

2. It is commonly situated a little in front of and above the angle of the jaw.
3. It is lobulated or smooth, firm, mobile, nontender and well-defined.
4. The overlying skin is free.
5. The ear lobule is displaced outward and upwards.
6. The facial nerve is normal.
7. The regional lymph nodes are not enlarged.

VIVA VOCE

1. **What is a pleomorphic adenoma?**
   It is a benign tumor of salivary tissue having a pleomorphic stroma.
2. **What do you mean by pleomorphic stroma?**
   This tumor has pseudocartilaginous, lymphoid, myxomatous and fibrous elements apart from epithelial cells.
3. **What is the cause of this tumor?**
   It is not known.
4. **What do you know about the origin of this tumor?**
   There are two views:
   - It arises from invagination of oral ectoderm into the salivary glands.
   - It is a true adenoma of salivary tissue and not a true mixed tumor.
5. **What are the sites of occurrence?**
   This tumor can arise from any salivary gland; 90 percent of the tumors occur in the parotid gland.
6. **What is its incidence in submandibular gland?**
   7 percent of adenomas occur in submandibular gland.
7. **What is the nature of this tumor?**
   It is a benign tumor.
8. **If it is a benign tumor, then why should it recur so frequently following excision?**
   It recurs because of the following reasons:
   - It has got an incomplete capsule.
   - There are tiny excrescences projecting from the tumor into the healthy glandular tissue which are left behind after enucleation.
9. **What is its gross appearance?**
   The tumor is a fleshy and rubbery resilient mass with bosselated surface. Cut surface shows a somewhat glistening, mucoid appearance with zones of apparent cartilage. It has a pseudocapsule and some fringe of tumor mass may protrude through the capsule and invade the adjoining areas.
10. **What is the microscopic picture?**
    Microscopically, it shows great variations. The epithelial elements are spheroidal, columnar,

squamous, basal or glandular while the stroma is fibrous or mucinous (pseudocartilage) (Fig. 18).

11. Why is it 'pseudocartilage'?

The 'cartilage' is not mesodermal in origin but is mucin or pseudomucin secreted by the epithelial cells which when stained resembles cartilage.

12. What is the commonest site of occurrence in the parotid gland?

Most of the tumors arise in the superficial lobe below the ear or in front of the ear.

13. Apart from major salivary glands does this tumor occur at other sites?

Yes, it can occur in the minor salivary glands of the oral mucosa.

14. What is the commonest site of occurrence in the minor glands?

The minor salivary glands of palate (Fig. 19).

15. What are the complications of this tumor?

It may undergo malignant transformation.

16. What are the signs of malignant change?

The signs of malignant transformation are:
- It becomes painful.
- It grows rapidly.
- It becomes hard in consistency.
- It loses its mobility by fixing to overlying skin and or underlying masseter.
- It involves facial nerve.
- The regional lymph nodes may be enlarged.
- It may ulcerate or fungate out.

17. How do you confirm the diagnosis?

Diagnosis is mostly clinical, but FNAC may be done.

18. Will you like to do incisional biopsy?

Incisional biopsy must not be done.

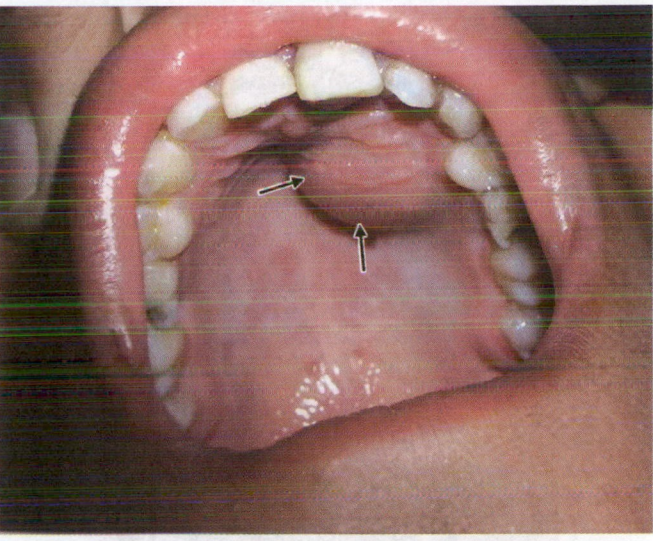

Fig. 19: Pleomorphic adenoma of minor salivary glands of palate (*Courtesy:* Professor Divya Mehrotra)

19. What is the role of CT scan/MRI?

These methods are used to see the anatomical details of the tumor, especially the tumors of the deep lobe.

20. How do you treat a pleomorphic adenoma of parotid?

It is treated by superficial parotidectomy.

21. What do you do in this operation?

After identifying the facial nerve and its branches (pes anserina) the superficial part of the gland is dissected from the underlying tissue and excised with the tumor (Figs 20 and 21).

22. What do you do to the facial nerve?

It is saved by careful dissection. A nerve stimulator may be used during the operation.

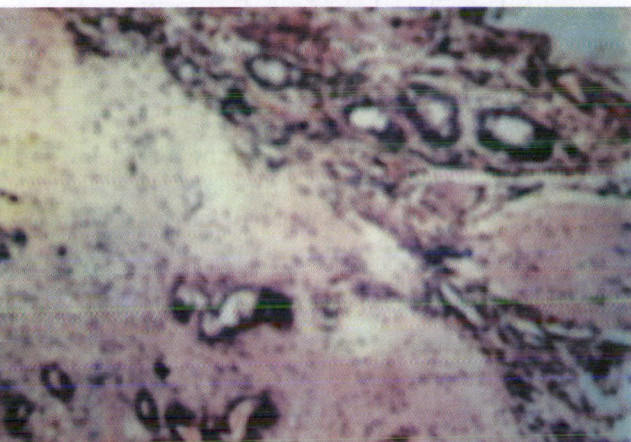

Fig. 18: Pleomorphic adenoma consisting of acini, myxomatous tissue and chondroid tissue (*Courtesy:* Professor PK Agarwal)

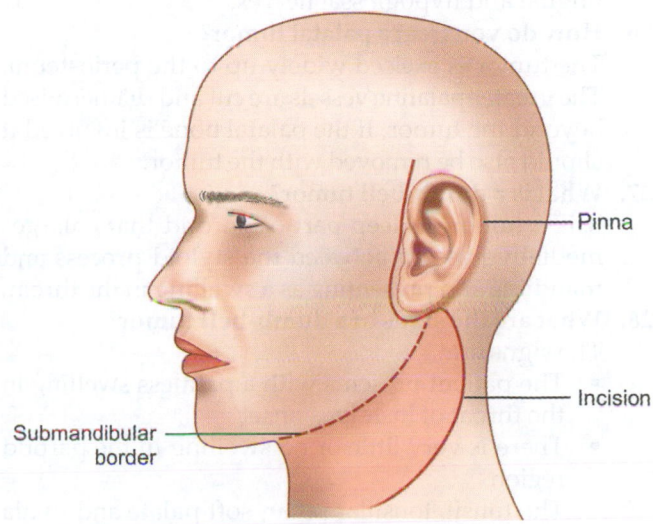

Fig. 20: Incision for superficial parotidectomy

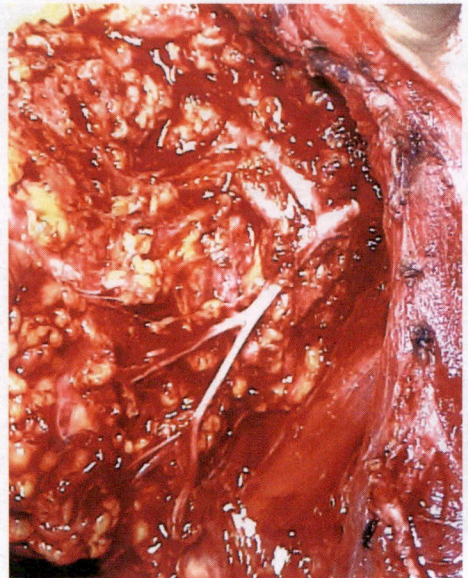

Fig. 21: Appearance of the wound after superficial parotidectomy with intact pes anserina (*Courtesy:* Professor Sandeep Kumar)

23. How do you make sure of that the whole tumor has been removed?

The excised tissue is examined histologically immediately by frozen section to make sure of complete excision of tumor.

24. What are the complications of this operation?

The complications are:

- Facial nerve injury
- Salivary fistula
- Auriculotemporal syndrome (Frey's).

25. How do you treat a submandibular tumor?

The whole gland is removed with care to preserve the lingual and hypoglossal nerves.

26. How do you treat a palatal tumor?

The tumor is excised widely up to the periosteum. The greater palatine vessels are cut and diathermised beyond the tumor. If the palatal bone is involved it should also be removed with the tumor.

27. What is a dumb-bell tumor?

It is a tumor of deep part of parotid that enlarges medially passing between the styloid process and mandible and presenting as a swelling in the throat.

28. What are the signs of a dumb-bell tumor?

The signs are:

- The patient presents with a painless swelling in the throat of insidious onset
- There is very little or no swelling in the parotid region
- The tonsil, tonsillar pillar, soft palate and uvula are pushed to the opposite side

- The swelling is firm, nontender and smooth or lobulated
- The pharyngeal mucosa is mobile on the swelling
- Bimanual examination may confirm its presence in parotid.

29. How do you treat this tumor?

This tumor is excised through a parotidectomy incision with a submandibular extension. The access to the tumor is obtained by dividing mandible anterior to mental foramen and styloid process.

30. What is an auriculotemporal syndrome?

In this syndrome, there is flushing and sweating of the skin innervated by auriculotemporal nerve whenever salivation is stimulated.

DISCUSSION

Pleomorphic adenoma is the commonest tumor of the major salivary glands. It has marked histologic diversity and composed of cartilage besides epithelial cells, hence called pleomorphic or mixed tumor.

Etiology: Not known.

Pathology:

Site: In about 90 percent of cases this tumor occurs in the parotid where the commonest site is the tail of the gland. About 7 percent of cases occur in submandibular gland. It may occur in the minor salivary glands of the palate, upper lip and buccal mucosa in that order.

Nature: It is basically a benign tumor but if it is removed by enucleation as was being done earlier, it has 45 percent recurrence rate. It is because of two reasons:

- It has got an incomplete capsule
- There are tiny excrescences projecting from the tumor into the healthy glandular tissue.

Macroscopic features: The tumor is a rubbery, resilient mass with bosselated surface. Cut section shows a somewhat glistening, mucoid appearance with zones of apparent cartilage.

Microscopic features consist of:

- Differentiated epithelial cells arranged in acini, cords or sheets. A trabeculated or tubular pattern may also be present. In about 25 percent of cases islands of squamous epithelium are present representing squamous metaplasia.
- Spindle or stellate cells usually separated by abundant intercellular mucoid material that appears like cartilage at places. The spindle cells are myoepithelial in nature. Both epithelial and spindle cells secrete the mucoid material which looks like cartilage. Thus this tumor has a 'pleomorphic stroma' with pseudocartilaginous, lymphoid, myxomatous and fibrous elements apart from epithelial cells (Fig. 18).

Origin: There are two views:
- It arises from embryonic rests from invagination of oral ectoderm.
- It is an adenoma of the salivary tissue and the cartilage is pseudocartilage.

Clinical Features

1. Age: It can occur at any age but more commonly seen around 40 years of age.
2. Sex: It is little more common in females.
3. Symptoms: A painless and slow growing swelling commonly in the parotid region.
4. Signs of a parotid tumor are:
   - The swelling is typically situated below the lobule of the ear, anterior and superior to the angle of mandible
   - It is hemispherical or hemioval
   - The surface is smooth or lobulated (Figs 16 and 17)
   - It is firm or variable in consistency
   - It is nontender and very well defined
   - It is mobile
   - The facial nerve is normal
   - The regional lymph nodes are not enlarged.

   Rarely, a tumor arises from the deep part of parotid gland (dumb-bell tumor). The examination of the oral cavity shows medial displacement of tonsil and the pillar of fauces.

Complications

This tumor may undergo malignant transformation, after 10, 20 or 30 years perhaps, in 3 to 5 percent of patients. The signs of this change are:

- It becomes painful, grows rapidly, becomes hard in consistency, loses its mobility by fixing to overlying skin and or underlying masseter.
- It involves facial nerve (very important sign), may involve the regional lymph nodes and may ulcerate or fungate out.

Investigations

Diagnosis is usually clinical but FNAC may be done. Incisional biopsy should never be done.

Treatment

1. *Parotid tumor:* It is treated by superficial parotidectomy (Patey's operation). After identifying the facial nerve and its branches (pes anserina) the superficial part of the gland is dissected from the underlying tissues and excised with the tumor (Figs 20 and 21).

   The excised tissue must be examined histologically immediately by frozen section. If there is some discrepancy further treatment must be done accordingly.
2. *Submandibular tumor:* The whole gland is removed with care to preserve the lingual and hypoglossal nerves.
3. *Palatal tumor:* The tumor is excised widely up to the periosteum. The greater palatine vessels are cut and diathermized beyond the tumor. If the palatal bone is involved, it should also be removed with the tumor.

CASE 5: CAVERNOUS HEMANGIOMA

CLINICAL DIAGNOSIS

1. The patient is usually young and presents with a painless and very slow growing swelling of insidious onset.
2. It can occur anywhere but commonly in the lip, face, cheek and tongue.
3. It is bluish and smooth or lobulated (Figs 22 and 23).

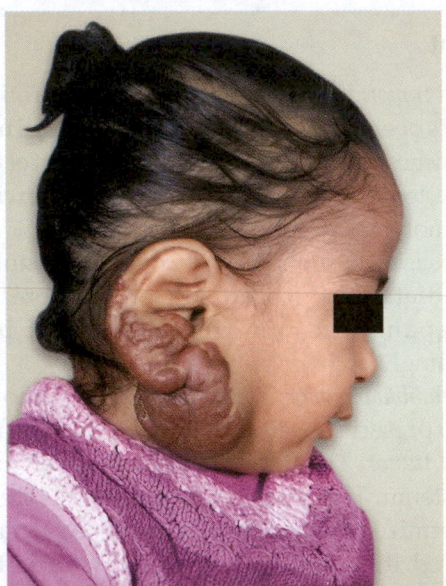

Fig. 22: Hemangioma of right parotid region involving lower half of pinna (*Courtesy:* Professor Rajiv Agarwal)

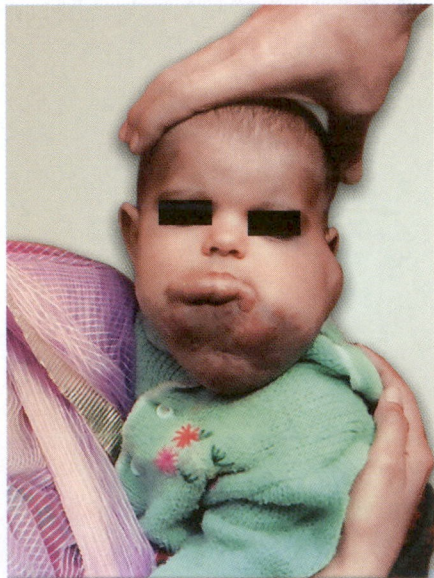

Fig. 23: Hemangioma of lower half of face, mainly on the left side

4. It is nontender and opaque.
5. It is soft and compressible.

VIVA VOCE

1. **What is a hemangioma?**

   It is a tumor-like swelling containing blood. Most of the hemangiomas are malformations of normal vascular structures, i.e. hamartomas. Some of them are true tumors arising from endothelial cells and other vascular elements.

   Sixty percent of hemangiomas occur in the region of head.

2. **How do you classify hemagiomas?**

   A simple classification is as given below:
   - Involuting hemagiomas
     - Superficial: Strawberry nevus, nevus vasculosus, capillary hemangioma
     - Combined superficial and deep: Strawberry nevus, capillary hemangioma, capillary and cavernous hemangioma (Figs 22 and 23)
     - Deep: Cavernous hemangioma
   - Noninvoluting hemagiomas
     - Port wine stains: Port wine stain, capillary hemangioma, nevus flammeus
     - Cavernous hemangioma
     - Venous racemose aneurysm
     - Arteriovenous fistula (Fig. 24).

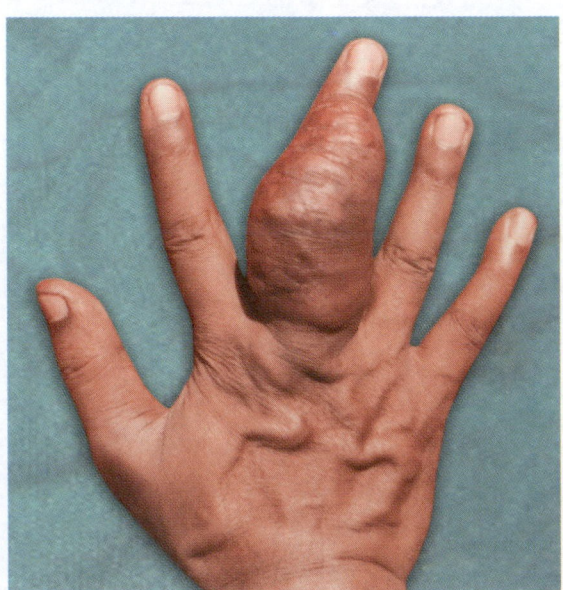

Fig. 24: Arteriovenous fistula

3. **What do you mean by an involuting hemangioma?**
It is a true tumor of endothelial cells that undergoes complete spontaneous involution with time.

4. **What are the features of an involuting hemangioma?**
It is the most common tumor that occurs during childhood. It constitutes 95% of hemangiomas.

5. **What is the time of occurrence of an involuting hemangioma?**
Usually it is present at birth or appears during the first 2–3 weeks of life.

6. **What is the chronology of involution?**
It grows at a rather rapid rate for 4–6 months, and then stops to grow. Subsequently, involution begins and progresses slowly till it is complete by 5–7 years of age.

7. **What are the clinical signs of a sup erficial involuting hemangioma?**
It is a sharply demarcated, bright-red and slightly raised lesion with an irregular surface resembling a strawberry.

8. **What are the signs of a deep involuting hemangioma?**
It presents as a deep bluish swelling extending deeply into subcutaneous tissue covered by normal appearing skin.

9. **What are the clinical features of a combined superficial and deep involuting hemangioma?**
It has combined characteristics of both superficial and deep involuting hemangiomas.

10. **What is the micropathology of an involuting hemangioma?**
   - In the growing phase, it consists of solid fields of closely packed round or oval endothelial cells. Cellular division and mitotic figures are seen
   - In the involution phase, the solid fields of endothelial cells appear breaking up into closely packed, capillary-sized, vessel-like structures composed of several layers of soft endothelial cells supported by a sparse fibrous stroma. The vascular structures gradually become fewer and spaced more widely apart in a loose, edematous fibrous stroma. The endothelial cells continue to disappear so that by the time involution is complete the histological picture is completely normal with no trace of endothelial cells.

11. **How do you treat an involuting hemangioma?**
No treatment is usually required as most of these lesions disappear spontaneously.

12. **What are the disadvantages if surgical excision is done?**
Surgical excision also cures the lesion but it has the following disadvantages:
   - It leaves a scar the appearance of which is poorer as compared to the scar of spontaneous disappearance
   - During excision of the lesion a part of the involved structure may have to be excised that may be difficult to reconstruct.

13. **What are the indications for operation?**
The indications are:
   - Large lesions causing functional problem, e.g. a large hemangioma of eyebrow or eyelid obstructing vision
   - Thin wrinkled or redundant skin ('crepe paper') left after involution of a large lesion.

14. **What is the nature of operation in the above situations?**
   - The operation should be very conservative. The excision should be adequate to alleviate the functional problem. The remaining portions should be allowed to involute spontaneously
   - The thin wrinkled or redundant skin is excised to improve the cosmesis.

15. **What is the role of dry ice?**
A superficial lesion can be destroyed by dry ice but it has following demerits:
   - It has no effect on a deep hemangioma
   - It results in severe scarring.

16. **What is the role of corticosteroids?**
Systemic and intralesional corticosteroids (2 mg/kg for 3 weeks) have been used with varying success (60%).

17. **What is the role of sclerosing injection?**
The sclerotherapy has hardly any effect.

18. **What is the role of radiotherapy?**
It has no place in the treatment.

19. **What are the newer methods of treatment?**
Laser therapy with insertion of a laser probe deep into the lesion reduces the size of the lesion. A life-threatening hemangioma of the head and neck region obstructing the airways and resistant to steroids can be treated by systemic interferon with some dramatic results.

20. **What are the complications of a hemangioma?**
Following complications can occur:
   - Infection
   - Ulceration
   - Bleeding.

21. What is Kasabach-Merritt syndrome?

When a large hemangioma causes disseminated intravascular coagulopathy due to platelet trapping, it is known as Kasabach-Merritt syndrome.

22. What are the differences between an involuting and a noninvoluting hemangioma?

The differences are:

Features	Involuting hemangioma	Noninvoluting hemangioma
Rate of growth	Grows rapidly for 4–6 months of early life	Grows slowly in proportion to the growth of child
Spontaneous disappearance	Disappears by 5–7 years of age	Does not disappear spontaneously

23. What are the features of a noninvoluting hemangioma?

This tumor is present at birth, grows rapidly during first 4 to 6 months of life and does not involute. It may cause cosmetic and functional problems.

24. What is a port wine stain?

It is the most common type of noninvoluting hemangioma occurring anywhere in the body but more commonly on the face as a flat patchy lesion that is reddish to purple in color.

25. What are the syndromes associated with a port wine stain?

The associated syndromes are : Sturge-Weber syndrome, Klippel-Trenaunay-Weber syndrome and Proteus syndrome.

26. What is the microscopic picture of a port wine stain?

There are thin-walled capillaries that are arranged throughout dermis, lined by flattened endothelial cells. In a lesion that produces surface growth, groups of round proliferating endothelial cells and large venous sinuses are seen.

27. How do you treat a port wine stain?

The treatment is uniformly disappointing. It is usually treated by camouflaging. Unfortunately, this is difficult because the port wine stain is darker than the surrounding lighter skin.

28. What is the role of tattooing?

Tattooing with skin-colored pigments may offer some measure of disguise in a lighter lesion but usually is unsatisfactory because the pigment deposited in the skin looks artificial and tends to be absorbed unevenly producing a mottled appearance.

29. What is the role of surgery in port wine stains?

If the lesion is small surgical excision with primary closure is possible. Unfortunately, most of the lesions are too big for excision.

30. What is the role of radiation treatment?

All types of radiations have been used but not recommended because of the following reasons:

- Damage to the surrounding tissues and overlying skin
- Increased incidence of malignancy.

31. Can you treat this lesion with laser?

It can be treated by pulsed-dye laser that produces a light with a specific wave length of 585 or 595 nanometers. The beam is selectively absorbed by red pigment (hemoglobin) in the blood vessels of the lesion. It produces selective heat destruction (selective photothermolysis) of these structures and the treated area appears whiter. Multiple treatments are required. It is good for early lesions.

In darker and advanced nodular lesions, it is less effective and may cause severe scarring and hyperpigmentation.

32. Can you treat this lesion by embolization?

Some fast growing or primarily arterialized hemangiomas are treated by super-selective embolization, either alone or in conjunction with surgery. It is performed under fluoroscopic control.

33. What are the complications of this procedure?

The most important complication of this procedure is sloughing of tissues.

34. What is the micropathology of a cavernous hemangioma?

It is composed of large dilated closely packed vascular sinuses that are engorged with blood, lined by flat endothelial cells and may have muscular walls like normal veins.

35. How do you treat a cavernous hemangioma?

- If the lesion is small, localized and/or superficial it may be excised.
- If the lesion is extensive, deep and involving many structures (muscles, bone) it can only be excised by radical surgery. Since most of these hemangiomas are no more than an aesthetic problem, radical surgery is rarely indicated.

36. What is the role of sclerotherapy?

Occasionally, injection of sclerosing agents directly into the venous sinuses may lead to some involution or may make the surgical excision easy.

DISCUSSION

Involuting Hemangioma

They are the most common hemangiomas constituting about 50 percent of all hemangiomas. They are the true tumors of the endothelial cells. They grow rapidly for 4 to

6 months, stop growing and then start involuting that continues slowly and is completed by 5 to 7 years of age.

They are seen shortly after birth or appear during the first 2 to 3 weeks of life. They occur anywhere on the body surface but more commonly on the head and neck.

They are of three types: superficial, combined superficial and deep.

- Superficial hemangiomas are sharply demarcated, bright-red, somewhat raised lesions with an irregular surface like a strawberry
- Combined superficial and deep hemangiomas have the same features but below the surface a firm, bluish swelling is present going into the subcutaneous tissue
- Deep hemangioma (e.g. cavernous hemagioma) is a deep blue tumor covered by normal looking skin.

Micropathology

During the growth phase, it consists of solid fields of closely packed round or oval endothelial cells. Cellular division and mitotic figures are present as seen in a hemangioendothelioma. During involution the solid fields break up into closely packed, capillary-sized, vessel-like structures consisting of many layers of soft endothelial cells in a sparse fibrous stroma. These structures and endothelial cells gradually disappear till the involution is complete when the picture is completely normal.

Complications

- Ulceration accompanied by infection occurs in 8 percent of patients
- Bleeding
- Kasabach-Merritt syndrome: It is disseminated intravascular coagulopathy due to platelet trapping by the hemangioma.

Treatment

No treatment is required as most of the lesions involute completely with a better result than that can be obtained by surgical excision. Further complete excision of the tumor may result in disfigurement that may be difficult to repair. If a lesion of eyelid or lip causing some functional disturbance partial resection of the lesion is done. After involution, the skin of the lesion may be thin, wrinkled or redundant. This defect is corrected by plastic surgery. Other methods of treatment that have been tried and discarded are dry ice and radiotherapy.

Corticosteroids may help in the involution process. Insertion of a laser probe deep into the lesion and heating the lesion reduces its size. Systemic interferon has been used in life-threatening hemangiomas resistant to steroids with some good results.

Noninvoluting Hemangiomas

Majority of these hemangiomas are present at birth. They are different from the involuting hemangiomas as described below:

- They do not grow rapidly in early life but grow in proportion to the growth of the child
- They do not involute and disappear and cause aesthetic and functional problems
- The treatment is difficult and results are not good.

Port wine Stains

They arise from capillary malformations and from defective maturation of cutaneous sympathetic innervations. They are the commonest noninvoluting hemangiomas and may occur anywhere on the body but most commonly on the face as flat patchy lesions, reddish to purple in color, often within the maxillary and mandibular dermatomes. They persist into adulthood and become keratotic and nodular. **Micropathology:** They are composed of thin-walled capillaries in the dermis, lined with mature flat endothelial cells. Surface growth producing lesions have groups of round proliferating endothelial cells and large venous sinuses. The port wine stain may be associated with Sturge-Weber syndrome, Klippel-Trenaunay-Weber syndrome and Proteus syndrome.

Treatment: Tattooing with skin colored pigments is the simplest treatment but looks artificial and tends to be absorbed unevenly producing a mottled appearance. Dry ice, liquid nitrogen, electrocoagulation, dermabrasion and radiotherapy – all have been tried and have failed.

Pulsed-dye laser gives the best results in early and intermediate lesions. It produces a light with a specific wave length of 585 or 595 nanometers that is absorbed by red pigmented material such as hemoglobin of the lesion. It produces selective heat destruction (selective photothermolysis) with treated area becoming whiter. It is less effective for darker and advanced lesions.

Capillary Hemangioma

Fast-growing capillary or arterialized hemangiomas can be treated by superselective embolization under fluoroscopic control.

Complications: Ulceration during proliferative phase, hemorrhage, thrombocytopenia, consumptive coagulopathy,

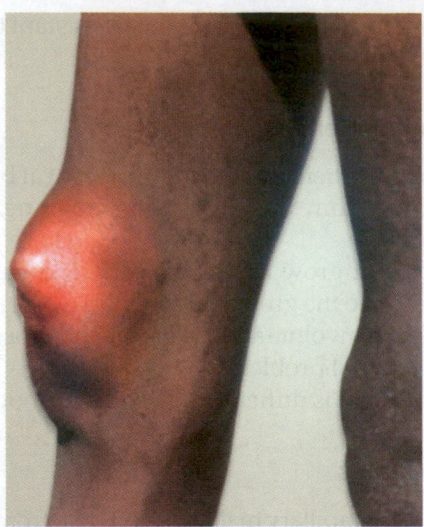

Fig. 25: Hemangioma knee region

high-output heart failure, visual field encroachment, airway obstruction and skeletal distortion.

Cavernous Hemangioma (Venous Angioma)

It is present at birth and grows with the normal growth of body. It may occur anywhere in the body but more common on the head and neck. It consists of a bunch of thin-walled, dilated, tortuous, fully-formed venous structure like a bag of worms (Fig. 25). It is lined by flat endothelial cells and may have muscular walls like normal veins. It is bluish or purplish lesion that empties on pressure. It may cause massive hemorrhage if injured or septicemia, if infected.

Surgery: A small superficial lesion may be completely excised; otherwise most of these lesions are not amenable to excision. Sclerotherapy may reduce its size, when it may be possible to excise it. If angiography detects the feeding vessel, therapeutic embolization may be tried.

CASE 6: SACROCOCCYGEAL TERATOMA

CLINICAL DIAGNOSIS

1. The patient is an infant more commonly a female who presents usually within 3 months of birth.
2. There is a large swelling projecting out between the rectum and sacrum.
3. It is irregular, nontender and variable in consistency (Fig. 26).
4. It is firmly attached to the coccyx.

VIVA VOCE

1. **What is a sacrococcygeal teratoma?**
   It is a congenital tumor derived from all the germ layers of early embryo. It may be considered a fetus in fetu (including fetus).
2. **What is the cause of this lesion?**
   It is a developmental lesion, the cause of which is not known. It occurs in the precoccygeal region which is the site of the 'primitive knot', a group of totipotent cells that retain their totipotentiality longer than any other except the sex anlage.
3. **What are the anatomical attachments of this tumor?**
   This tumor which arises between the rectum and sacrum is firmly attached to the coccyx, and occasionally to the last piece of sacrum.
4. **What is the nature of this tumor?**
   This tumor is usually large but has a benign nature. Sometimes, it may be small enough to pass unnoticed till it enlarges or complicates. The latter type may become malignant at about 10 months of age.
5. **What are the types of this tumor?**
   It is of four types: The type I is predominantly external (46%) and type IV is predominantly internal, type II and III are in between.
6. **What are the complications of this neoplasm?**
   The complications are:
   - Ulceration
   - Infection
   - Malignant change
   - Rectal and urinary obstruction.
   These complications can result in a fatality.
7. **What are the investigations?**
   - X-ray of sacrococcygeal region (Fig. 27).
   - MRI is done to define its exact extent and its relationship with the neighboring structures.
8. **Will you not like to do a biopsy?**
   It is usually not required, the clinical diagnosis is enough. Further, it may cause ulceration and infection.
9. **What do you look for in the radiograph?**
   We look for any change in the local bones. It shows the soft tissue shadow of the tumor (Fig. 27).
10. **How do you treat this condition?**
    The lesion is excised completely.
11. **What is the age of excision?**
    Soon after birth.

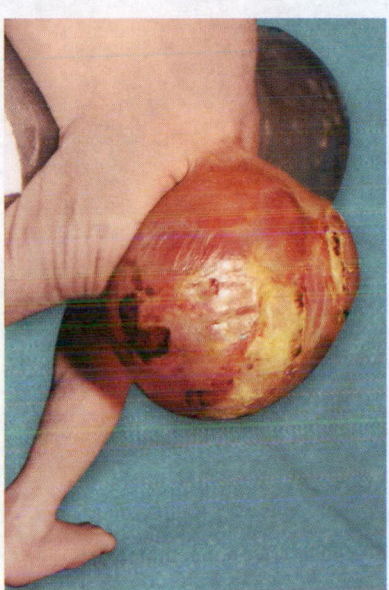

Fig. 26: Sacrococcygeal teratoma
(*Courtesy:* Professor Ashish Wakhlu)

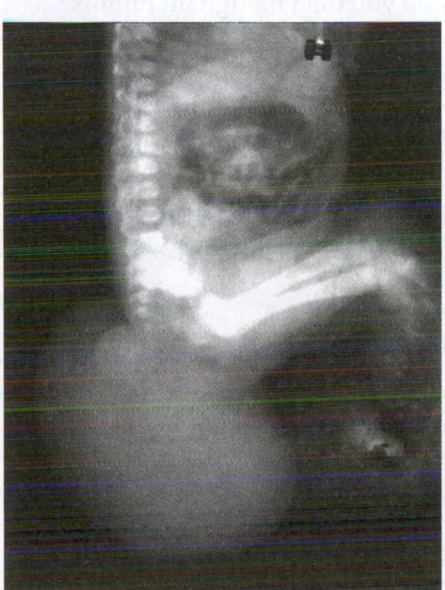

Fig. 27: Radiography of a sacrococcygeal teratoma

12. **What is the technique of excision?**
    Through a longitudinal elliptical incision the tumor is mobilized all round till the coccygeal attachment is defined. Then the tumor is removed with coccyx and sometimes with the last piece of sacrum. The wound is closed in layers leaving a drain.

13. **What is its relationship with rectum?**
    Sometimes, there is a fistula between the tumor and rectum.

14. **How do you deal with this fistula during operation?**
    As it is small, it is excised along with the tumor and the rectal opening is closed.

15. **Do you need a colostomy for its management?**
    No.

16. **What are the complications of operation?**
    The complications are:
    • Wound infection
    • Flap necrosis
    • Hemorrhage.

17. **Do you ever need abdominoperineal approach?**
    It is sometimes required to excise type III and IV tumors.

18. **What is the prognosis?**
    If the excision is done soon after birth, it is good. If it is delayed, the child may die due to complications.

19. **Can it recur?**
    It can recur. Hence, the patient has to be followed-up.

20. **What is a malignant sacrococcygeal teratoma?**
    Majority (97%) of these tumors are benign. If the treatment is delayed by 2 months, 50 to 60 percent of the tumors turn malignant.

21. **How do you treat malignant tumors?**
    They are treated by surgery (wide excision) and chemotherapy.

DISCUSSION

Sacrococcygeal teratoma is a tumor of precoccygeal region arising from the 'primitive knot'. It is the most common among the large tumors that are seen in neonates (Fig. 29).

Etiology

The 'primitive knot' consists of a group of totipotent cells that retain their totipotentiality longer than other cells except the sex anlage. This tumor arises from these cells.

A history of twins is common. This lesion can be detected by prenatal ultrasonography. Such pregnancy may be complicated by fetal high-output cardiac failure due to arteriovenous shunting in the tumor, maternal polyhydramnios and hydrops fetalis that may cause fetal death.

Types of Tumor

It is of four types depending upon its site (Fig. 28):
Type I: Predominantly external (46%)
Type II: External mass with a presacral component (35%)
Type III: Visible externally but predominantly internal (9%)
Type IV: Entirely presacral, not visible externally (10%)

Clinical Features

This tumor is usually present at the time of birth and is quite big. Twenty percent of newborns are born dead. The

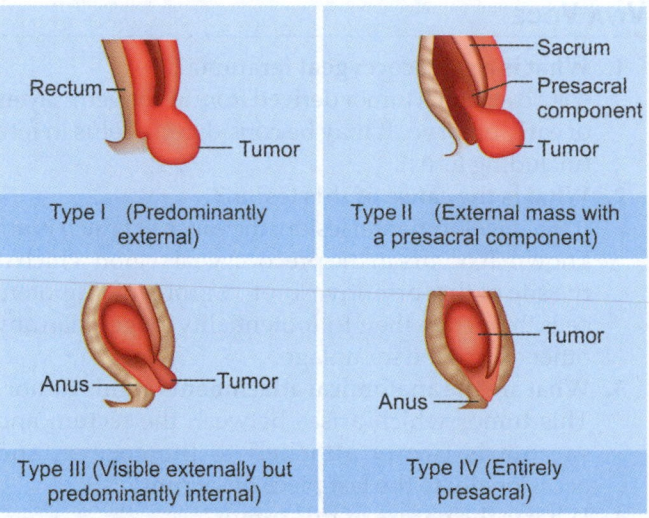

Fig. 28: Types of sacrococcygeal teratoma

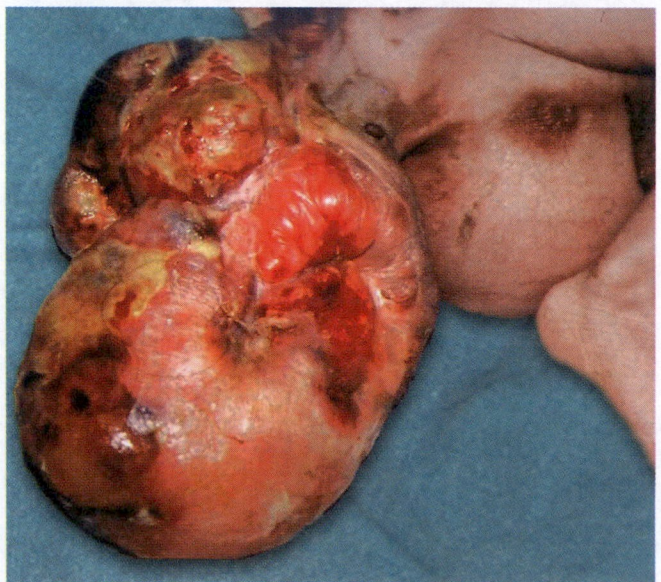

Fig. 29: A large sacrococcygeal teratoma
(*Courtesy:* Professor Ashish Wakhlu)

swelling is present between the rectum and sacrum, and firmly attached to the last piece of coccyx. It occurs more commonly in female infants than males. Sometimes, the swelling is so small that it is not identified at birth and only recognized later when it grows or develops some complication. This type may be malignant usually at about 10 months of age. A digital rectal examination (DRE) is done to assess its retrorectal extent.

Complications

If not treated early, it may have the following complications: infection, ulceration (Fig. 29) rectal or urinary obstruction and malignant change and the infant may die of these complications.

Investigations

- Radiography: It shows the soft tissue shadow of this tumor in the sacrococcygeal region (Fig. 27)
- MRI shows the extent of the lesion and its relationship with the structures in the vicinity
- Biopsy is not required although FNAC may be done.

Treatment

It should be excised along with the coccyx as early as possible after birth. Through a longitudinal elliptical incision, the tumor is mobilized all round except the coccygeal attachment, as the coccyx is excised with the tumor. Sometimes, the last piece of sacrum is also resected. Sometimes, there is a small fistula between the tumor and the rectum which has to be closed at the time of surgery. Usually, a colostomy is not required. The wound is closed around a drain. Type III and type IV tumors may require an abdominoperineal approach.

Malignant Sacrococcygeal Teratoma

Ninty-seven percent of tumors of the newborn are benign. The greatest risk of malignancy is age at diagnosis which is about 50 to 60 percent after 2 months of age. The malignant tumors are treated with surgery and chemotherapy.

Prognosis

- If the excision is done soon after birth, the prognosis is good
- The patient is followed-up by serial AFP levels and physical examination including DRE, as recurrence can occur
- The 5-year survival rate of malignant tumor is 50 percent.

CASE 7: CERVICAL TERATOMA

CLINICAL DIAGNOSIS

1. The patient is usually an infant who presents with a large swelling in the neck.
2. The swelling is smooth, firm or variable with prominent surface veins (Fig. 30).
3. It may ulcerate and bleed.
4. There may be respiratory difficulty due to large size of the swelling.

VIVA VOCE

1. **What is a teratoma?**
   A teratoma is an embryonal tumor that arises in the pleuripotent cells and composed of a wide variety of tissues foreign to the organ or the anatomic site of occurrence and derived from at least two of the three germ layers.
2. **What is the cause of this tumor?**
   It is not known. It is a developmental defect.
3. **What is the incidence of cervical teratoma?**
   Teratoma of the neck constitute 3 percent of all teratomas.
4. **Which is the commonest teratoma?**
   Sacrococcygeal teratoma is the commonest teratoma that constitutes 57% of all the teratomas.
5. **What are the other sites of occurrence?**
   The next common site is gonads where 29 percent of tumors occur. The other sites are mediastinum, retroperitoneum, cranial cavity and other places (Fig. 31).
6. **What is the nature of this tumor?**
   Most of these tumors are benign, only 27 percent are malignant.
7. **What are the harmful effects of this tumor?**
   The harmful effects of this tumor are:
   - A large tumor may cause respiratory embarrassment
   - The tumor may ulcerate and bleed
   - It has a terrorist-look. Thus, it has an appropriate name
   - It may become malignant.
8. **What are the investigations?**
   X-ray shows a soft-tissue mass having calcification. Ultrasonography reveals a mixed cystic and solid lesion. The diagnosis can be confirmed by biopsy (needle biopsy). Serum levels of AFP and β-hCG are usually elevated. They are used as tumor markers to detect recurrence after excision.
9. **How do you deal with respiratory embarrassment?**
   It is treated by rapid establishment of an endotracheal airway. To do a tracheostomy is risky due to distortion of landmarks for operation.
10. **How do you treat this tumor?**
    - A benign tumor is cured by complete excision.
    - A malignant tumor is excised, if resectable. It is treated adjunctively with a combination of

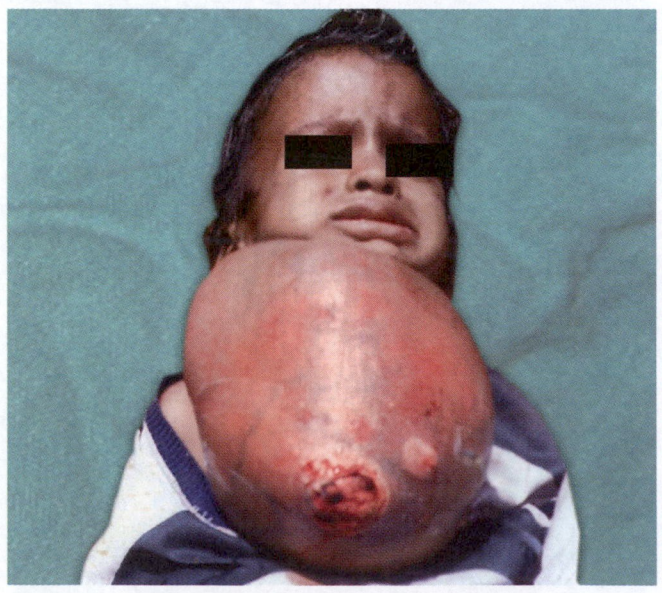

Fig. 30: Cervical teratoma
(*Courtesy:* Professor Ashish Wakhlu)

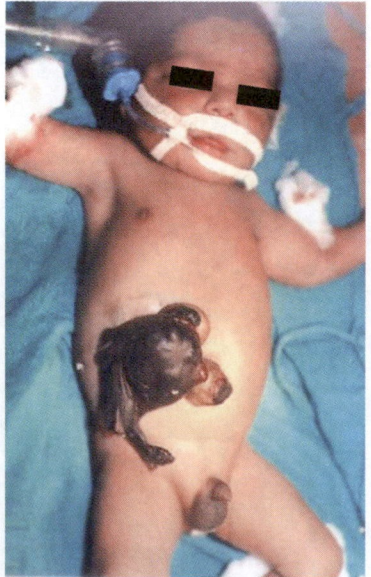

Fig. 31: Teratoma of abdominal wall
(*Courtesy:* Professor Ashish Wakhlu)

cisplatin, vinblastine and bleomycin, or with dactinomycin, cyclophosphamide and vincristine.

11. **What is the role of radiotherapy?**

A malignant teratoma responds to radiotherapy. Hence, it may be given postoperatively or in a non-resectable tumor.

DISCUSSION

The word teratoma is derived from the Greek word, teraton that means a monster as most of these tumors are large and have a ferocious look. It is an embryonal tumor that arises in the pleuripotent cells and composed of a wide variety of tissues foreign to the organ or the anatomic site of origin and derived from at least two of the three germ layers: ectoderm, mesoderm and endoderm.

The teratomas are usually midline or para-axial tumors and are distributed in the body as given below: sacrococcygeal 57 percent, gonadal 29 percent, mediastinal 7 percent, retroperitoneal 4 percent and cervical 3 percent. Other sites are rare (Fig. 31). Most of these tumors are benign, only 27 percent are malignant.

Depending on the age of occurrence these tumors are put into two broad groups:

1. Non-gonadal that constitute 71 percent of all tumors. They occur during infancy.
2. Gonadal constitute 29 percent of tumors. They are seen during adolescence.

Cervical Teratoma

It usually occurs in neonates and may be very large as to cause respiratory distress. It is usually smooth, firm or variable in consistency, has large surface veins and tends to ulcerate (Fig. 30).

Investigations

- X-ray shows a soft-tissue mass having calcification
- Ultrasonography reveals a mixed cystic and solid lesion
- Serum levels of AFP and β-hCG are usually elevated. They are used as tumor markers to detect recurrence after surgery
- Biopsy may be done. Most of the tumors are benign. The most common malignant type is a yolk-sac tumor (endodermal sinus tumor).

Treatment

- Respiratory difficulty is treated by rapid establishment of an endotracheal airway. The tracheostomy is risky because of distortion of landmarks for operation
- The tumor is excised completely. It cures a benign tumor
- A malignant tumor responds to radiotherapy. It is treated adjunctively with a combination of cisplantin, vinblastine and bleomycin, or with dactinomycin, cyclophosphamide and vincristine.

CASE 8: NEUROFIBROMA

CLINICAL DIAGNOSIS

1. Solitary neurofibroma (Fig. 32)
   - The patient presents with a subcutaneous nodule of insidious onset (Fig. 32).
   - It is firm, mobile and may be nontender or tender with the pain radiating along the course of the nerve from which it is arising.
2. Neurofibromatosis (Fig. 33)
   - The patient is usually a middle-aged or elderly person who presents with multiple nodules on the skin all over the body
   - The nodules are mostly subcutaneous but some are pedunculated
   - They may be firm or soft
   - There may be multiple hyperpigmented spots (café au lait).
3. Plexiform neurofibromatosis (Figs 34 and 35)
   - The patient presents with a large, firm and smooth swelling arising from the branches of trigeminal nerve
   - It may rarely occur in the extremities.

VIVA VOCE

1. **What is a neurofibroma?**

   It is a benign tumor of nerves that contains both neural (ectodermal) and fibrous (mesodermal) elements (Fig. 36).

2. **What are the types of neurofibroma?**

   It is of the following types:
   - Solitary neurofibroma
   - Neurofibromatosis
   - Plexiform neurofibromatosis
   - Elephantiasis neurofibromatosis

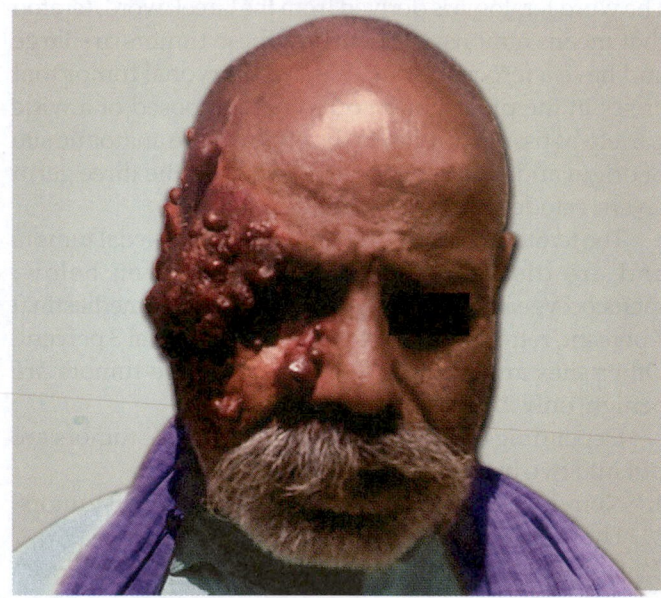

Fig. 33: Neurofibromatosis of right half of face

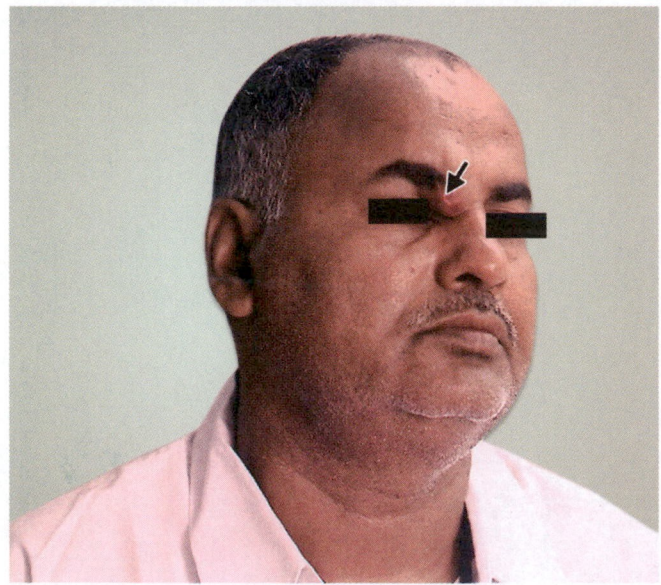

Fig. 32: Recurrent neurofibroma near the medial canthus of the right eye. Excision biopsy revealed it to be a neurofibrosarcoma

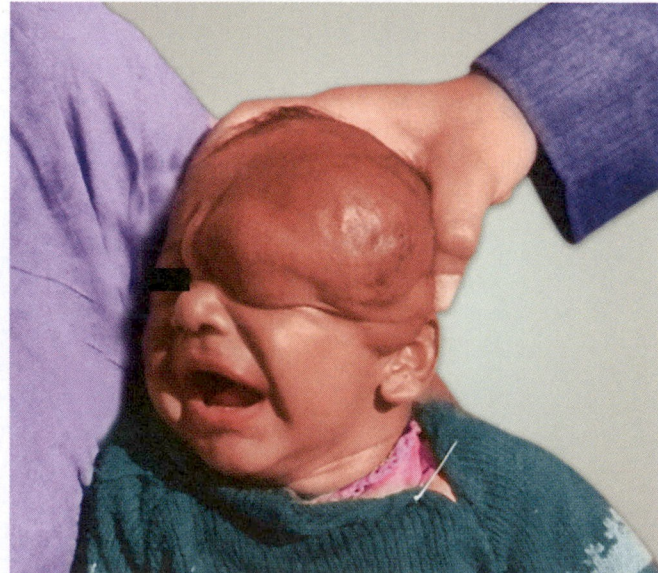

Fig. 34: Plexiform neurofibroma occurring in connection with the ophthalmic division of trigeminal nerve

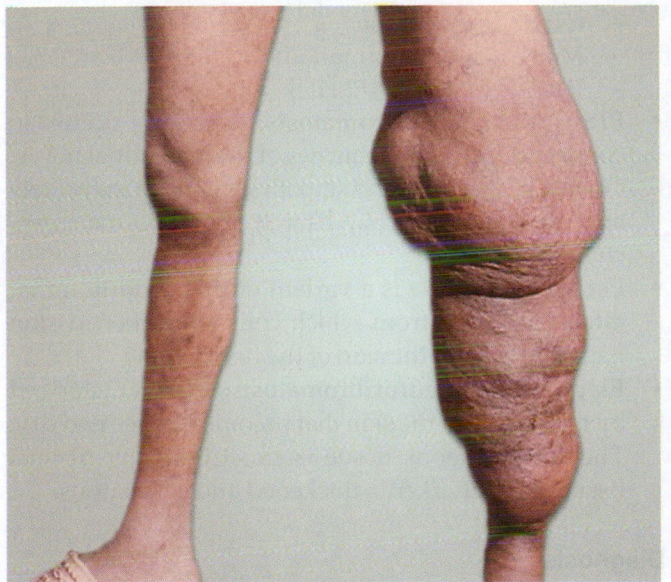

Fig. 35: Plexiform neurofibroma of left leg

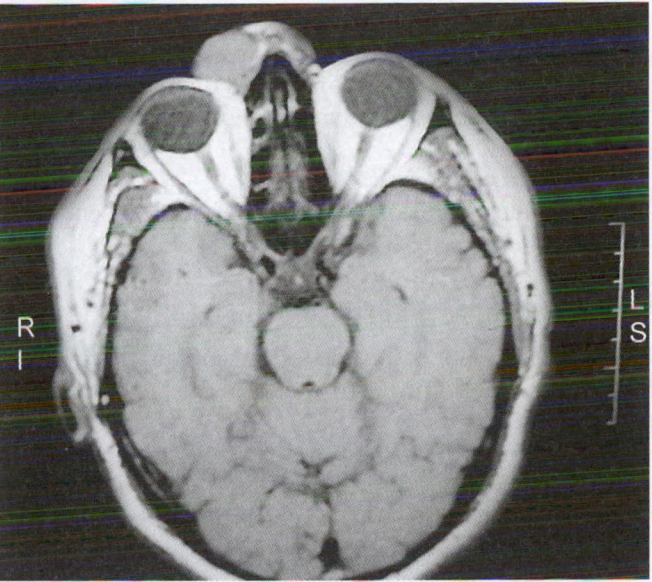

Fig. 37: MRI: Enhancing mass lesion right medial canthus (neurofibrosarcoma). It is the picture of the patient shown in Figure 32

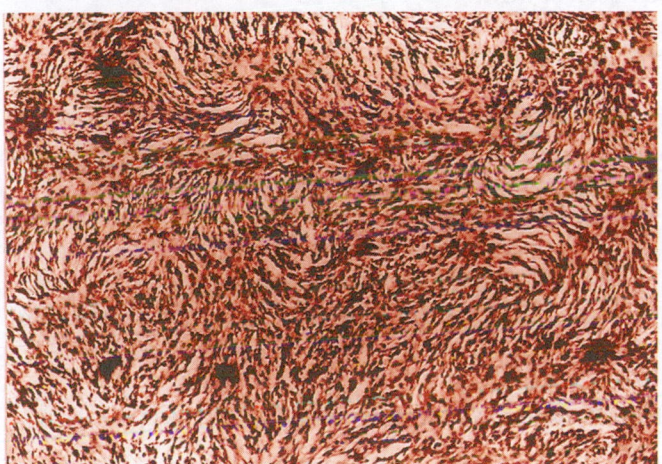

Fig. 36: Micropathology of a neurofibroma showing fibrous connective tissue

3. What is neurofibromatosis?

It is characterized by occurrence of multiple neurofibromas. It may either occur sporadically or on a familial basis with autosomal dominant inheritance.

4. What are the types of neurofibromatosis?

It is of two types:

Type I (von Recklinghausen's disease): It is characterized by multiple hyperpigmented macules (café au lait) and multiple neurofibromas all over the body.

Type II: It is characterized by auditory (8th cranial nerve) tumors and may be associated with other intracranial or intraspinal tumors.

5. What is the genetics of familial neurofibromatosis?

In familial disease the gene for type I is located on chromosome 17 and that for type II on chromosome 22.

6. What is the etiology?

The cause of a neurofibroma is not known.

7. What are the complications?

- Pressure symptoms, e.g. deafness in an acoustic neuroma, spinal compression by a dumb-bell tumor and mediastinal syndrome by a mediastinal tumor
- Cystic degeneration
- Malignant transformation
- Cosmetic problem.

8. What are the investigations?

- In a subcutaneous neurofibroma, FNAC may be done
- Deep-seated tumors can be seen in detail by CT scan or MRI (Fig. 37).

9. How do you treat a neurofibroma?

- No treatment is required in an asymptomatic neurofibroma
- A symptomatic or enlarging neurofibroma is treated by complete excision. Recurrences are rare
- Neurofibromatosis: A symptomatic tumor or the one that is increasing in size may be excised. The rest are left as such
- Plexiform neurofibromatosis and elephantiasis neurofibromatosis: They are excised with the help of a plastic surgeon to improve the looks.

10. **What is a neurilemmoma?**
    It is a benign tumor of Schwann cells of neurilemma. It is an encapsulated tumor that displaces the nerve fibers to one side. The commonest site of occurrence is acoustic nerve.

11. **How do you treat it?**
    It is enucleated from the affected nerve preserving its function.

DISCUSSION

It is a benign tumor of the nerves that contains both neural (ectodermal) and fibrous (mesodermal) elements. It is of many types:

- **Solitary neurofibroma:** It is a very common benign tumor that can occur at any age but usually seen in adults. It occurs in the subcutaneous tissue. The patient presents with a painless or slightly painful subcutaneous nodule of insidious onset. It is firm, smooth and can be moved from side to side but not in the direction of nerve from which it is arising. Pressure on it may cause paresthesia and tingling along the course of the nerve. It may affect the eighth cranial nerve (acoustic tumor). The complications are rare, and they are cystic degeneration and malignant change (Fig. 32).

- **Neurofibromatosis (Fig. 33):** Neurofibromatosis is characterized by multiple tumors. It may occur either sporadically or on a familial basis with autosomal dominant inheritance. It is of two types:

  Type I (von Recklinghausen's disease): It is characterized by multiple hyperpigmented macules (café au lait spots) and neurofibromas.

  Type II: It is characterized by eighth nerve tumors and may be associated with other intracranial or intraspinal tumors. In familial disease, the gene for type I is located on chromosome 17 and that for type II on chromosome 22. The patient presents with multiple neurofibromas occurring all over the body and affecting the cranial, spinal and peripheral nerves. Multiple nodules may be present at birth. The whole body is almost covered with tumors of various sizes. Most of the nodules are subcutaneous but some are pedunculated and may be firm or soft. The complications are:
  - Pressure symptoms: Deafness in an acoustic neuroma, spinal compression by a dumb-bell tumor and mediastinal syndrome by a mediastinal tumor
  - Cystic degeneration
  - Malignant transformation
  - It may be part of MEN II B.

- **Plexiform neurofibromatosis:** It usually occurs in connection with the branches of the trigeminal nerve. There is a large, firm and smooth swelling. It may rarely affect the upper extremity. It rarely undergoes malignant change (Fig. 33).

- Pachydermatocele is a variant of this condition that affects the neck from which coils of thickened skin hangs down like the skin of the neck of cow.

- **Elephantiasis neurofibromatosis:** It is characterized by thickening of the skin that becomes coarse and dry. The subcutaneous tissue is substituted by fibrous tissue that is markedly thickened and edematous.

Diagnosis

The diagnosis can be confirmed by biopsy. The deep-seated lesions and the extent of the large lesions can be seen by CT scan or MRI.

Treatment

- An asymptomatic neurofibroma may be left as such
- A symptomatic or enlarging neurofibroma is excised and the whole specimen is sent for histopathology.
- Plexiform neurofibromatosis and elephantiasis neurofibromatosis: They are excised with the help of a plastic surgeon to improve the cosmetic looks
- Neurofibromatosis: A symptomatic neurofibroma or the one that is increasing in size may be excised.

Neurilemmoma (Schwannoma)

It is an uncommon benign tumor that arises from the Schwann cells of neurilemma which is ectodermal in origin. It presents as a solitary, round or fusiform firm mass along the course of a large nerve. There may be radiating pain. The commonest site of occurrence is acoustic nerve but it can also occur in posterior mediastinum or retroperitoneum. This tumor does not have any tendency to malignant transformation. It is an encapsulated tumor that displaces the nerve fibers to one side. Hence, it can be shelled out with preservation of function of the affected nerve.

CASE 9: RASPBERRY TUMOR (ENTEROTERATOMA)

CLINICAL DIAGNOSIS

1. The patient is usually an infant or child who presents with a weeping umbilicus since birth.
2. There is a small moist, pink, smooth and soft raspberry-like swelling in the umbilicus (Fig. 38).
3. It may be pedunculated or sessile.
4. It discharges serous or mucoid fluid.

VIVA VOCE

1. **What is raspberry tumor?**
   It is a raspberry-like 'tumor' arising from the mucosa of the patent distal segment of the vitellointestinal duct that is near the umbilicus. The mucosa of unobliterated vitellointestinal duct prolapses through the umbilicus which gives rise to this lesion that bleeds on touch.

2. **Is it really a tumor?**
   Truly speaking it is not a tumor. It is a developmental defect.

3. **What is the micropathology?**
   Microscopically, it consists of columnar epithelium of small bowel rich in goblet cells.

4. **How do you treat this condition?**
   If the lesion is pedunculated a ligature is tied around its base. The tumor falls off in a few days with a cure. If the lesion is sessile or recurs after ligature umbilectomy is indicated.

5. **What is the indication for doing laparotomy?**
   If there is some evidence or suspicion of existence of a vitellointestinal duct or band along with a Meckel's

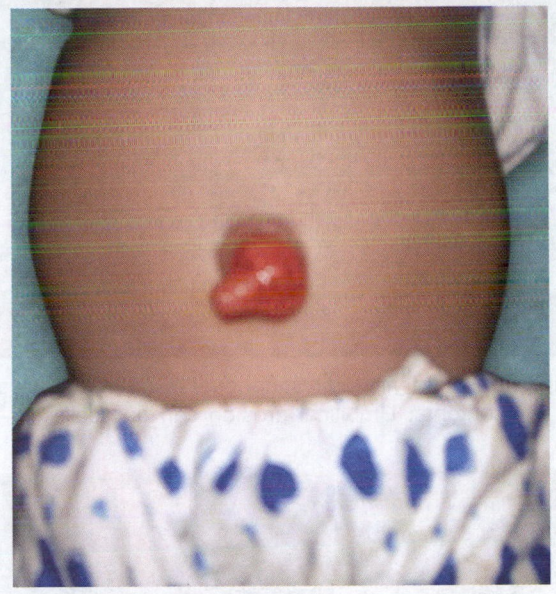

Fig. 38: Raspberry tumor of umbilicus (*Courtesy:* Professor Sandeep Kumar)

diverticulum, exploration of abdomen should be done and the anomaly is completely excised.

6. **What are the clinical presentations of persistent vitellointestinal duct?**
   A persistent vitellointestinal duct may present in the following manners (Fig. 39):
   • Patent duct at umbilicus discharging mucus and rarely feces (Figs 40 and 41)
   • A small segment of duct remaining patent at umbilicus giving rise to raspberry tumor

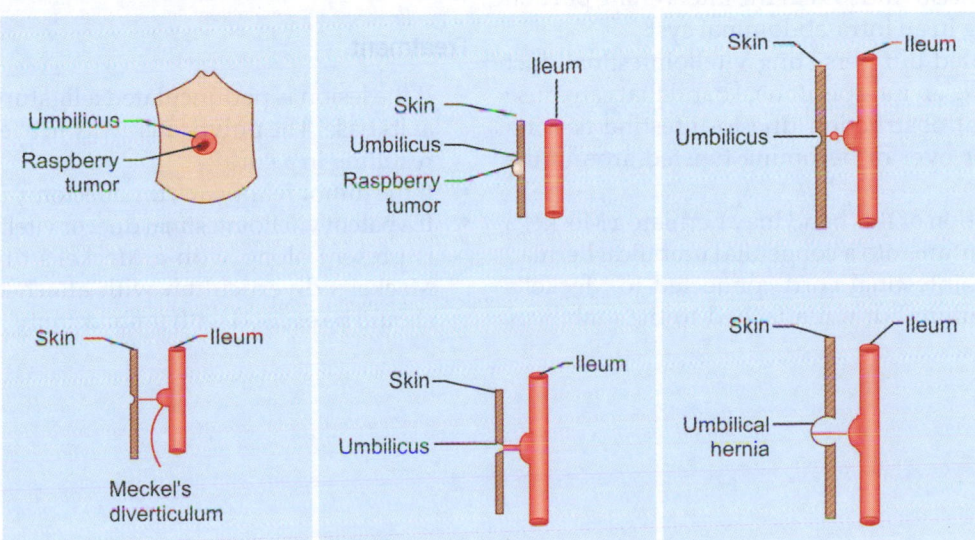

Fig. 39: Fate of vitellointestinal duct

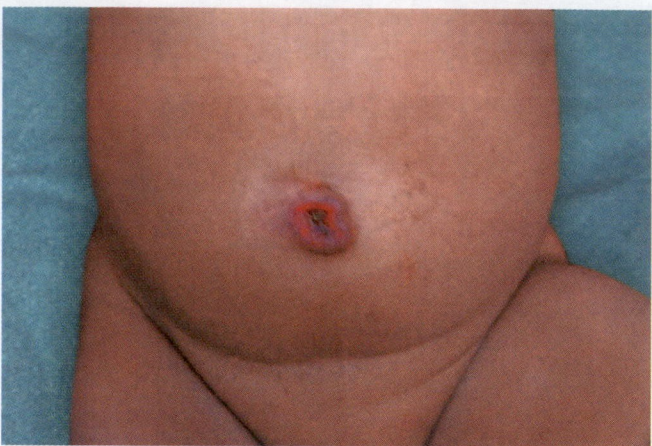

Fig. 40: Patent vitellointestinal duct discharging bowel contents. Umbilical erosion can be seen

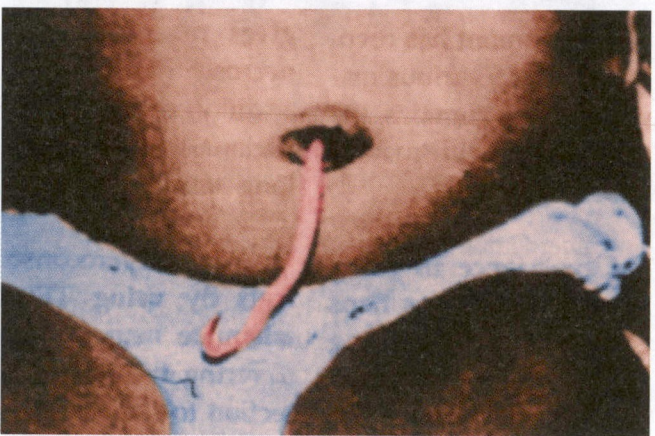

Fig. 41: Ascaris coming out of patent vitellointestinal duct

- Closure of both umbilical and intestinal ends with persistence of mucosa in the intervening portion resulting in an intra-abdominal cyst
- Obliterated but persisting vitellointestinal duct providing an intraperitoneal band that can cause intestinal obstruction due to intestine passing under or over or becoming twisted around the band
- Contraction of this band may herniate a Meckel's diverticulum into a congenital umbilical hernia
- A vitellointestinal cord connected to Meckel's diverticulum but not attached to the umbilicus becoming adherent to or knotted around another loop of small bowel may present as intestinal obstruction.

7. **What is an umbilical granuloma?**
   It is the presence of pouting granulation tissue in the umbilicus due to chronic infection.
8. **How do you treat it?**
   It is destroyed by silver nitrate application. One application is enough.
9. **What is an umbolith?**
   It is a stone-like structure present in the umbilicus that is usually black, soft and is composed of desquamated epithelial cells.
10. **How do you treat it?**
    The umbilical orifice is enlarged and the umbolith is removed.
11. **What is Sister Joseph's nodule?**
    It is a secondary carcinoma situated at umbilicus. The primary cancer may be in the stomach, colon, ovary or breast.

DISCUSSION

Umbilical adenoma is a tumor-like small swelling of umbilicus commonly seen in infants due to a partially unobliterated vitellointestinal duct (Fig. 38). Sometimes, it is due to completely unobliterated duct.

The patient is usually an infant who is brought with a small, pinkish swelling in the floor of the umbilicus that discharges a small amount of mucus and may at times bleed. The swelling looks like a raspberry. It is actually prolapsing mucosa of vitellointestinal duct which comes through the umbilicus. It is moist and bleeds on touch.

Microscopically the tumor consists of columnar epithelium rich in goblet cells.

Treatment

- If the lesion is pedunculated a ligature should be tied at its base. The polyp falls away in a few days by itself resulting in a cure
- If the tumor reappears, umbilectomy is indicated
- If a patent vitellointestinal duct or vitellointestinal band is present along with a Meckel's diverticulum, the Meckel's diverticulum with attached band or duct should be excised with umbilectomy

CASE 10: DESMOID TUMOR

CLINICAL DIAGNOSIS

1. The patient is commonly a middle-aged female who has given birth to many children and presents with a painless and slow growing swelling of abdominal wall of insidious onset (Fig. 42).
2. It is smooth or lobulated, firm or hard, nontender and well-defined.
3. It varies in size and often quite big.
4. It is fixed to the muscle layer, and often arises from the abdominal wall below the level of umbilicus.

VIVA VOCE

1. **What is a desmoid tumor?**
   It is a tumor arising from musculo-aponeurotic structures of abdominal wall particularly from rectus sheath and looks like a tendon in appearance and texture (GK desmos = tendon, eidos = appearance)
2. **What is the etiology of this condition?**
   The exact cause of this lesion is not known but a few facts are known about its etiology as given below:
   - It may be caused by repeated trauma as stretching of muscle fibers during pregnancy. This tumor is commonly seen in middle-aged multiparous women
   - It may occur in scars of operations, especially those of operations of hernia
   - A small traumatic hematoma of abdominal wall may be a precipitating factor.
3. **What is the gross pathology of this tumor?**
   This tumor is a hard fleshy mass that cracks on cutting. It does not have a capsule and it infiltrates into the surrounding muscles.
4. **What is the microscopic appearance?**
   Microscopically, it is composed of fibrous tissue and multinucleated plasmodial masses resembling foreign body giant cells.
5. **Does this tumor metastasize?**
   No.
6. **What are the complications of this tumor?**
   The complications are:
   - Infiltration of surrounding muscles. Rarely, it may extend through the abdominal wall to involve the bowel or the urinary bladder
   - Myxomatous change: If this tumor increases in size rapidly it may undergo myxomatous degeneration
   - Recurrence in spite of wide excision (Fig. 42).

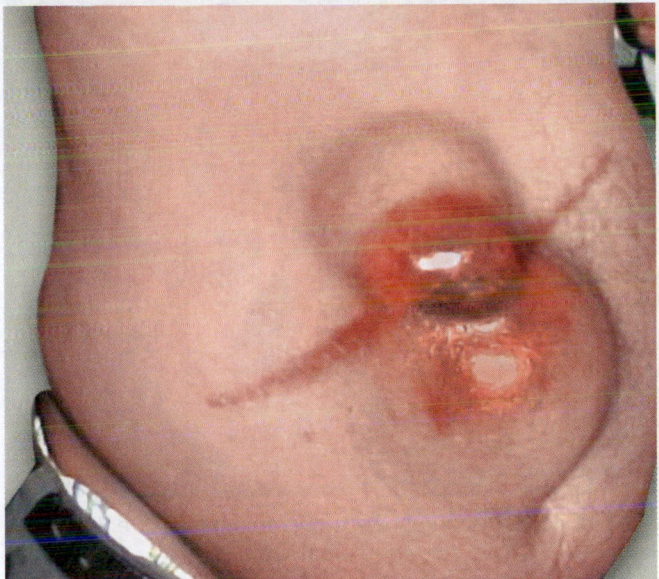

Fig. 42: Recurrent desmoid tumor. It was excised in the part the scar of which is visible
(*Courtesy:* Professor Sandeep Kumar)

7. **Does it ever undergo malignant change?**
   No.
8. **What are the investigations?**
   The investigations are:
   - Biopsy (Trucut needle biopsy will do)
   - CT scanning to see the extent, depth and infiltration (Fig. 43).
9. **How do you treat this disease?**
   It is treated by wide excision with a surrounding margin of at least 2.5 cm of healthy tissue. The abdominal wall may need reconstruction by polypropylene mesh and skin grafting.
10. **Can you treat this lesion by radiotherapy?**
    It is usually not treated by radiotherapy. But if it cannot be excised then it can be treated by radiotherapy as this tumor is moderately radiosensitive.
11. **Can this tumor recur?**
    This tumor can recur even after wide excision.

DISCUSSION

The desmoid tumor is a slow-growing tumor of the abdominal wall of unknown etiology and usually characterized by a massive swelling.

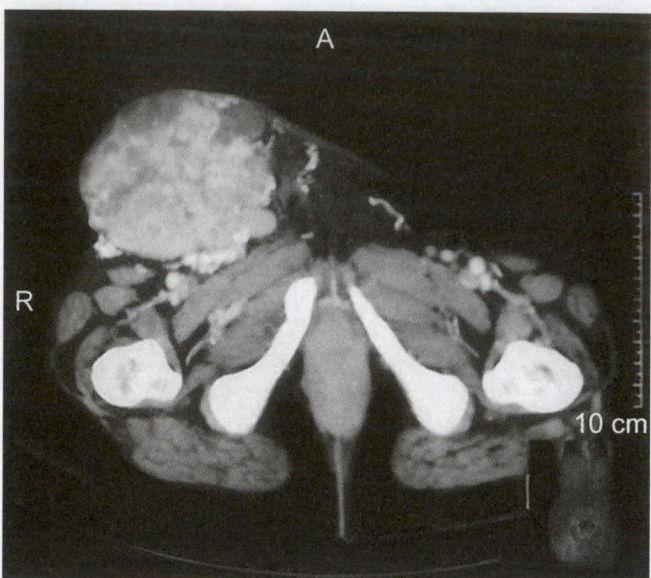

Fig. 43: CT scan shows a desmoid tumor of anterior abdominal wall

Etiology

Most of these tumors (80%) occur in women, many of whom have given birth to many children. Sometimes, this tumor occurs in the scars of hernia and other abdominal operations. Hence, trauma, e.g. stretching of muscle fibers during pregnancy or may be a small parietal hematoma may be the causative factor.

This tumor may occur in patients of familial adenomatous polyposis.

Pathology

This tumor originates in the musculoaponeurotic tissue of the abdominal wall, especially below the umbilicus. It does not have a capsule. It is very hard and cuts like an unripe pear with creaking. The term desmiod is derived from Greek word *desmos* that means a band or tendon.

Microscopically, it consists of fibrous tissue having multi-nucleated plasmodial masses looking like foreign body giant cells. It may look like a low-grade fibrosarcoma. It is infiltrative in nature but does not metastasize. It grows to a large size and may undergo a myxomatous change.

Treatment

This tumor is excised widely with a surrounding margin of at least 2.5 cm of healthy tissue. The abdominal wall defect is reconstructed by polypropylene mesh. This tumor is likely to recur, especially if wide excision is not done. It is moderately radiosensitive but radiation is not used in therapy usually.

CASE 11: CARCINOMA OF PAROTID GLAND

CLINICAL DIAGNOSIS

Carcinoma of parotid (Figs 44 and 45) occurs in two ways—
(a) As a malignant change in a pleomorphic adenoma, or
(b) As a de novo carcinoma.

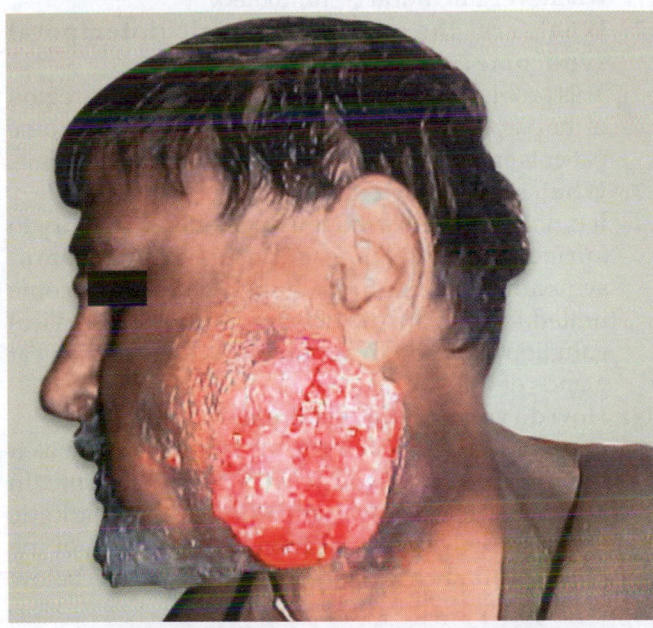

Fig. 44: Squamous cell carcinoma of left parotid
(*Courtesy:* Professor Sandeep Kumar)

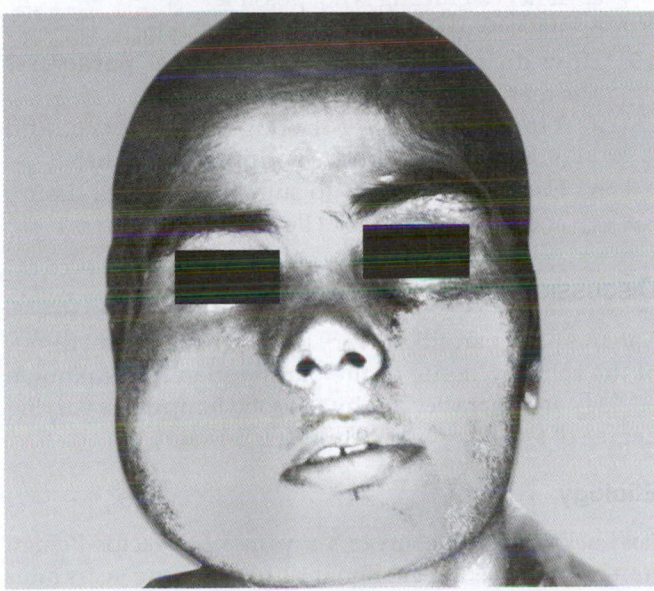

Fig. 45: Carcinoma of right parotid gland associated with paresis of facial nerve

a. Malignant change in a pleomorphic adenoma
The patient is a middle-aged or elderly person who had a swelling in the parotid region for many years. It has undergone the following changes recently:
1. The swelling is growing rapidly.
2. It has become painful.
3. The facial nerve is paralysed partially or completely.
4. It may be fixed to underlying masseter or mandible, or overlying skin.
5. It may be ulcerated and fungated.
6. The regional lymph nodes may be enlarged.
b. De novo carcinoma
1. The patient is a middle-aged or elderly person who presents with a rapidly growing swelling in the parotid region of recent onset.
2. It may be painful and tender.
3. It is variable in size, hard, irregular and ill-defined.
4. The facial nerve is paralysed partially or completely.
5. It may be fixed to masseter or mandible, or overlying skin.
6. It may have ulceration or fungation.
7. The regional lymph nodes may be enlarged.

VIVA VOCE

1. **What is carcinoma of parotid?**
   It is a malignant tumor of parenchyma of parotid salivary gland.
2. **How do you classify parotid tumors?**
   The tumors are classified as given below:
   a. Adenoma
      • Pleomorphic adenoma
      • Monomorphic – Adenolymphoma (Warthin's tumor).
   b. Carcinoma
      • Low grade – Acinic cell carcinoma
                     Adenoid cystic carcinoma
                     Mucoepidermoid carcinoma, low grade
      • High grade – Adenocarcinoma
                      Squamous cell carcinoma
                      Mucoepidermoid carcinoma, high grade.
   c. Others
      • Nonepithelial tumors – Hemangioma, lymphangioma
      • Lymphoma – Hodgkin's lymphoma, lymphoma in Sjogren's syndrome

- Secondary tumors
- Unclassified tumors.

3. How does this carcinoma produce facial nerve palsy?

As this tumor infiltrates the perineural tissues the nerve is irritated initially as can be seen by producing muscle spasm if the tissues over the nerve are tapped. As the infiltration and pressure of growing tumor continues paralysis is produced.

4. What are the investigations you will do in this tumor?

The investigations are:

a. X-ray of parotid region to see for any erosion of underlying bone.

b. CT scan to see the extent of disease including the cervical nodal involvement.

c. FNAC may be done.

d. Routine investigations – Hgb, blood counts, blood sugar, urine.

5. Will you like to do biopsy to confirm the diagnosis?

It is not done because:

a. The cancer cells may seed the incision readily to cause recurrence.

b. The facial nerve may be damaged.

6. What is the micropathology?

The adenoid cystic carcinoma consists of myoepithelial cells and duct epithelial cells. The former form sheets of cells within which basophilic material accumulates in blobs to give them a cribriform or lace-like appearance. The duct epithelial cells form strands and cords but tend also to form duct-like structures and microcysts in which some eosinophilic material accumulates. They also add to cribriform appearance.

In an adenocarcinoma, the cell arrangement resembles various glandular elements seen in a salivary gland.

7. How will you treat a carcinoma of parotid?

It is treated by radical excision of parotid with excision of the segment of facial nerve traversing the gland. The neural defect is bridged by a graft taken from great auricular nerve.

8. What is the role of radiotherapy?

The radiotherapy as a primary method of treatment cannot be used, as this tumor is not fully responsive. It is used to improve the results of surgery, especially in high grade tumors.

9. What are the limitations of radical excision of parotid?

The radical excision of parotid is limited by the internal carotid artery on its deep aspect and the cranial cavity posterosuperiorly. The excision of parotid including the mandible is straight forward, but inclusion of temporal bone requires special surgical expertise.

10. What are the complications of parotidectomy?

The most important complication is facial paralysis. The other complications are – hemorrhage, wound infection, sialocele, flap necrosis, auriculotemporal syndrome (Frey's syndrome).

11. What is auriculotemporal syndrome?

In this syndrome, there is flushing and sweating of the skin innervated by the auriculotemporal nerve whenever salivation is stimulated.

12. What are the causes of auriculotemporal syndrome?

This problem follows surgery or trauma in the region of the parotid gland or temporomandibular joint. Some patients are congenital and may be due to birth trauma.

13. What is the mechanism of this syndrome?

It is not known. It is thought that following injury to auriculotemporal nerve, postganglionic parasympathetic fibers from the otic ganglion become united to sympathetic fibers from superior cervical ganglion destined to supply the vessels and sweat glands of the skin.

14. How do you treat this syndrome?

In most of cases it does not need any treatment as it disappears spontaneously with passage of time. In severe cases an intratympanic parasympathetic neurectomy is done which involves division of the tympanic branch of glossopharyngeal nerve below the round window in the middle ear.

15. What are the causes of persistent facial paralysis after radical parotidectomy?

The causes are:

a. If nerve grafting is not possible.

b. If nerve graft fails to take up function.

16. How do you treat persistent facial paralysis?

The therapeutic measures are:

a. Transposition of hypoglossal nerve and anastomosing it to the peripheral branches.

b. Use of facial slings to support the facial tissues and to mask the facial deformity.

DISCUSSION

Carcinoma of parotid salivary gland is a malignant tumor of the salivary tissue of the parotid gland of unknown etiology and characterized by a parotid lump and a varying degree of facial nerve paralysis (Figs 44 and 45).

Etiology

It is not known. Exposure to X-rays may be a factor. Benign tumors may become malignant 10, 20 or more years after their onset. In half of all malignant tumors, a more benign variety of tumor can be detected somewhere in the specimen.

Pathology

Various forms are described, i.e. adenocarcinoma, squamous cell carcinoma, undifferentiated carcinoma, etc. Often there is little apart from the site to indicate that they arise from the salivary tissue. The different types have little relationship to the behavior of tumor.

The frankly malignant carcinoma is very malignant, killing its victim sometimes by local invasion and sometimes by widespread metastases. Local invasion of base of skull, cranial nerves, sinuses and major blood vessels produces distressing symptoms. The death from metastases, often in lungs, is kinder.

It spreads by local invasion and by lymphatics to the cervical lymph nodes. Hematogenous spread is rare and late.

The malignant tumors of the parotid are of two types depending upon their behavior:

1. Low-grade tumors, e.g. acinic cell carcinoma. Clinically, these tumors cannot be differentiated from benign tumors.
2. High-grade tumors: These tumors present as painless, rapidly growing swelling of insidious onset. Cervical nodal metastases may be present.

Investigations

1. Open biopsy: It is usually not done for the real danger of implantation of cancer cells in the wound, but in malignant lesions, it may be done when preoperative tissue diagnosis is needed as a prelude to radical excision.
2. FNAC: Some authorities recommend this procedure, but this carries the following disadvantages:
   - The sample is so small that it is difficult to interpret
   - The nature of lesion may vary between one area and another
   - There is a risk of implantation or recurrence which may be theoretical. It should be further noted that prior knowledge of the histology of lump rarely alters the management which in most of the cases in wide excision.
3. CT scan: This investigation is done to determine the exact site and extent of the tumor and metastases, MRI is also useful.
4. Radiography: The mandible may be radiographed to see for any bony involvement. X-ray of the chest may be done if there is clinical suspicion of pulmonary metastases.

Treatment

There are three clinical situations, the treatment of each is described below:

a. Unremarkable swelling

Here the definitive clinical diagnosis cannot be made. If the duration of illness is very short, the possibility that the lump is a reactive lymph node is always there. Here, the action should be delayed until at least 3 months.

If the lump persists after 3 months, it should be excised with a wide margin of normal tissue to avoid recurrence.

b. Clinical carcinoma

The patient should be prepared for radical parotidectomy and a generous open biopsy and frozen section should be done. If the tumor is malignant, a radical parotidectomy is done. Ideally, it should be combined with some sort of radiotherapy.

Radical parotidectomy: All branches and or the trunk of the facial nerve are removed alongwith the parotid gland.

Facial nerve damage: There is a gap which is usually bridged by a segment of great auricular nerve.

One method of treatment (Corcoran et al, 1983) is to give a course of radiotherapy of two thirds of the total dose, a wide local excision including some or all of the following—mandibular ramus, pinna, zygoma, external ear, middle ear and mastoid, the whole temporal bone plus a block dissection with reconstruction usually by a latissimus dorsi flap; then to give remaining one third of radiotherapy.

c. Lump unexpectedly reported to be histologically malignant

As the lump is widely removed in the previous operation no further treatment is done immediately. The patient is kept on a regular follow-up.

Prognosis

The carcinoma of parotid is one of the most lethal tumor, as the five-year survival rate rarely exceeds 20 percent in most series. Wide local excision in combination with preoperative and postoperative radiotherapy, achieves reasonable local control.

CASE 12: OSTEOSARCOMA

CLINICAL DIAGNOSIS

1. The patient is usually a young person between 10 to 20 years of age who presents with pain and a rapidly enlarging swelling of a bone.
2. There is persistent pain which has preceded the swelling.
3. The swelling can affect any bone but it commonly arises from the lower end of femur, upper end of tibia and upper end of humerus, radius or ulna (Figs 46 and 47).
4. It is usually situated in the metaphyseal region of a long bone.

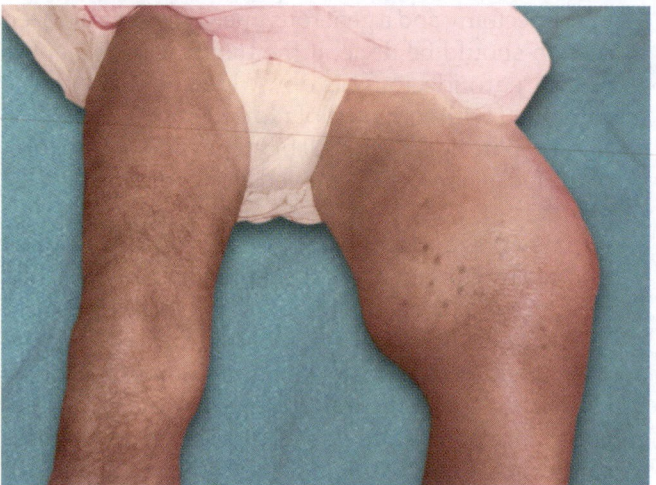

Fig. 46: Osteosarcoma of lower metaphysis of left femur

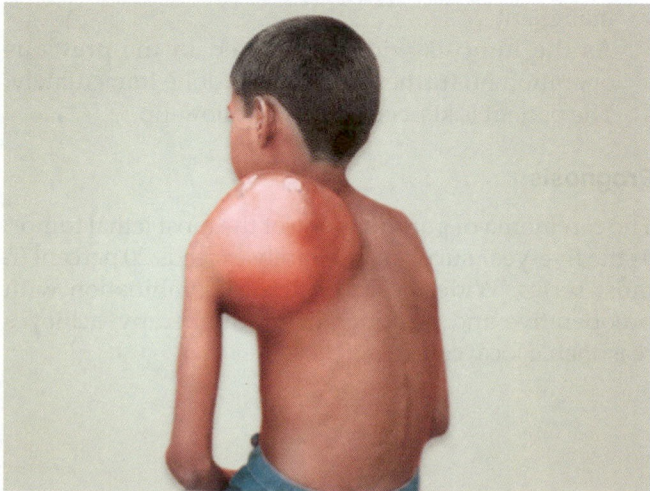

Fig. 47: Osteosarcoma of left scapula

5. The overlying skin is shiny, tense and red with prominent veins.
6. The surface is usually smooth or may be uneven.
7. It is asymmetrical and tends to be more on one side of the bone.
8. It is tender, hot and variable in consistency.
9. The joint in the vicinity may be stiff and may have effusion.
10. The patient may present with signs of pulmonary metastases, i.e. chest pain, cough and hemoptysis.

VIVA VOCE

1. **What is an osteosarcoma?**
   It is the second most common primary malignant tumor of bone of unknown etiology characterized by pain and swelling of recent onset near a joint.
2. **What is the cause of this tumor?**
   The cause is not known but the following facts are known:
   a. The Paget's disease of bone predisposes to develop a sarcoma of bone about 60 percent being osteosarcomas. Such tumors develop late in life.
   b. Excessive exposure to radiation can produce this disease.
   c. It can occur in fibrous dysplasia, multiple enchondromatosis and osteochondromata.
3. **What is the incidence of this tumor?**
   It is 2.8 patients per 1,00,000 population per year.
4. **What is the gross pathology?**
   The tumor starts in the medullary cavity of the metaphyseal area of a long bone. It elevates or perforates the periosteum. The angle between the elevated periosteum and the bone is known as Codman's triangle. The epiphysis may be invaded if it has fused. The tumor varies in vascular, fibrous, cartilaginous and osseous contents.
5. **What is the microscopic picture?**
   It consists of pleomorphic cells, the pattern is that of a sarcoma with osteoid production, recognized by its faint eosinophilic and glossy appearance. Usually, tumor cells are small, spindle-shaped with hyperchromatic nuclei and mitotic figures. They are arranged in palisades, columns or alveoli. There are numerous thin walled blood vessels and sinusoids (Fig. 48).
   Variants range from extremely well-differentiated tissue with abundant bone production or highly anaplastic lesions.

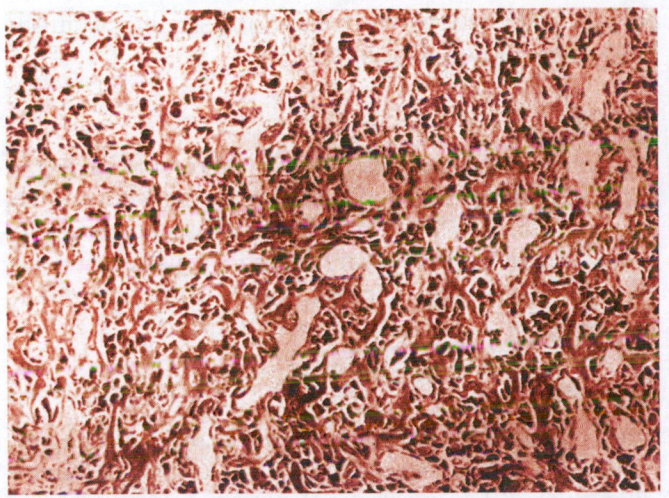

Fig. 48: Osteosarcoma showing intercellular osteoid matrix

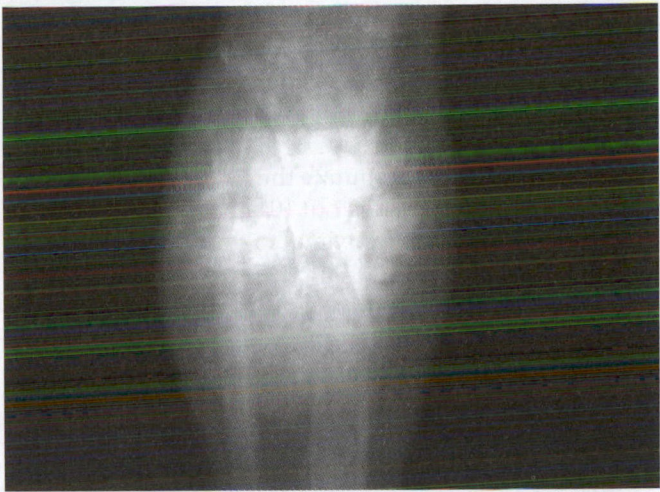

Fig. 49: Sun-ray appearance of osteosarcoma of upper metaphysis of tibia

6. How does this tumor spread?
This tumor spreads early to lungs by blood stream. It may spread to liver, bones and brain.
Locally, it spreads by continuity and contiguity to the neighboring structures.

7. What are the investigations?
The investigations include:
a. X-ray of the affected part.
b. X-ray of chest.
c. CT scan.
d. Others: Serum alkaline phosphatase, bone scan, MRI.

8. What are the radiographic signs of this tumor?
The radiographic signs are:
a. There is an irregular bone destroying lesion in the metaphyseal region of a bone.
b. 'Sunray' (or sunburst) appearance due to the presence of thin radio-opaque spicules of the bone radiating away from the cortex of bone.
c. The periosteum may be raised off the bone by the tumor mass, forming reactive bone at the periosteal margin (Codman's triangle).
d. Soft tissue shadow around the tumor (Fig. 49).

9. Why do you want to do CT scan of chest?
To accurately evaluate for pulmonary metastases.

10. What is the role of CT scan of affected part?
It is done to plan resectional surgery after adjuvant therapy.

11. When do you do MRI?
Instead of CT scan MRI can be done for better and sharper delineation of the lesion, especially soft tissue invasion for planning operation.

12. What is the indication for bone scan?
When there is suspicion of metastases in bone.

13. What happens to serum alkaline phosphatase?
It may be significantly elevated in cases where there is considerable osteogenic activity.

14. How do you treat this disease?
This lesion is treated by neoadjuvant chemotherapy followed by resection or amputation.

15. Can the limb be conserved?
If the lesion is small and early the limb can be conserved by local resection of the tumor.

16. How do you make up for resected bone?
The bone resected in the limb salvage surgery can be reconstructed by custom prosthetic replacement, arthrodesis or allografting.

17. What are the contraindications of limb salvage surgery?
An advanced lesion or when there is a pathological fracture with contamination of all compartments or involvement of neurovascular bundle precludes salvage surgery and indicates an amputation.

18. What are the drugs used?
Various regimes have been employed using high dose methotrexate with citrovorum rescue, doxorubicin and vincristine. Other drugs are cyclophosphamide, ifosfamide, bleomycin, dacarbazine, cisplatin and dactinomycin.

19. How long is chemotherapy continued?
Chemotherapy is usually continued for one year after operation.

20. **How do you deal with the problem of length of limb in a pediatric patient after resection?**
   The prosthetic designs that can be periodically lengthened by a minor operation allow limb salvage in pediatric patients.

21. **Where will you amputate the limb?**
   Amputation is carried out 10 cm above the tumor or joint immediately proximal to the bone involved by the tumor.

22. **How do you treat solitary pulmonary metastasis?**
   It is treated by lobectomy.

23. **What are the results of treatment?**
   The results are better now with 50 to 70 percent 5-year survival rates.

24. **How do you treat a tumor of pelvis or spine?**
   These tumors are treated by chemotherapy, local excision and perhaps radiation therapy.

25. **Why do you give chemotherapy before surgery?**
   The treatment with amputation alone is seldom successful because micrometastases are presumed to have occurred by the time of diagnosis. Chemotherapy is effective against most of these micrometastases and cure rates have markedly improved with this treatment.

26. **What do you mean by limb salvage surgery?**
   The aim of limb salvage is to resect the tumor and to provide the patient with a useful and functional limb with an equal chance of cure compared with amputation.

27. **What are the indications for prosthetic replacement?**
   The most common indication is after resection of a tumor of the distal femur and proximal tibia.

28. **What are the advantage of prosthetic replacement?**
   The advantages are:
   a. Early mobilization and weight bearing.
   b. Low rate of early complications.
   c. Cost effective.
   d. Readily available.

29. **What are the surgical options for osteosarcoma?**
   Surgical options for sarcomas of bone:
   a. Amputation.
   b. Limb salvage.
   c. Simple excision alone, e.g. tumor of fibula.
   d. Excision and reconstruction with autograft, e.g. tumors of mid tibia.
   e. Excision and arthrodesis, e.g. tumors of ankle joint
   f. Excision and allograft.
   g. Excision and arthroplasty.

DISCUSSION

Osteosarcoma is the second most common primary malignant bone tumor (after myeloma) of unknown etiology and characterized by pain and swelling. It affects 2.8 persons in 1,00,000 population.

Etiology

- Primary osteosarcoma: Majority of tumors belong to this group where the cause of the disease is not known.
- Secondary osteosarcoma which is secondary to malignant transformation in Paget's disease of bone, multiple enchondromatosis, fibrous dysplasia, irradiation of bone and osteochondroma.

Pathology

Sites: Usually, this lesion is metaphyseal. Any bone may be involved but it is extremely rare in small bones of distal extremities and spine. The common sites of involvement in a decreasing order of frequency are lower end of femur (52%), upper end of tibia (20%) and upper end of humerus (9%).

Gross pathology: An osteoblastic tumor is grayish white, hard and cuts with a gritty sensation. A chondroid tumor may appear opalescent and bluish gray.

A fibroblastic tumor has a typical fish-flesh sarcomatous appearance. A telangiectatic tumor may have large areas of tumor necrosis and blood-filled spaces in the tumor.

Micropathology: It has anaplastic mesenchymal parenchyma with tumor cells surrounded by osteoid.

Cartilage formation is a prominent feature of periosteal and parosteal variants of osteosarcoma.

Telangiectatic variants are lytic and expansile, have prominent vascular spaces and very little bone formation (like an aneurysmal bone cyst).

Clinical Features

The pain is first symptom which is constant and boring. It is soon followed by a swelling which increases the pain. It is often worse at night, sometimes the patient may present with a pathological fracture.

The swelling is metaphyseal. The skin over the swelling is shiny with prominent veins. The swelling is hot, tender and ill-defined.

It spreads usually by blood stream to lungs where it may be asymptomatic or cause chest pain, cough, wheezing or hemoptysis.

Investigations

Radiography: There is an evidence of irregular bone destruction, soft tissue shadow and new bone formation. The cortex overlying the lesion is eroded.

The periosteum is lifted by growing tumor resulting in irregular periosteal reaction. At the ends of the tumor, at the tumor-host cortex junction, a triangular area of subperiosteal new bone is seen called Codman's triangle.

The tumor grows into the overlying soft tissues in which the new bone is laid along the blood vessels centrifugally giving rise to sunray appearance.

The X-ray of the chest may show metastases. CT scan of the chest may be required.

Biopsy: It is the most important part in the work-up of the tumor and should be carried out at the center where the definitive treatment is going to be done.

The appropriate part of the tumor is sampled to ensure viable and representative material. The uncontaminated compartment should not be violated while doing biopsy. Needle biopsy (core biopsy) via a small incision usually gives sufficient representative material which is sent for histologic and cytogenetic studies.

CT scan, MRI of the affected part is required to assess the extent of lesion for limb saving surgical planning.

Others: Serum alkaline phosphatase may be elevated. It has no diagnostic value but may be used in follow-up.

Bone scan may be done to find the intramedullary spread (skip lesions).

Treatment

- **Limb saving surgery:** With early diagnosis, exact assessment of local extent and control of systemic micrometastases with neoadjuvant chemotherapy, it is now possible to do limb saving surgery. The bone resected can be reconstructed by custom made prosthesis, arthrodesis and bone grafting.
- **Chemotherapy:** In most of the patients, the systemic micrometastases have already occurred by the time the diagnosis is made. They are controlled by preoperative (neoadjuvant) and/or postoperative (adjuvant) chemotherapy. Many drugs or drug combinations are in use, e.g. high dose methotrexate with citrovorum factor, doxorubicin and vincristine. Other drugs are cyclophosphamide, ifsofamide, bleomycin, dacarbazine, cisplatin and dactinomycin. These drugs are very toxic, hence given in the supervision of an oncophysician.
- **Radiotherapy:** It can be used for the local control of disease occurring at surgically inaccessible sites or in patients who refuse surgery. It is not given as a routine preoperative treatment.
- **Amputation:** It can be both palliative or definitive. The palliative amputation is done in advanced disease for pain relief and avoiding ulceration. It is also done when there is a pathological fracture.

The definitive amputation is done with the aim of cure. In the past disarticulation through the joint proximal to the affected bone was done to avoid stump recurrence. Now, due to effective chemotherapy the amputation can be performed through the affected bone, 10 cm above the tumor margin.

- **Immunotherapy:** It is a new concept in which a portion of tumor is implanted into a sarcoma survivor (if agrees) which is removed after two weeks. Now, the sensitized lymphocytes are infused into the patient. They kill the cancer cells selectively.

Prognosis

- Without treatment the patient dies within 2 years, and within 6 months, if metastases are detected.
- The 5-year survivals with surgery are 20 percent and with surgery and chemoitherapy 70 percent.
- A telangiectatic sarcoma has worst prognosis.

Parosteal Osteosarcoma

It occurs in a slightly older age group and starts adjacent to the periosteum rather than in the bone. The most frequent sites are posterior aspect of femur and proximal humerus and tibia.

The lesion is usually well circumscribed, slow growing with late metastases usually to the lungs.

Microscopically, it consists of spindle cells with woven bone formation, fibrous and focal cartilage formation.

Treatment: This tumor is not sensitive to chemotherapy hence it is resected with reconstruction or treated by amputation.

Prognosis: It is better than usual osteosarcoma.

Periosteal Osteosarcoma

It arises from the surface of the diaphysis most commonly distal tibia or femur. It is considered to be a variant of parosteal osteosarcoma with significant cartilage component.

Secondary Osteosarcoma

It occurs in elderly people. The most common cause is Paget's disease where it occurs in 1 to 10 percent of patients. It can occur in fibrous dysplasia and following radiation.

5 to 10 percent of patients treated by high intensity radiation for other cancers (sarcoma, lymphoma, etc.) may develop this lesion 10 to 20 years later.

This tumor is an invariably high grade aggressive tumor with extremely poor prognosis and tendency for early metastases.

Most patients (because of age) do not tolerate the toxicity of intensive chemotherapy, hence treated by excision or amputation.

Management of Osteosarcoma

- Patient 15 to 20 years of age having rapidly growing metaphyseal swelling lower end of femur, upper end of tibia, upper end of humerus or other sites
- Shiny skin, prominent veins, warm, tender and firm or variable consistency
- Radiography: Irregular bone destruction in metaphysis, soft tissue shadow and may be new bone formation of sun-ray pattern
- Biopsy: Anaplastic mesenchymal parenchyma with cells surrounded by osteoid tissue.

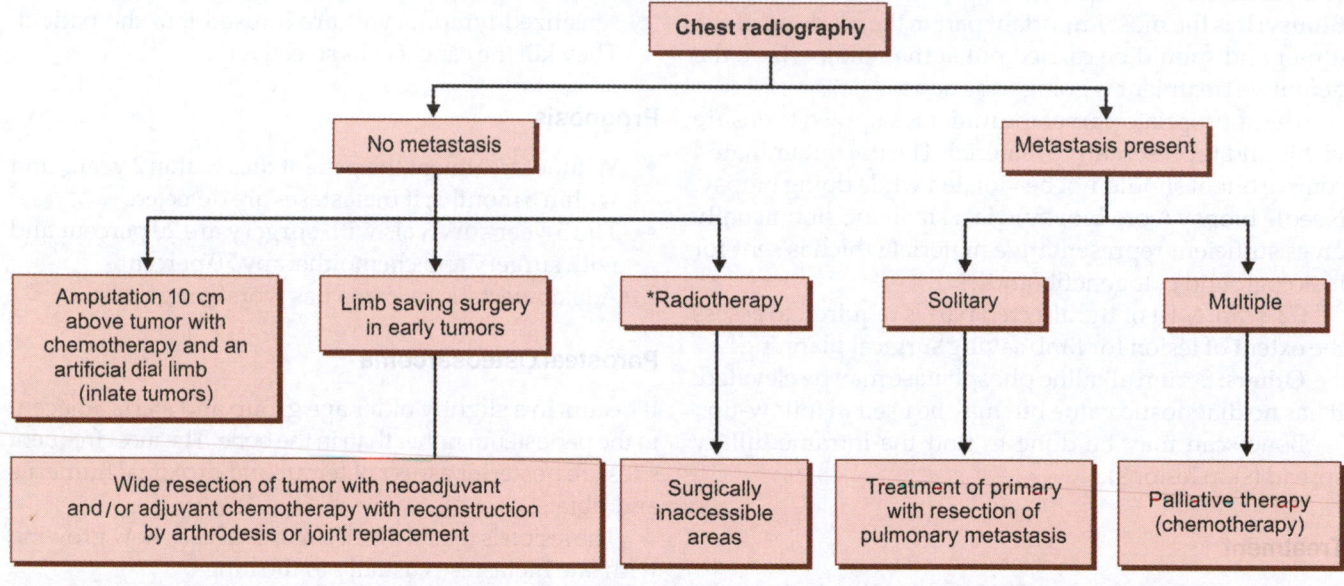

CASE 13: GIANT CELL TUMOR (OSTEOCLASTOMA)

CLINICAL DIAGNOSIS

1. The patient who is between 20 to 45 years of age, presents with a slow growing swelling of a bone of insidious onset.
2. A dull ache is commonly present in the lesion.
3. The swelling usually arises in the epiphysis of long bones (Figs 50 and 51) most commonly in the distal femur, proximal tibia, proximal femur and distal radius.
4. It may occur in sacrum, ribs, pelvic bones or vertebral column.

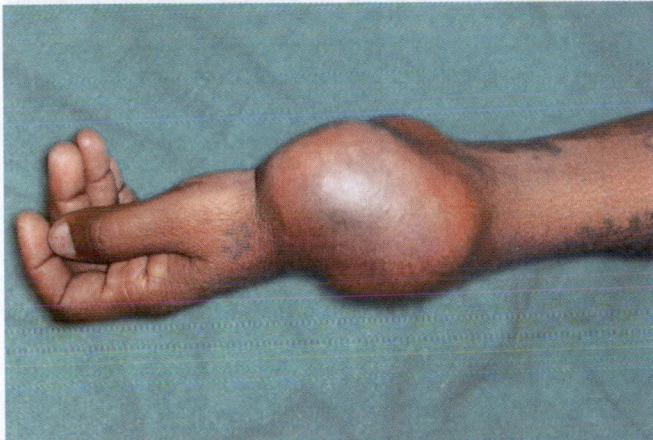

Fig. 50: Osteoclastoma of lower end of left radius
(*Courtesy:* Dr Uttam Garg)

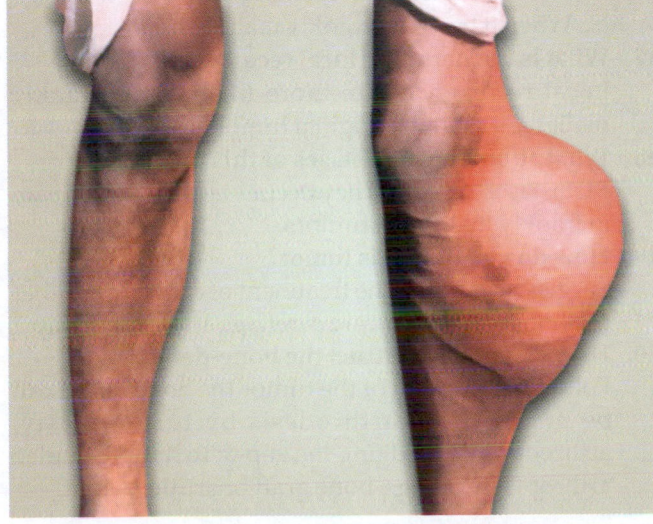

Fig. 51: Osteoclastoma of upper end of left fibula

5. It is either a diffuse expansion of epiphysis or an asymmetrical swelling noticeable on one side only.
6. It is smooth or lobulated.
7. It is firm or variable in consistency; egg-shell crackling may be present.
8. The regional lymph nodes are not enlarged.

VIVA VOCE

1. **What is an osteoclastoma?**
   Osteoclastoma is a locally malignant tumor of unknown etiology occurring in the epiphyses of long bones in young persons (Figs 50 and 51).
2. **What is the nature of this tumor?**
   This tumor is often classified as a benign bone tumor, but only one third of the tumors are benign, and of the rest one third invade the local tissues and one third produce metastases.
3. **What is the cell of origin?**
   It is not yet clear from which cell this tumor takes its origin.
4. **What are the common sites of this lesion?**
   The commonest site of this tumor is around the knee joint. The other common sites are upper end of humerus, upper end of femur and lower end of radius.
5. **What is the site of origin in the bone?**
   It probably arises in the metaphysis but grows so rapidly involving the epiphysis towards the joint surface that by the time it is seen clinically, it is almost an epiphyseal tumor.
6. **What is the gross appearance of this tumor?**
   The tumor is large, lobulated and reddish brown in color due to hemorrhages inside and patches of fat. When the tumor grows inside the medulla it causes expansion and thining of cortex.
   There is no new bone formation. As thinning continues the lesion may have egg-shell crackling.
7. **What is the microscopic picture?**
   Microscopically, it consists of monocytic stromal cells, vascular tissue and sheets of large multinucleated osteoclast-like cells (giant cells) (Fig. 52).
8. **What are the other giant cell lesions?**
   The other giant cell lesions are:
   a. Eosinophilic granuloma
   b. Brown tumor of hyperparathyroidism
   c. Aneurysmal bone cyst
   d. Chondroblastoma
   e. Osteoblastoma
   f. Nonossifying fibroma

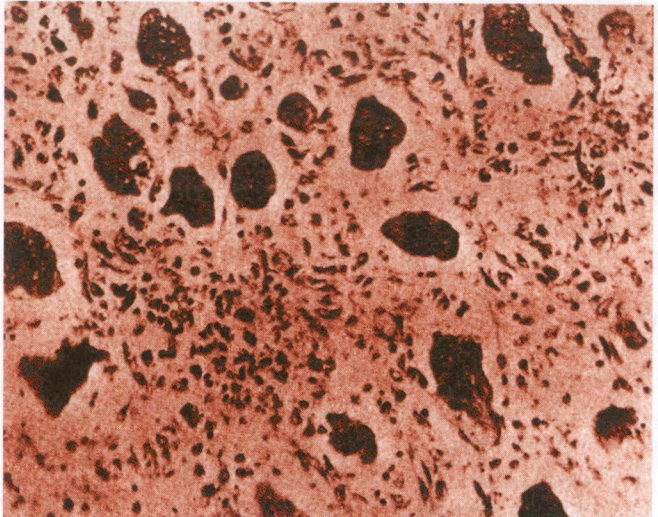

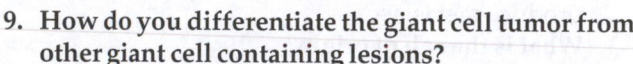

Fig. 52: Microscopic picture of a giant cell tumor showing many giant cells

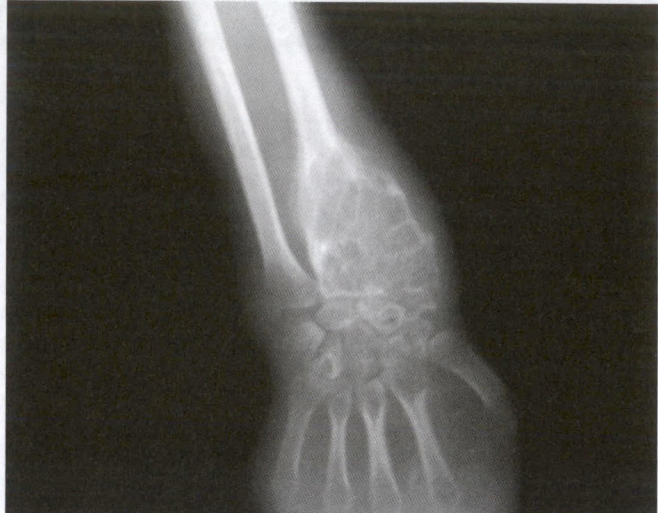

Fig. 53: Osteoclastoma of lower end of radius having classical "soap bubble" appearance

9. **How do you differentiate the giant cell tumor from other giant cell containing lesions?**
   In a giant cell tumor, the oval nuclei of monocytic stroma resemble those of giant cells suggesting a common origin. This features is absent in other giant cell containing lesions.

10. **What is osteoclastoma alba?**
    Osteoclastoma occurring at the lower end of radius is often whitish in color, hence called osteoclastoma alba.

11. **Can this tumor involve a joint?**
    Joint involvement is not uncommon as the tumor may invade the articular cartilage resulting in joint stiffness.

12. **What are the investigations?**
    The investigations include:
    a. X-ray of affected part.
    b. X-ray of chest.
    c. Biopsy.
    d. CT scan of the lesion may be done if it is involving sacrum, pelvic bones or vertebral column.

13. **What are the X-ray signs?**
    The X-ray signs are:
    a. The end of a long bone is expanded eccentrically or asymmetrically.
    b. The tumor is almost abutting against the articular cartilage.
    c. The expansion has septa and spaces giving a typical 'soap bubble' appearance.
    d. There is no evidence of new bone formation.
    e. A soft tissue shadow is seen, but there is no soft tissue invasion (Fig. 53).

14. **What are the signs of a frankly malignant osteoclastoma?**
    The following signs favor malignancy:
    a. Breach in the outer outline of thin expanded cortex.
    b. Soft tissue invasion.
    c. Loss of demarcation with healthy bone.
    d. Hazy look of the tumor.

15. **What are the complications?**
    The complications include:
    a. Pathological fracture.
    b. Transformation into a frankly malignant lesion (sarcoma).

16. **What are the causes of tissue invasion by this tumor?**
    The causes of tissue invasion are:
    a. When pathological fracture occurs.
    b. When it becomes frankly malignant.

17. **What is the nature of local recurrence?**
    Local recurrences are more likely to be frankly malignant than the original tumor.

18. **What about the metastases of this tumor?**
    Metastases are rare. They occur via the blood stream in frankly malignant tumors.

19. **How do you treat this tumor?**
    Surgical excision is the treatment of choice. The other methods of treatment are curettage and radiotherapy.

20. **How do you reconstruct the bone-defect?**
    Following excision of the tumor the bone defect can be made up by arthrodesis by turn-o-plasty, arthrodesis by bridging the gap with double fibulae arthroplasty using a bone graft or artificial joint.

21. **What do you do in turn-o-plasty procedure?**
   The joint end of healthy bone is split in two halves for the required length and one half is turned upside down and fixed in the defect left after excision of the tumor, and the joint is immobilized to arthrodese.

22. **What is the disadvantage of curettage?**
   Curettage alone is followed by 25 to 50 percent recurrence rate. Hence, it must be supplemented by some other procedure.

23. **What are the supplementing procedures?**
   The supplementing procedures are:
   - Cryotherapy where liquid nitrogen is used to produce freezing to kill residual tumor cells
   - Burning with cauterization
   - Thermal effect of bone cement (methyl methacrylate).

24. **What are the advantages of cementation technique?**
   The main advantage of cementation technique is that if local recurrence occurs, it can be easily detected by radiography as luceny next to cement.

25. **What are the disadvantages of cementation technique?**
   The main disadvantage of cementation is that the presence of cement next to the articular cartilage (tumor being epiphyseal) may predispose to cartilage degeneration.

26. **What do you do in such a situation?**
   The cement is removed and bone grafting is done after 2 years, if there is no evidence of recurrence.

27. **What are the results of cementation technique?**
   This method of treatment is successful in 90 percent of cases.

28. **What is the role of radiotherapy?**
   It is the method of treatment of a tumor of vertebral and other surgically inaccessible areas.

29. **What is the dose of radiotherapy?**
   5000 to 6000 rad in 5 to 6 weeks

30. **What is the major risk of radiotherapy?**
   It may cause post-radiation sarcoma.

31. **How do you manage the joint during wide excision?**
   The joint is managed by arthroplasty or arthrodesis.

32. **When do you do an amputation?**
   The amputation is indicated in:
   a. Persistent recurrence of tumor.
   b. Malignant osteoclastoma.

DISCUSSION

Osteoclastoma is a locally malignant tumor of bone of unknown etiology consisting of monocytic stromal cells, vascular tissue and large osteoclast-like giant cells.

Although this tumor is often classified under the group of benign bone tumors, it is not a true benign tumor. One third of these tumors are benign, one third invade the local tissues and about one third metastasize.

Pathology

This tumor usually arises in the epiphyses of long bones most commonly in the distal femur, proximal tibia, proximal femur and distal radius.

The tumor is large, lobulated and reddish brown in color due to hemorrhages inside and patches of fat. When the tumor grows inside the medulla it causes expansion and thinning of cortex. There is no new bone formation. As thinning continues, it gives rise to 'egg-shell crackling' when the bone is pressed upon.

This tumor often extends to the subchondral surface and can even invade the joint.

Microscopically, it consists of monocytic stromal cells, vascular tissue and sheets of large multinucleated osteoclast-like cells. The oval nuclei of monocytic stroma resemble those of giant cells suggesting a common origin.

Clinical Features

The patient is between 20 to 45 years of age and presents with a slow growing swelling of a bone of insidious onset. It may be painless but local dull ache is commonly present.

The swelling is either a diffuse expansion of epiphysis, or an asymmetrical swelling noticeable on one side only. It is smooth or lobulated and firm or variable in consistency. Egg-shell crackling may be present.

Investigations

1. *Radiography:* The affected part must be X-rayed. The radiographic picture shows a purely lytic, well circumscribed and occasionally expansile lesion with cortical destruction with trabeculae of the remnants of bone traversing it (soap-bubble appearance). The perforation of the cortex is a sign of malignancy.
2. Biopsy, either Trucut needle biopsy or open biopsy is mandatory.

Complications

1. Pathological fracture.
2. *Malignant transformation:* This usually occurs when the benign giant cell tumor is treated by radiotherapy.

Treatment

1. Excision: If possible excision is the best method of treatment. If it causes significant functional impairment, some reconstructive procedure is combined with excision, for example, in a tumor of

knee region the post-excision defect is made up by arthrodesis of the knee or arthroplasty.

- Arthrodesis by turn-o-plasty: After excision of the tumor of lower end of femur, the upper end of tibia is split into two halves for the required length. One half of split tibia is turned up and fixed in the femoral defect left after excision of the tumor. A similar procedure may be done for a tibial tumor by taking on half of split femur
- Arthrodesis by double fibulae: Two grafts of fibula taken from both limbs are fitted in the defect
- After excision the joint can be reconstructed by bone graft or a joint prosthesis.

2. *Curettage:* It is done when tumor has not yet involved the joint and not gone beyond the cortex. Curettage alone is associated with 25 to 50 percent recurrence rate as some tumor cells are always left along the wall of the cavity. Hence, it is supplemented by some other procedure, e.g. cryotherapy using liquid nitrogen, thermal burning using cauterization or filling the cavity with bone cement (methyl methacrylate) which kills the tumor cells by the heat it produces.

3. *Amputation:* Amputation is rarely required for an aggressive or recurrent tumor.

4. *Radiotherapy:* A tumor of the vertebrae is treated by radiation treatment.

The treatment of common sites of an osteoclastoma is given below:

- Upper end of tibia and lower end of femur is treated by excision and turn-o-plasty.
- Lower end of radius is treated by excision with fibular grafting
- Upper end of fibula and lower end of ulna is treated by excision.

Prognosis

This tumor can recur when the tumor becomes more aggressive.

CASE 14: EWING'S SARCOMA

CLINICAL DIAGNOSIS

1. The patient is usually a child between 5 to 20 years of age who presents with recurrent attacks of pain and swelling in the shaft of a long bone of recent onset.
2. It commonly affects tibia, fibula, humerus or femur.
3. The pain is throbbing type, increases at night and made worse by movement.
4. The swelling is circumferential and fusiform.
5. It is red, hot, smooth, firm and tender.
6. The upper and lower limits are not well defined.
7. It is usually associated with pyrexia (Fig. 54).
8. The regional lymph nodes may be enlarged.

VIVA VOCE

1. **What is an Ewing's tumor?**
   It is a highly malignant tumor of unknown etiology arising from midshaft or metaphysis of long bones.
2. **What is the origin of this tumor?**
   There is some controversy regarding the origin of this tumor. It is probably derived from primitive mesenchyme.
3. **What is its incidence?**
   0.1 case per 1,00,000 population per year.
4. **What is male/female ratio?**
   3:2.
5. **What are the most common sites of occurrence of this tumor?**
   Femur, tibia and pelvis.
6. **What is the pathology of this tumor?**
   - It is nonspecific with neoplastic tissue permeating bone and muscles with consistency varying from firm connective tissue to liquefaction necrosis.
   - Microscopically, there are sheets of small cells resembling lymphocytes. The tumor cells surround a central clear area (Fig. 55).
7. **What are the sites of metastases?**
   The metastases are most common in the lung but can occur in bones and bone marrow.
8. **What are the investigations?**
   The investigations are:
   - X-ray of affected bone or part (Fig. 56)
   - X-ray of chest
   - Biopsy
   - Culture of biopsy specimen
   - CT scan or MRI
   - Bone scan.
9. **What are the radiographic signs of this tumor?**
   The radiographic signs are:
   - There is irregular destruction of bone (moth eaten)
   - There is subperiosteal new bone formation giving the appearance of a cut onion (onion-peel appearance) (Fig. 56).
   - It is usually a lesion of diaphysis.
10. **What is the role of CT scan?**
    It is done to find the extent of the lesion.

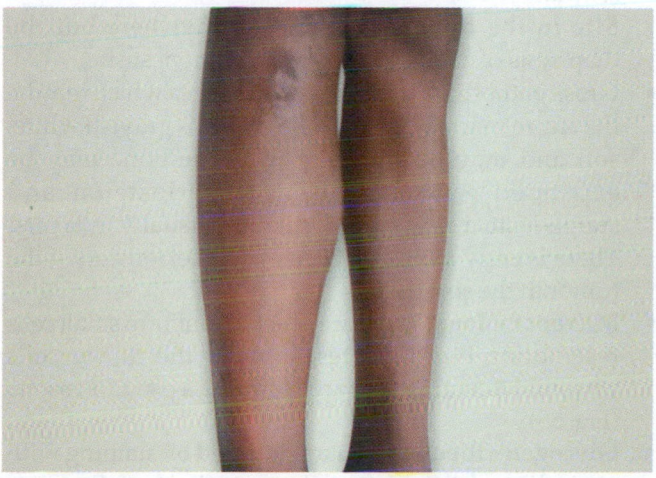

Fig. 54: Ewing's sarcoma of right tibia in an eleven-year-old boy having pain diffuse swelling and sometimes fever

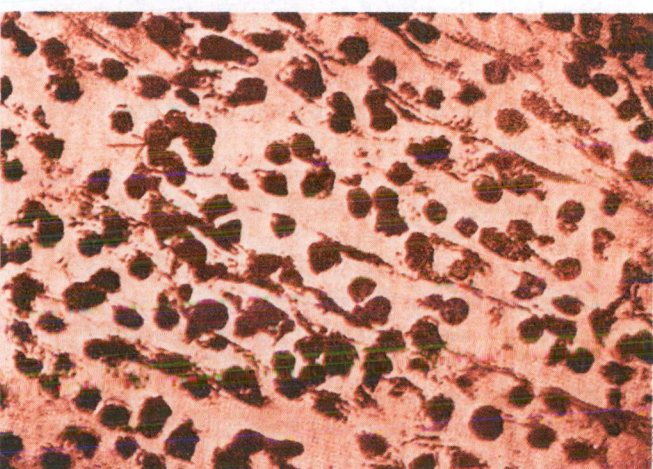

Fig. 55: Microscopic picture of an Ewing's sarcoma showing sheets of small cells resembling lymphocytes

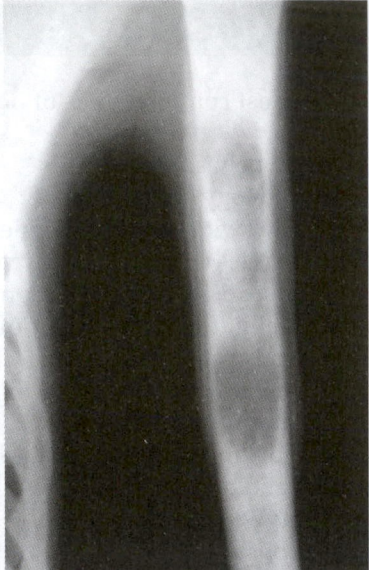

Fig. 56: Onion-peel appearance of an Ewing's sarcoma of humerus as seen on radiography

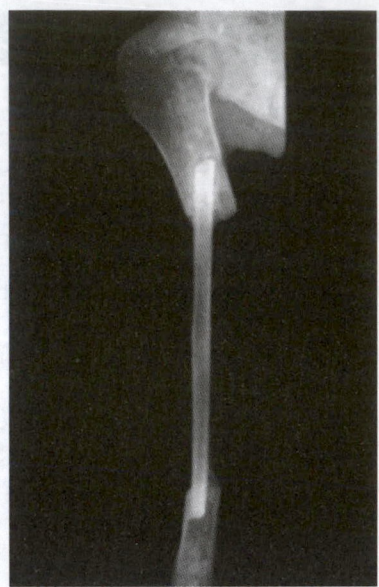

Fig. 57: Fibular grafting following resection of humeral shaft for an Ewing's sarcoma

11. **What is the role of MRI?**

    It is nearly the same as CT scan but it gives better information of soft tissue invasion.

12. **Why do you want to do bone scan?**

    It is done to find bony metastases and extent of bone involvement.

13. **What are the findings in the blood?**

    The blood may show leukocytosis, raised ESR and elevated lactic dehydrogenase.

14. **How will you differentiate it from acute osteomyelitis?**

    By investigations – the biopsy tissue is examined histologically as well as by bacteriological culture.

15. **How do you treat this condition?**

    It is treated by systemic chemotherapy followed by surgical resection with limb salvage or radiotherapy.

16. **What are the drugs used?**

    The drugs used are doxorubicin, cyclophosphamide or ifosfamide, etoposide, vincristine and dactinomycin.

17. **How do you reconstruct for the loss of bone?**

    The gap is filled with bone graft and the segments are internally supported with plate and screws or nail (Fig. 57).

18. **What is the prognosis?**

    - With the modern methods the prognosis has improved remarkably with 80 percent at 5-year survival rates
    - It is a curable tumor in children below 11 years of age.

DISCUSSION

Ewing's tumor, the fourth most common primary malignant tumor of the bone, is a tumor of unknown etiology occurring in children between 5 to 20 years of age that tends to arise in the diaphysis of the long bones (60%) and flat bones (40%).

Pathology

- **Bones affected:** Femur is the most common bone affected, followed by tibia, fibula, humerus, pelvis, and scapula
- **Site in the bone:** It may occur anywhere but the diaphysis of a long bone is the commonest site
- **Gross pathology:** It involves a large area which may be the entire marrow cavity. The tumor is grayish white, soft and may be thin like pus. The bone may be expanded with elevation of periosteum and subperiosteal new bone formation, usually in layers. There is early rupture of cortex with extension of the tumor in the soft tissues
- **Micropathology:** There are sheets of uniform small cells resembling lymphocytes. Usually the tumor cells surround a central clear area forming a pseudo-rosette (Fig. 55)
- **Glycogen-filled cytoplasm detected** by staining with periodic acid-Schiff is characteristic of Ewing's sarcoma cells. p 30/32, the product of the mic-2 gene is a cell surface marker

- **Spread:** This tumor grows rapidly and aggressively and spreads through the blood stream to produce metastases in lungs, bones and bone marrow.

Clinical Features

Ewing's sarcoma constitutes 10 to 15 percent of all bone sarcomas and occurs during adolescence with a peak incidence in the second decade of life.

The patient presents with pain, fever and swelling. Hence, it may be confused with osteomyelitis. The pain is throbbing type increasing at night and made worse by movement.

Investigations

Radiography: There is a lytic lesion in the medullary zone of midshaft with cortical destruction and new bone formation in layers producing an onion-peel appearance (Fig. 56).

In the flat bones, it produces a lytic lesion with hardly any new bone formation.

The chest is radiographed to see for any pulmonary metastasis.

Biopsy: It is done either by open method or by a biopsy needle (core biopsy). If there is suspicion of osteomyelitis, the specimen may be sent for bacterial culture.

CT scan is done to find the extent of the lesion. MRI defines the soft tissue invasion better.

Bone scan may be done to find the extent of bone involvement.

Blood may show leukocytosis, raised ESR and elevated lactic dehydrogenase.

Treatment

As this tumor is very aggressive, it is considered a systemic disease. Hence, systemic chemotherapy is the mainstay of treatment. The drugs used are doxorubicin, cyclophosphamide or ifosfamide, etoposide, vincristine and dactinomycin.

The local treatment of the tumor includes surgical resection or radiotherapy (6000 rad). Following resection the gap is filled with bone and the segments are internally supported with plate and screws or nail.

Prognosis

With the modern methods, the prognosis has improved significantly.

Tumors below the elbow or mid calf have a 5-year survival rate of 80 percent.

It is a curable tumor even in the presence of metastases especially in children below 11 years of age.

CASE 15: AMELOBLASTOMA (ADAMANTINOMA)

CLINICAL DIAGNOSIS

1. The patient is usually in third decade of life and presents with a painless and slow growing swelling of the jaw, commonly of the lower jaw of insidious onset.
2. It is usually situated in the horizontal ramus of mandible in the second or third molar region.
3. Both the tables of the mandible are expanded, the outer being more than the inner table (Fig. 58).
4. The swelling is variable in consistency and may have egg-shell crackling.
5. The overlying mucosa may be ulcerated.
6. The alignment of the related teeth may be disturbed.

VIVA VOCE

1. **What is ameloblastoma?**
   It is an epithelial tumor of the jaw of unknown etiology arising from dental lamina and characterized by a painless and slow growing swelling of insidious onset.
2. **What are the other places where this lesion can occur?**
   This tumor can occur rarely in tibia or fibula.
3. **What is the origin of this lesion in leg?**
   This tumor may be arising from:
   • Embryonic inclusion of tooth germ epithelium within the developing bones of the leg
   • Accidental inclusion of surface epithelium under the periosteum due to trauma.
4. **What are the types of ameloblastoma?**
   It is of two types:
   • Cystic form (common)
   • Solid form (rare).
5. **What is the microscopic appearance?**
   This lesion is a multilocular cyst lined by tall columnar epithelium with islands of osseous and fibrous tissues (Fig. 59).
6. **What is the nature of this tumor?**
   It is usually a locally malignant tumor.
7. **What are the investigations?**
   The investigations include:
   • X-ray of mandible (orthopantomogram of mandible), CT scan
   • Biopsy (needle)
   • Others: Hemoglobin, blood counts, X-ray chest, blood sugar, urine examination.
8. **What are the radiographic signs?**
   There is a well defined radiolucent area which is characteristically multilocular with small daughter cysts on the periphery (soap bubble or honey-comb appearance) (Figs 60 and 61).
9. **What are the causes of soap bubble appearance?**
   The causes are:
   • Giant cell tumor (osteoclastoma)
   • Ameloblastoma
   • Brown tumor of hyperparathyroidism
   • Giant cell reparative granuloma
   • Fibrous dysplasia of bone.

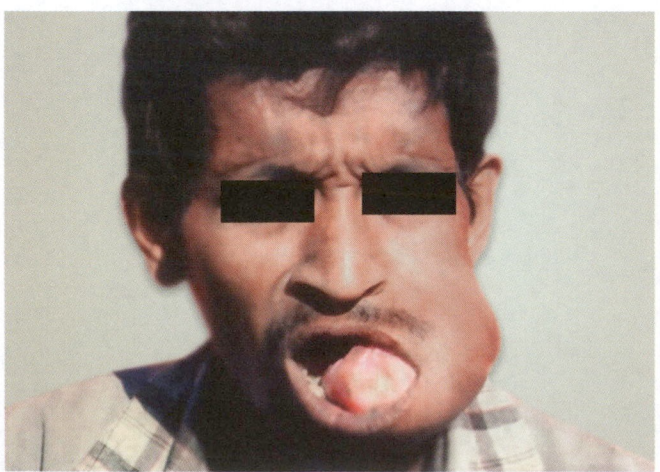

Fig. 58: A large ameloblastoma of mandible on left side

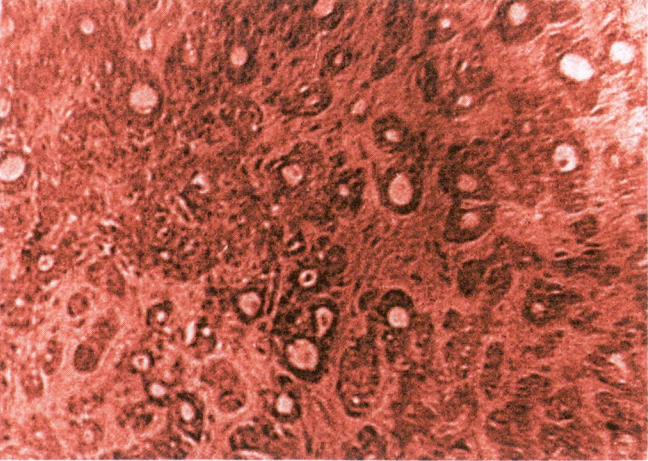

Fig. 59: Micropathology of an ameloblastoma

10. **How do you treat this tumor?**
    - If the cortical plate is not invaded (early disease), subperiosteal excision is done with a margin of up to 1 cm of cancellous bone
    - If the cortical plate is penetrated, extraperiosteal excision is done, including an adequate amount of soft tissue
    - Some cases need a full thickness excision of the affected part of the jaw and restoration with a bone graft.

11. **How do you determine the types of surgical treatments?**
    This tumor tends to penetrate medullary spaces, hence should be removed with a margin of up to 1 cm of cancellous bone. The cortical plate is less readily invaded, and a subperiosteal excision can be done with little chance of recurrence.

12. **Can you treat this tumor by enucleation and curettage?**
    No, as these methods will invariably lead to recurrence.

13. **Can you treat it by radiation or drugs?**
    No, the adjuvant therapies are not effective.
    Radiation therapy can be given in multiple surgical failures.

14. **What are the results of treatment?**
    The results of adequate excision of the lesion are good, but follow-up should be indefinite as recurrences may occur upto 20 years or more.

DISCUSSION

Ameloblastoma constitutes 1 percent of all the tumors of the jaws. 80 percent occur in the mandible with the molar ramus region most commonly involved (Fig. 58).

It is an epithelial tumor of unknown etiology arising from dental lamina. It is a multilocular lesion with the loculi lined by tall columnar epithelium with islands of osseous and fibrous tissues. This tumor is slow growing but may become very big and erode the adjacent bone.

Rarely, it occurs in the diaphysis of bones of leg.

Clinical Features

The patient is usually in third decade of life and presents with a painless and gradually increasing swelling of insidious onset. Both the tables of the jaw are expanded, the outer more than the inner. The mucosa overlying the swelling may get ulcerated (Fig. 58).

It causes gradually increasing deformity of face or loosening of teeth.

It is a locally invasive or malignant tumor which extends into the adjacent areas by contiguous growth. Rarely regional and pulmonary metastases may occur.

Radiography: There is a radiolucent area in the jaw with some of the following features—expansion of overlying cortical plate, a scalloped margin, a multilocular or soap-bubble appearance, more like a honey-comb, and resorption of adjacent teeth (Figs 60 and 61).

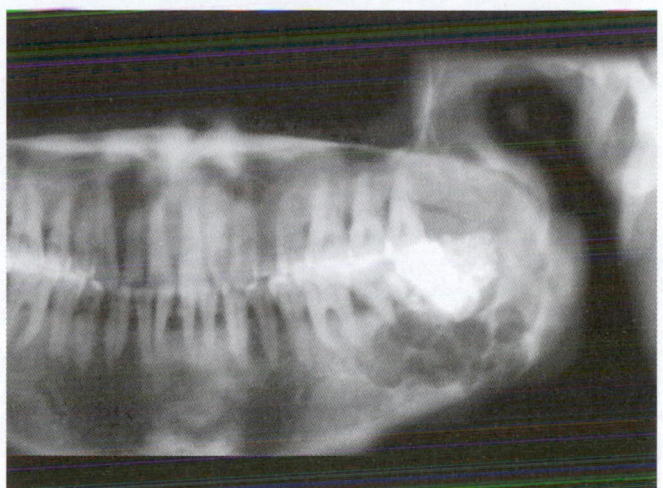

Fig. 60: Orthopantomogram showing a multilocular lytic lesion near the left angle of mandible—ameloblatoma (*Courtesy:* Professor GN Agarwal)

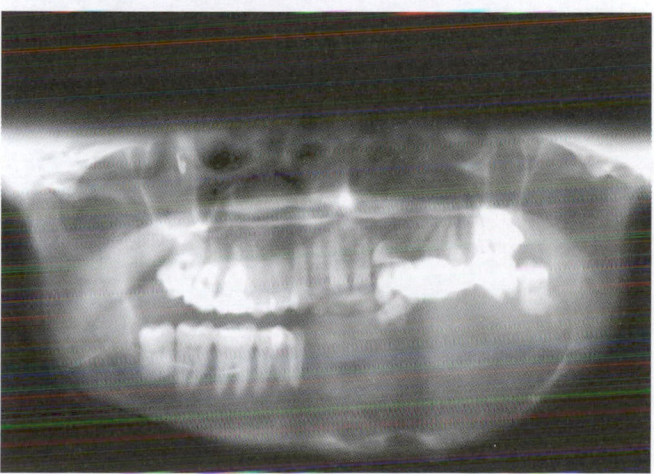

Fig. 61: Orthopantomogram showing a large ameloblastoma of mandible involving the left half of mandible (lytic lesion) (*Courtesy:* Professor Divya Mehrotra)

Biopsy is required (needle or core biopsy) to confirm the diagnosis (Fig. 59).

Treatment

It is treated by wide resection. Early small lesions can be excised with a margin of up to 1 cm of cancellous bone.

It may respond to radiation but it is usually employed after multiple operative failures and in advanced disease. Its curative ability is not clear. Chemotherapy has no role.

The results are good but the follow-up should be indefinite as recurrences may occur up to 20 years or more.

CASE 16: SARCOMA OF MAXILLA

CLINICAL DIAGNOSIS

1. The patient is commonly a woman about 40 years of age who presents with a painful and rapidly growing swelling of the upper jaw (Fig. 62).
2. It is smooth or lobulated, firm or variable with prominent veins on the surface.

3. As the disease advances, the swelling becomes painful and may cause nasal obstruction, epiphora, proptosis and fungation.
4. The regional lymph nodes are not enlarged.

VIVA VOCE

1. **What is this tumor?**
   It is one of the most common and highly malignant bone tumor but it occurs less commonly in jaws as compared to long bones (Figs 62 and 63).
2. **What is the cause of this tumor?**
   The cause is not known but it may occur after irradiation in elderly people.
3. **What is the cause of epiphora?**
   It is because of obstruction of nasolacrimal duct.
4. **What is the cause of proptosis?**
   It is because of expansion or extension of the tumor into the orbit pushing the eyeball upwards and outwards.
5. **How does this cancer spread?**
   It spreads both by local extension and blood stream thereby producing pulmonary metastases.
6. **What are the investigations done in this disease?**
   The investigations are:
   - Radiography of maxilla (Fig. 64)
   - Biopsy
   - X-ray chest
   - CT scan of maxillary region (Fig. 65).

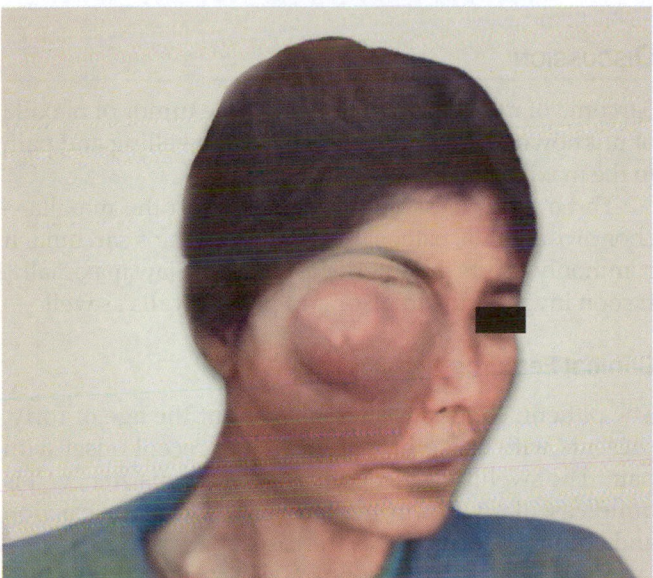

Fig. 62: Osteosarcoma of right maxilla

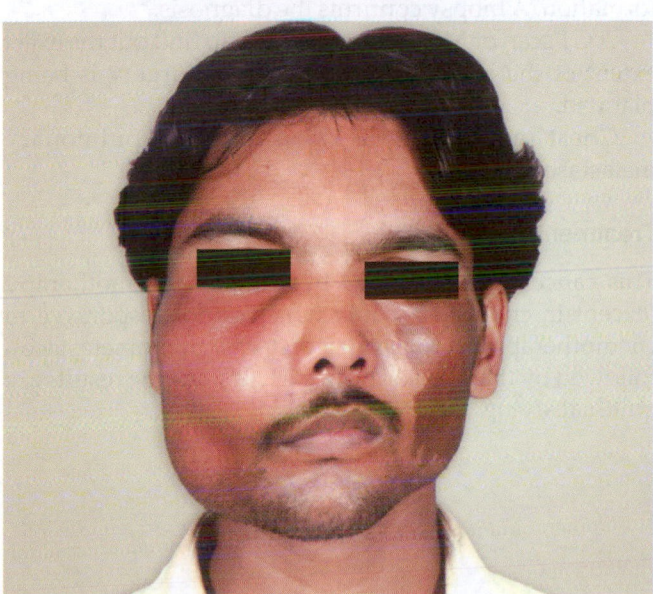

Fig. 63: Sarcoma of right maxilla
(*Courtesy:* Professor Rajiv Agarwal)

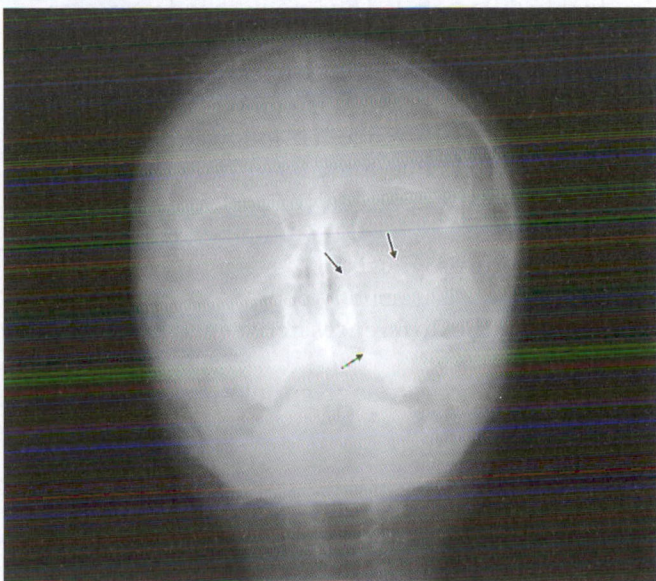

Fig. 64: Sarcoma of left maxilla—there is opacity with expansion. There is marked deviation of lateral nasal wall medially

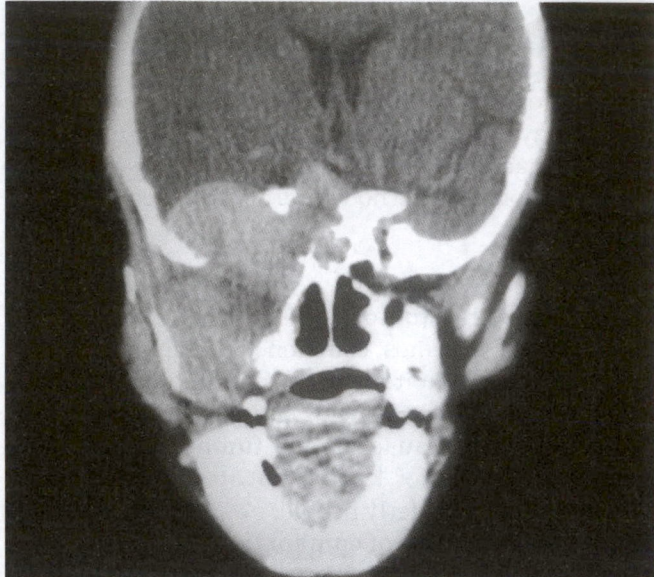

Fig. 65: CT scan showing a sarcoma of right maxilla which is extending into temporal region and into the cranium with extension into sella and erosion of anterior clinoid process. It is a soft tissue mass with attenuation
(*Courtesy:* Dr Divya Mehrotra)

7. **Which aspect of the jaw is maximally affected?**
   Usually, the anterior aspect of the jaw is maximally affected.

8. **What are the X-ray signs?**
   There is resorption of normal bone with expansion and occasional radio-opacities due to irregular bone formation throughout the lesion (Fig. 63).

9. **What is the micropathology?**
   Usually it is a round cell sarcoma. Rarely it may be a highly differentiated fibromyxochondrosarcoma.

10. **How do you treat this tumor?**
    Like sarcomas of long bones it is treated by preoperative adjuvant chemotherapy (it does not work in chondrosarcoma) followed by wide local excision or maxillectomy.
    Radiotherapy is given for residual or recurrent disease.

11. **What is the prognosis?**
    The prognosis is usually poor.

12. **What are the differences between a carcinoma and sarcoma?**
    The differences are as given below:

Features	Carcinoma	Sarcoma
Age	Middle-aged or elderly	About 40 years
Sex	More common in males	Commonly in females
Incidence	Very common (80% of cancers of jaw)	Less common
Rate of growth	Slow or variable	Usually rapid
Swelling	Indurated, irregular	Firm, variable with prominent veins
Lymphatic spread	May occur	Does not occur
Hematogenous spread	Very rare	Can occur
Prognosis	Better than sarcoma	Worse

DISCUSSION

Sarcoma of maxilla is a malignant bone tumor of maxilla of unknown etiology characterized by swelling and pain in the maxillary region.

Three types of sarcomas can occur in the maxilla—chondrosarcoma, osteosarcoma and Ewing's sarcoma. It commonly affects the anterior aspect of the jaw maximally. It soon involves the inferior and palatal walls as well.

Clinical Features

The patient, commonly a female about the age of forty, presents with a swelling of maxilla of recent onset with pain. The swelling is firm or variable in consistency. It is quite vascular with prominent veins. Nasal obstruction and epiphora occur late as the disease advances.

The diagnosis can be confirmed by radiography which shows expansion of maxilla, soft tissue shadow, irregular bone destruction and may be some evidence of new bone formation. A biopsy confirms the diagnosis.

A CT scan or MRI should be done to find out the exact extent of the lesion, especially before surgery is being planned.

Chest radiography is done to detect pulmonary metastases.

Treatment

This cancer is first treated by adjuvant chemotherapy (except in chondrosarcoma which is not responsive to chemotherapy) to look after systemic micrometastases, followed by maxillectomy. In early lesions the results are quite satisfying.

CASE 17: CARCINOMA OF MAXILLARY ANTRUM

CLINICAL DIAGNOSIS

1. The patient is usually a middle-aged or elderly person who may present with pain and loosening of upper teeth, unilateral epistaxis and upper cervical lymphadenopathy of recent onset.
2. There may be unilateral nasal obstruction, proptosis and epiphora.
3. There may be a swelling of one side of face (Fig. 66), palate (Fig. 67) or inside the nose which is ill-defined, indurated, irregular and nontender.
4. The upper deep cervical lymph nodes may be enlarged, hard, nontender, mobile or fixed.

VIVA VOCE

1. **What is an antral carcinoma?**
   It is the commonest malignant tumor of maxilla of unknown etiology arising from the mucosa of maxillary antrum.
2. **How do you correlate the clinical manifestations with the site and direction of growth of the tumor?**
   The clinical manifestations of this tumor depend upon the site and direction of spread of tumor, i.e.
   * Posterior wall tumor: Hardly any change in the contour of face
   * Medial wall tumor: Nasal obstruction, epiphora
   * Anterolateral wall tumor: Swelling of face

* Inferior wall (floor) tumor: Bulge in hard palate (Fig. 67)
* Invasion of roof: Proptosis, diplopia, chemosis

3. **What is the micropathology of this tumor?**
   Histologically, it is of two types—squamous cell carcinoma and adenocarcinoma.
4. **What is the frequency of lymph node involvement?**
   Lymph node involvement is uncommon and is present only in 5 percent of patients when first seen.
5. **Can a patient present with an oroantral fistula?**
   Yes, tumors of lower half of antrum may invade the alveolus or palate and produce an oroantral fistula.
6. **Can a dental surgeon be accused of producing an oroantral fistula?**
   A patient with antral carcinoma may present with loosening of teeth. If a dental surgeon unwaringly extracts such a loose tooth, he may produce an oro-antral fistula.
7. **What are the investigations done in this tumor?**
   The investigations include:
   * X-ray of maxilla
   * Biopsy (needle or endoscopic)
   * CT scan (3D)
   * Others: Routine investigations, cervical lymph node biopsy or FNAC, if indicated.
8. **What are the findings in X-ray of maxilla?**
   In early stage there may be haze or opacity and increase in the size of the antrum (nonspecific signs).

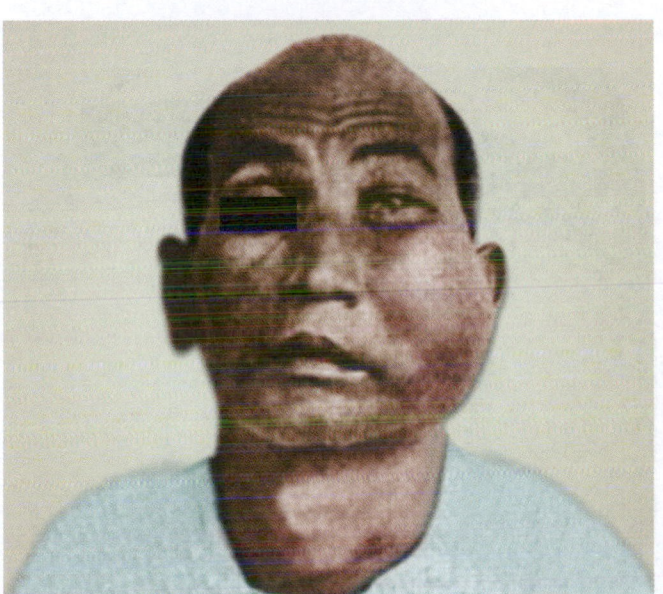

Fig. 66: Carcinoma of maxillary antrum. The lymph nodes of the neck (left side) are also enlarged

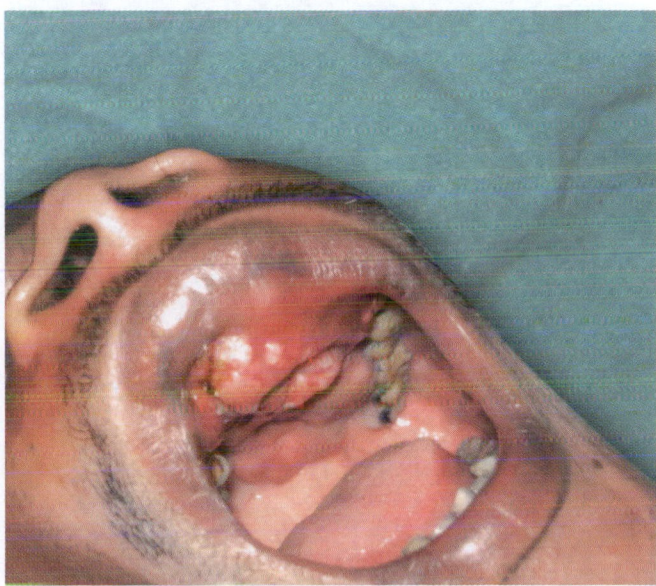

Fig. 67: Advanced carcinoma of maxillary antrum showing the tumor involving the hard and soft palate, upper alveolus and lip (*Courtesy:* Professor Sandeep Kumar)

Subsequently, there is irregular erosion or destruction of maxilla.

9. **What is the role of CT scan?**
   It is done to see the exact extent and size of the lesion. It also reveals the invasion of nasopharynx and base of skull (Fig. 68).

10. **How do you do biopsy?**
    The biopsy may be carried out via the intranasal route.

11. **Why do you want to do it via intranasal route?**
    It is done via the nasal route as the lateral wall of the nose will subsequently be removed during excision of maxilla.

12. **How do you treat this tumor?**
    It is treated by surgical resection, the extent of resection depending on the extent of disease:
    - If the floor of orbit is free then the eye and the orbital rim may be left undisturbed
    - If the floor of orbit is involved a maxillectomy with resection of orbital floor with or without orbital exenteration in done.

13. **What will you do if lymph nodes are involved?**
    A block dissection of the lymph nodes is done.

14. **What is the incision used for maxillectomy?**
    Weber Fergusson incision is most commonly employed.

15. **Describe the incision.**
    The incision begins in the midline of the upper lip and then skirting the ala runs upwards along the lateral border of the nose to the medial canthus and continues laterally about 5 mm below the lower lid to end over the zygoma.

16. **How do you approach an extensive lesion involving ethmoid cells?**
    It can be extirpated by a craniofacial approach.

17. **What do you do in this approach?**
    The tumor is approached from above through the anterior cranial fossa.

18. **Does maxillectomy cause a significant deformity?**
    No, especially if a prosthesis is made by a dental expert and fitted as soon as the wound is healed (Figs 69 to 71).

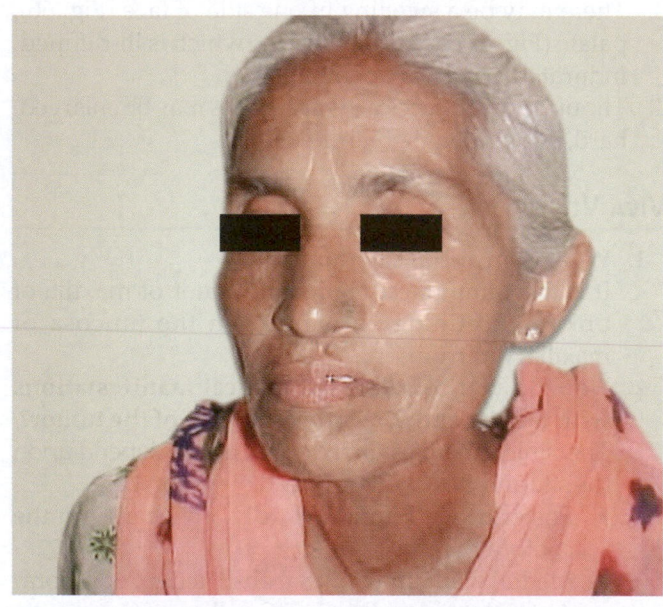

Fig. 69: Appearance of the face after maxillectomy for carcinoma of maxillary antrum (*Courtesy:* Professor Sandeep Kumar)

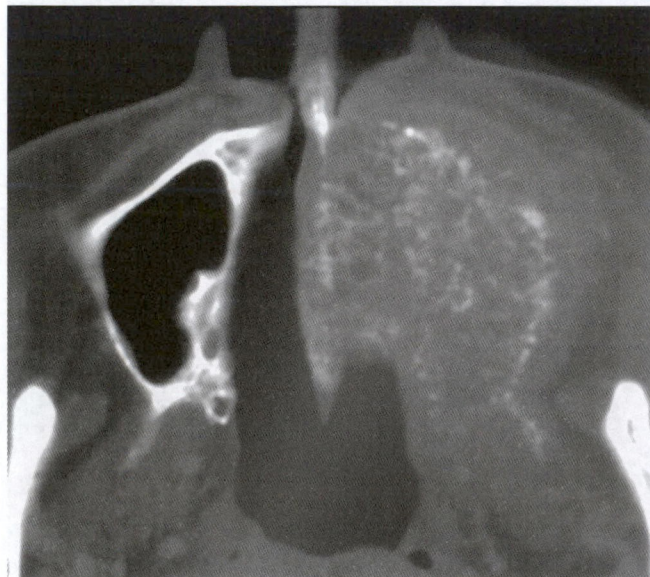

Fig. 68: CT scan showing carcinoma of maxilla with bone destruction (*Courtesy:* Dr SS Sarkar of Sarkar Diagnostics)

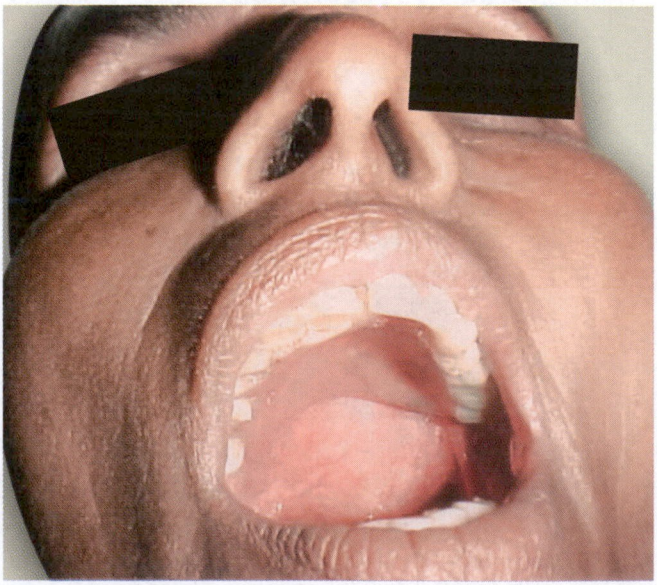

Fig. 70: Appearance of face, upper lip, teeth and palate after fitting a prosthesis after maxillectomy (*Courtesy:* Professor Sandeep Kumar)

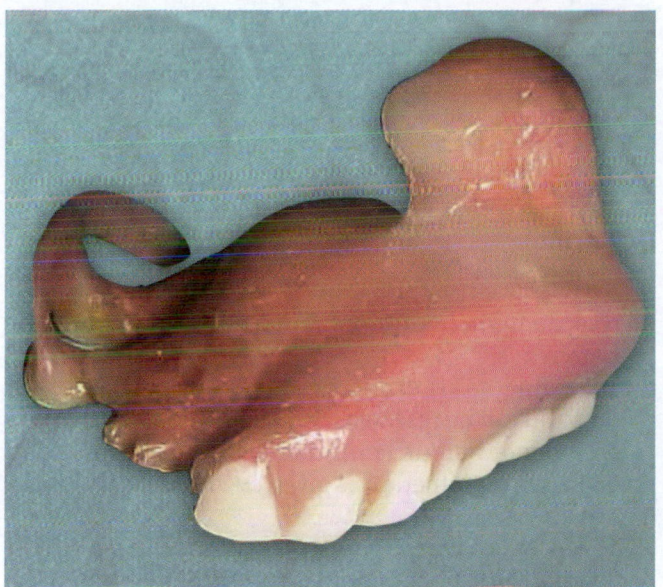

Fig. 71: Maxillary prosthesis with teeth for use after maxillectomy (*Courtesy:* Professor Sandeep Kumar)

19. **What is the role of cytotoxic drugs?**

    These drugs may be tried if the lesion persists or recurs after radiotherapy and excision. Overall they have hardly any role.

20. **What is the prognosis?**

    The overall prognosis is poor. Of those who are operated a 5-year cure rate of approximately 42 percent is reported.

21. **What is the role of radiotherapy?**

    It can be given preoperatively to downstage the tumor or postoperatively to reduce the chances of local recurrence.

22. **What are the results?**

    The 5-year survivals after local control are 42 to 43 percent.

DISCUSSION

Each maxilla is a hollow bone which has a single pyramidal cavity (sinus). Its medial wall is the lateral wall of nasal cavity and has one or two openings communicating with the middle meatus under the middle turbinate. The inferior wall is hard palate. The posterolateral wall is related to the zygomatic process and the pterygomaxillary space. The superior wall is orbital floor. The maxillary antrum is lined by ciliated epithelium. Two types of the cancer occur in the maxilla:

1. Carcinoma arising from the lining of maxillary antrum, usually a squamous cell carcinoma.
2. Sarcoma arising from the bony wall which is usually a chondrosarcoma, osteosarcoma or Ewing's sarcoma.

Spread

- Both the tumors grow locally and extend to involve the local tissues. The pattern of spread and bone destruction depend on the site of origin:
  1. Cancers arising from anterolateral infrastructure invade through the lateral inferior wall or grow through the dental sockets causing loosening of teeth, improper seating of a denture or an oroantral fistula.
  2. Cancers of medial infrastructure extend into the nasal cavity which may be obstructed.
  3. Cancers of posterior infrastructure extend through the posterolateral wall into the infratemporal fossa and superiorly to the base of skull.
  4. Cancers of the roof of the sinus extend into the orbit, though the ethmoids and lamina papyracea or by way of infratemporal fossa and then through infraorbital fissure.
  5. Cancers of the suprastructure may extend laterally invade the malar bone and produce a lump just below the lateral border of orbit and may ulcerate on the skin. The lateral invasion of orbit displaces the eye upwards and inwards. The temporal fossa and the zygomatic bone may be involved (Fig. 72)

  The medial suprastructural cancers invade the nasal cavity, ethmoid and frontal sinuses, lacrimal apparatus and medial inferior orbit.

- Lymphatic spread occurs in carcinoma. A cancer that invades the oral cavity may spread to submandibular and level II lymph nodes

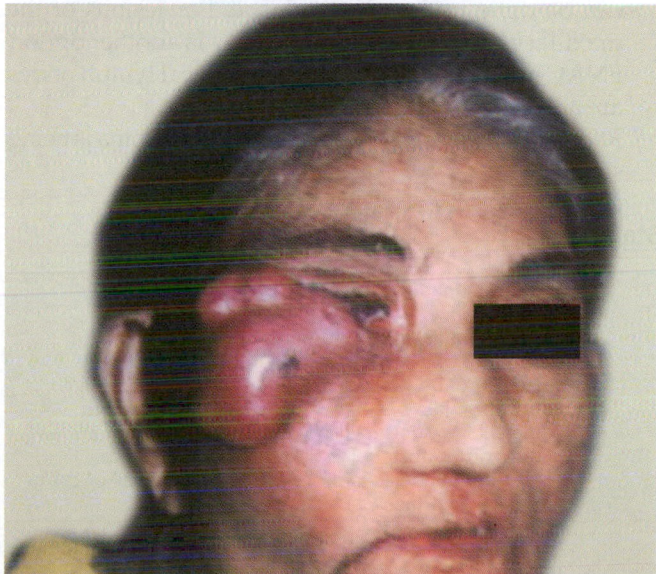

Fig. 72: Carcinoma of right maxilla with involvement of overlying skin (*Courtesy:* Professor RK Agrawal & Professor AK Khare, Udaipur)

A cancer that invades the nasal cavity or nasopharynx spreads to nasopharyngeal nodes and then to the level II nodes.

- Hematogenous spread occurs in sarcoma of maxilla, usually to the lungs.

Clinical Features

- So long as the tumor is confined to the sinus it is asymptomatic. It becomes symptomatic when it extends through the walls
- A cancer extending towards the oral cavity presents with pain and loosening and loss of teeth
- Posterior extension into the orbit is characterized by proptosis, diplopia and chemosis. There may be paresthesia in the distribution of infraorbital nerve
- Medial tumors produce nasal obstruction, bleeding, sinus pain or fullness over the antrum. They may lead to infected lacrimal sac, displacement of eye upward and laterally with proptosis, diplopia and chemosis.
- Cancers of lateral suprastructure are characterized by a mass below the lateral canthus with associated pain. The eye may be deviated medially and upward with narrowing of the palpebral aperture. The cancer may extend into the temporal fossa producing a diffuse fullness.

Investigations

- Radiography: The tumor may be seen by radiography. The CT scan (3D) shows the exact anatomy of the tumor
- Biopsy: For definitive diagnosis biopsy is required. It can be done under CT guidance. For lesions of the maxillary cavity endoscopic biopsy is another option FNAC may be done if the upper cervical lymph nodes are enlarged
- Radiography of the chest, especially if sarcoma is being suspected.

Staging

Tx	:	Tumor cannot be assessed
To	:	No evidence of primary tumor
Tis	:	Carcinoma in situ
T1	:	Limited to sinus mucosa, no erosion of bone
T2	:	Erosion of bone including extension into hard palate and/or middle nasal meatus, except extension to posterior wall of maxillary sinus and pterygoid plates
T3	:	Invasion of posterior wall of maxillary sinus or subcutaneous tissues, or floor or medial wall of orbit, or pterygoid fossa or ethmoid sinuses

Contd...

Contd...

T4a	:	Invasion of anterior orbital contents, skin of cheeks, pterygoid plates, infratemporal fossa, cribriform plate, sphenoid or frontal sinuses
T4b	:	Invasion of orbital apex, dura, brain, middle cranial fossa, cranial nerves other than maxillary nerve (V_2), nasopharynx, or clivus

Treatment

- Early infrastructure lesions are cured by surgical resection. The margin of surgical resection must be negative
- Other tumors are excised, even portions of the base of the skull can be resected. Extension into nasopharynx or sphenoid sinus contraindicates operation. Post-operative radiotherapy is given even if the margins are negative.

  The extent of the surgery depends upon the extent of disease. If the floor of orbit is free then the eye and the orbital rim may be left undisturbed

- If the floor of the orbit is involved, then a maxillectomy with resection of orbital floor with or without an orbital exenteration is done. If the posterior wall or pterygoid plates are involved they are included in resection. The raw area is covered by a split thickness graft to line the cavity which is filled by a dental prosthesis. The prosthesis is prepared preoperatively. It is placed in the cavity to act as a stent. A permanent prosthesis is made about 6 months after the maxillectomy (Fig. 71).
- If cervical lymph nodes are involved, a block dissection of the nodes is done
- Radiotherapy: The field of irradiation includes entire maxilla, adjacent nasal cavity, ethmoid sinus, nasopharynx and pterygopalatine fossa. All or part of the orbit is included if it was involved. CT at times combined with image-fusion MRI helps in planning the treatment.

  The dose of radiation is 74.4 Gy at 1.2 Gy per fraction twice daily. The dose of preoperative radiation is 50-60 Gy and of postoperative, 60-74.4 Gy.

  The 5-year survivals after local control are 42 to 43 percent.

  Recurrence: Recurrence is not common with these cancers. It is heralded by pain and cranial nerve palsies. Localized post-surgery recurrence is treated by radiation treatment, or craniofacial resection and postoperative radiotherapy.

  Radiotherapy failures may be treated by surgery including craniofacial resection whatever is possible.

CASE 18: FIBROUS EPULIS

CLINICAL DIAGNOSIS

1. The patient is usually a middle-aged women who presents with a painless and slow growing swelling of the gum (Fig. 73).
2. It is usually present between two incisors commonly of the lower jaw, on the labial (outer) surface.
3. It is longitudinal with a narrow base (Fig. 74).
4. It is pink, smooth, firm and nontender.
5. The oral hygiene is usually poor with calcareous deposits on the neck of related teeth.

VIVA VOCE

1. **What is an epulis?**
   It is a discrete swelling of the gum (Figs 73 and 74).
2. **What is the cause of this lesion?**
   It is a localized inflammatory hyperplasia of the gum arising in response to local irritation from the sharp

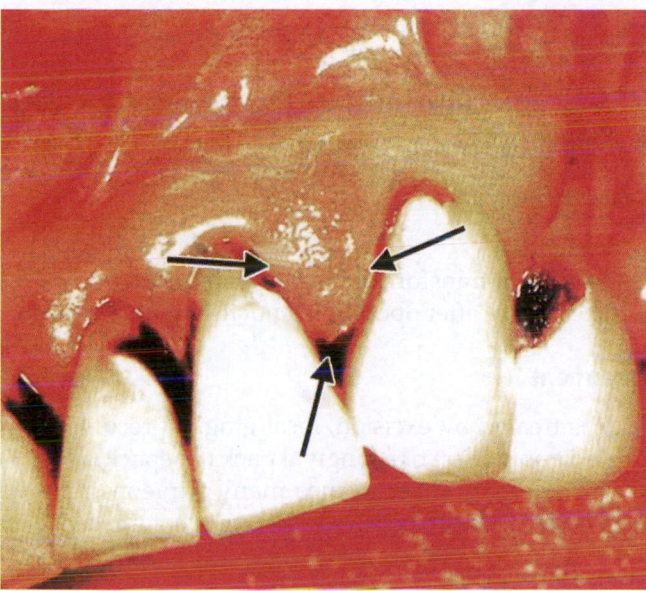

Fig. 73: Fibrous epulis (black arrows). Deposits on the neighboring teeth can be seen

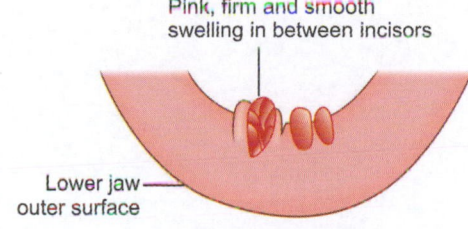

Pink, firm and smooth swelling in between incisors

Lower jaw outer surface

Fig. 74: Fibrous epulis

margin of a carious cavity or subgingival calcareous deposit (Fig. 73).
3. **What is the tissue of its origin?**
   It arises from interdental papilla.
4. **What is its histological structure?**
   It is mainly composed of collagen.
5. **What are its complications?**
   It may ulcerate due to trauma during mastication and then look like a malignant lesion.
6. **Is it a malignant lesion?**
   No, it is a benign lesion.
7. **What are the investigations?**
   Apart from routine, an X-ray of the jaw and FNAC may be done.
8. **How do you treat this condition?**
   It is treated by excision, local gingival recontouring and application of a gingival pack (Coepack).
9. **Can this condition recur?**
   Yes, if the cause is not eliminated.
10. **How do you prevent recurrence?**
    The source of irritation must be eliminated.
11. **What are the causes of generalized gingival hyperplasia?**
    The causes are:
    - Long-term phenytoin therapy
    - Familial condition, fibromatosis gingivae
    - Hormonal changes of adolescence
    - Acute leukemia.
12. **How do you prevent the gingival hyperplasia of phenytoin?**
    By maintaining meticulous oral hygiene.
13. **What is pregnancy epulis?**
    It is a pedunculated swelling of interdental papilla occurring during pregnancy.
14. **What is the cause of this condition?**
    It is probably a local response to calcareous deposit conditioned by hormonal changes of pregnancy.
15. **How does it differ from fibrous epulis?**
    Unlike the fibrous epulis, it grows rapidly and is soft, pink and vascular.
16. **How does it disturb the patient?**
    Apart from swelling and some pain, it may bleed during last months of pregnancy.
17. **How do you treat this condition?**
    The oral hygiene should be maintained with the help of a dental surgeon. If it bleeds it may be excised by a dental diathermy with a unipolar cutting electrode.
18. **What is a giant cell equlis?**
    It is now called giant cell reparative granuloma as it resembles an intrabony giant cell reparative granuloma histologically.

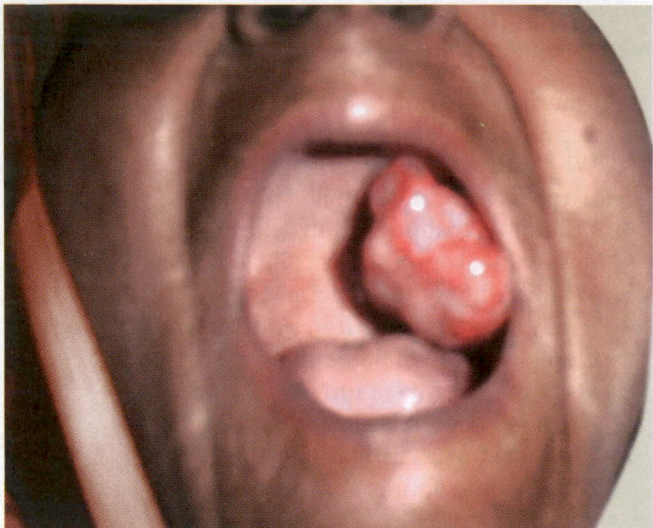

Fig. 75: A large epulis of the upper jaw
(*Courtesy:* Professor Divya Mehrotra)

19. **What is the site of origin?**
    It arises adjacent to an infected socket or the site of shed primary tooth.
20. **How does it differ from a fibrous epulis clinically?**
    Unlike a fibrous epulis it is purple and soft.
21. **How do you treat this condition?**
    By local excision and curettage of bony surface.

DISCUSSION

Epulis is a swelling situated on the gum (epulis means upon the gum) which consists of mainly the fibrous tissue (Fig. 75).

Etiology

It is a localized inflammatory hyperplasia of the gum arising from the periodontal membrane in response to local irritation from the sharp margin of a carious cavity or subgingival calcareous deposit.

Pathology

It arises from the interdental papilla and mainly composed of fibrous tissue, which contains fusiform cells and many blood vessels. As it grows the related teeth are separated and become loose.

Clinical Features

Age: It usually occurs in middle-aged persons.
Sex: It is commonly seen in females.
Symptoms: The patient presents with a painless slow growing swelling of the gum.
Signs:
- There is a polypoidal or longitudinal swelling situated at the junction of the gum and tooth
- It is usually present between two incisors commonly of the lower jaw, on the labial (or outer) surface
- It is pink, smooth, firm, sessile or pedunculated and nontender
- The oral hygiene is usually poor with calcareous deposits on the neck of related teeth
- The adjacent teeth may be slightly separated and be loose.

Investigations

1. X-ray of jaw to see if there are any changes in the bone.
2. Biopsy.

Complications

1. Ulceration.
2. Malignant transformation into a fibrosarcoma.
3. Recurrence after operation if not thoroughly excised.

Treatment

- It is treated by excision, local gingival recontouring and application of a gingival pack (Coepack)
- For preventing recurrence many surgeons remove adjacent tooth or teeth and a wedge of bone in between.

Cysts or Cystic Swellings

CASE 1: SCROTAL HYDROCELE

CLINICAL DIAGNOSIS

1. The patient presents with a unilateral or bilateral scrotal swelling of insidious onset (Fig. 1).
2. It is usually painless, but there may be slight pain or heaviness.
3. The upper limit of the swelling is reachable.
4. It is smooth, soft and nontender.
5. It is fluctuant.
6. It is usually translucent.
7. In a large hydrocele, the testis cannot be felt separately from the swelling.

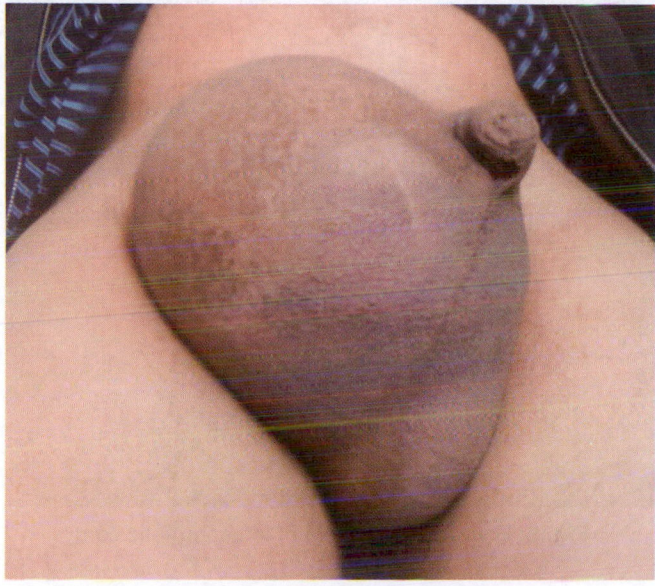

Fig. 1: Right-sided hydrocele

VIVA VOCE

1. **What is a hydrocele?**
   It is an abnormal accumulation of serous fluid within some part of processus vaginalis, commonly in the tunica vaginalis of testis (Fig. 1) .
2. **What are the causes?**
   Etiologically hydrocele is of two types:
   a. Primary or idiopathic.
   b. Secondary, where the cause is known, ie.
      – Trauma (post-traumatic)
      – Epididymo-orchitis (post-inflammatory)
      – Tumor
      – Filariasis (adenolymphatic obstruction).
3. **What are the types of primary hydrocele?**
   They are of four types (Fig. 2):
   • Scrotal or vaginal hydrocele
   • Infantile hydrocele
   • Congenital hydrocele
   • Encysted hydrocele of cord.
4. **Which one is the commonest type?**
   Scrotal or vaginal hydrocele.
5. **What is the commonest cause of hydrocele in our country?**
   Filariasis.
6. **What is scrotal or vaginal hydrocele?**
   In this type, the fluid accumulation is confined to scrotum only.
7. **What is an infantile hydrocele?**
   The tunica and processus vaginalis are distended with serous fluid upto internal inguinal ring but not communicating with the peritoneal cavity.

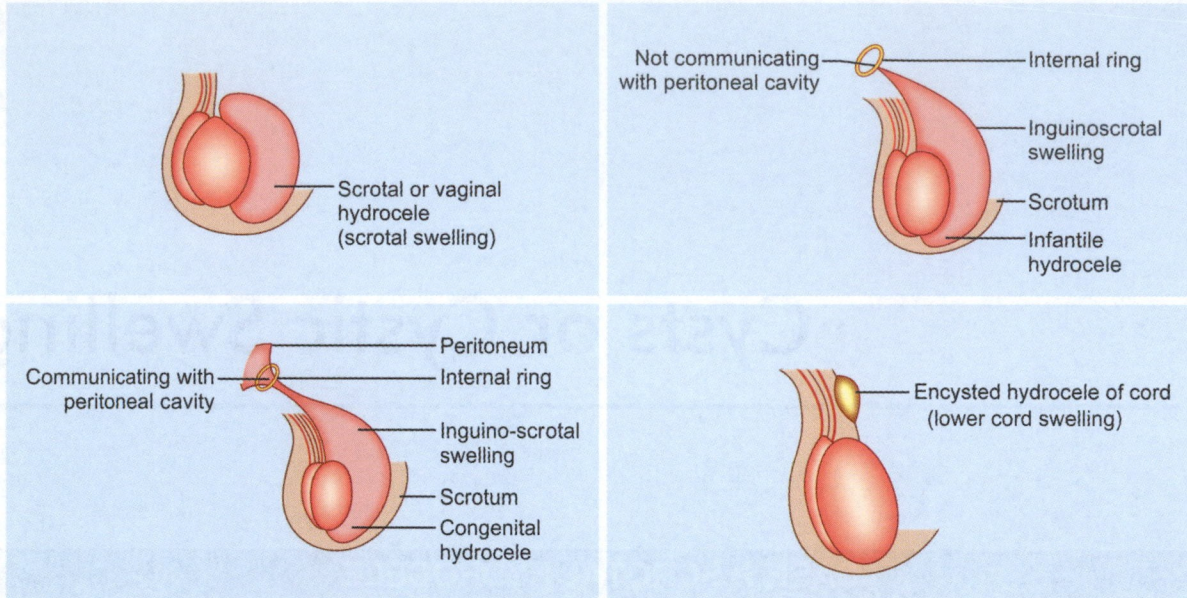

Fig. 2: Types of hydrocele

8. **What is a congenital hydrocele?**
   It is like an infantile hydrocele, but it is communicating with the peritoneal cavity at internal ring.

9. **Can this communication cause herniation of bowel?**
   The communication is so small that it allows only the peritoneal fluid to come out and not any other abdominal content.

10. **What is an encysted hydrocele of cord?**
    It is a cyst of spermatic cord derived from some portion of processus vaginalis neither communicating with tunica vaginalis nor with the peritoneal cavity (Fig. 3).

11. **What are the complications of a hydrocele?**
    The complications are:
    - Rupture
    - Secondary infection resulting in a pyocele
    - Herniation of hydrocele sac through dartos
    - Calcification
    - Testicular atrophy in late cases of large hydroceles

12. **Does it disturb the testicular function?**
    It may affect the testicular function but it is very uncommon.

13. **How do you treat a hydrocele?**
    A hydrocele is usually treated by eversion of sac (Jaboulay's operation).

14. **What do you do in eversion?**
    The tunica vaginalis is cut anteriorly and everted on the testis and stitched together at its back.

15. **What is Lord's operation?**
    It is an alternative to Jaboulay's operation. In this procedure, a series of interrupted absorbable sutures are employed to plicate the redundant tunica. When they are tied tunica is bunched into a ruff at its attachment to testis.

16. **What is the main advantage of this operation?**
    The chances of hematoma formation are less.

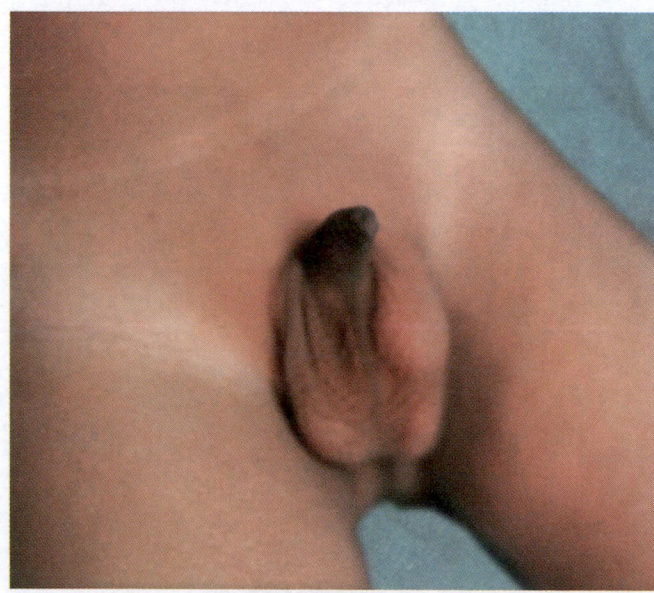

Fig. 3: Encysted hydrocele of left spermatic cord

17. **What is excision of sac?**
    In this operation, the parietal layer of tunica is excised and the cut edge is carefully sutured with a hemostatic suture.

18. **What is the indication of this operation?**
    It is indicated when the sac is thick-walled and not evertable.

19. **What are the complications of this operation?**
    The main complication is scrotal hematoma which is quite common and awful.

20. **Can you treat this disease by aspiration?**
    It can be treated by aspiration but the disease comes back within a week or so.

21. **Why do you not inject a sclerosant to prevent recurrence?**
    It is being done but it is usually very painful.

22. **What are the complications of tapping?**
    The complications are:
    - Infection
    - Hemorrhage
    - Perforation of bowel if associated with a hernia.

23. **How do you treat hydrocele of infants and children?**
    It is treated like an inguinal hernia by dissecting out the processus vaginalis and excising it after ligating at the internal ring.

24. **How do you treat an encysted hydrocele?**
    It is treated by excision.

25. **What are the complications of eversion of sac?**
    The complications are:
    - Scrotal hematoma
    - Wound infection
    - Torsion of testis.

DISCUSSION

Hydrocele is an abnormal collection of serous fluid in some part of processus vaginalis, commonly the tunica vaginalis of scrotum (Fig. 1).

Etiology

- Serous fluid in processus vaginalis can accumulate in the following four ways:
    1. Excessive production as occurs in a secondary hydrocele.
    2. Defective absorption as occurs in most of the primary hydroceles.
    3. Defective lymphatic drainage of scrotal contents.
    4. Peritoneal fluid coming into the tunica vaginalis through a patent processus vaginalis as occurs in a congenital hydrocele.

- Etiologically hydrocele can be of following types:
    1. Congenital hydrocele
    2. Acquired hydrocele
        a. Primary or idiopathic
        b. Secondary: The fluid accumulation is due to testicular disease, e.g. tumor, epididymo-orchitis.

Pathology

- Depending upon the type of tunica, hydrocele is of four types (Fig. 2):
    1. Vaginal or scrotal hydrocele: The fluid accumulation is confined to scrotum only.
    2. Infantile hydrocele: The tunica and processus vaginalis are distended with serous fluid upto the internal inguinal ring but not communicating with peritoneal cavity.
    3. Congenital hydrocele: Anatomically it is like an infantile hydrocele but communicating with the peritoneal cavity hence the fluid in hydrocele is peritoneal fluid.
    4. Encysted hydrocele of cord: It is a cyst of spermatic cord derived from lower part of processus vaginalis (Fig. 3).

- Fluid: It is straw-colored and contains albumin and fibrinogen, and no bacteria. As such it does not clot, but clots if it is mixed with even a small quantity of blood.

    In long standing hydroceles, the fluid may be opalescent with cholesterol and may sometimes contain crystals of tyrosine.

Clinical Features

This disease can occur at any age, and the patient presents with a painless and slow growing swelling of scrotum of insidious onset.

a. Scrotal hydrocele
    - The swelling is smooth and ovoid or spherical.
    - The upper limit is reachable.
    - It is nontender and fluctuant.
    - It is usually translucent.
    - The testis is usually not palpable.

b. Infantile hydrocele
    - The swelling is scroto-inguinal and extends up to the internal ring.
    - It is soft, cystic, fluctuant and translucent.
    - It cannot be reduced.
    - On making the patient cough, the scrotal swelling may become more prominent.

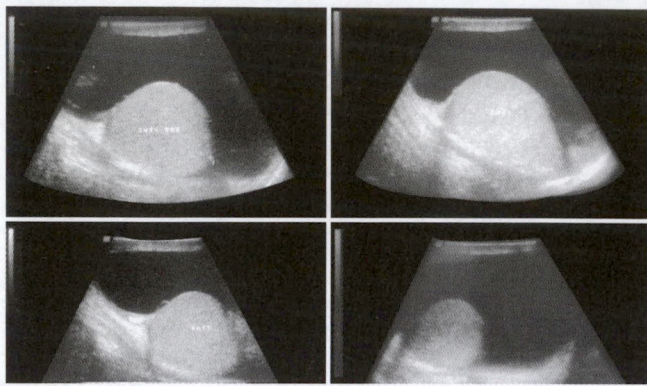

Fig. 4: Ultrasonography of scrotum showing collection of fluid around a normal testis

c. Congenital hydrocele
- The patient is usually a child who presents with a scroto-inguinal swelling of insidious onset.
- It is smooth, nontender, soft and translucent.
- It reduces on lying down, hence there is minimal or no swelling in the morning.
- It starts appearing when the erect posture is resumed, hence it is maximum in the evening.
- It cannot be emptied by digital pressure.
- There may be signs of ascites, especially in bilateral cases.

d. Encysted hydrocele of cord (Fig. 3)
- The patient presents with a painless and slow growing swelling of the spermatic cord of insidious onset.
- It is smooth, oval, well-defined , nontender, cystic and translucent.
- It is separated from the testis.
- On pulling the testis down the swelling moves down and becomes immobile. It returns to its original position on leaving the testis (traction test).

Complications

It may have the following complications:
1. Rupture: It may be traumatic or spontaneous. Rarely the hydrocele may heal following rupture.

2. Hematocele: Hemorrhage into the sac may occur following trauma or spontaneously.
3. Hernia of hydrocele: It occurs through the dartos in a long-standing case.
4. Calcification of sac.

Investigations

Ultrasound scanning: It may be required to see the testis, especially when it cannot be felt in a large tense hydrocele (Fig. 4).

Treatment

1. Acquired primary hydrocele: A variety of operations are done for treating acquired hydrocele:
   a. Jaboulay's operation: It is eversion of sac with placement of the testis in a pouch prepared by blunt dissection in the fascial planes of scrotum. This operation is done when the sac is thin walled.
   b. Lord's operation: This is good alternative to Jaboulay's operation. A series of interrupted absorbable sutures are employed to plicate the redundant tunica. When they are tied, the tunica is bunched into a 'ruff' at its attachment to the testis. In this operation, the chances of scrotal hematoma are minimal.
   c. Excision of sac: If the sac is thick walled, it cannot be everted. Hence, it is usually excised and the cut edge is carefully sutured with a continuous blanket suture. The hemorrhage from the cut edge is liable to cause a large scrotal hematoma, even if the wound is drained.
   d. Aspiration: It is a very simple procedure but the disease comes back within a week or so. It may be done in very elderly infirm men who are unfit for operation.

   Injection of sclerosants such as tetracycline is sometimes effective but is usually very painful.
2. Congenital hydrocele: It is treated by herniotomy and the excision of processus vaginalis.
3. Encysted hydrocele: It is treated by excision.
4. Secondary hydrocele: The cause must be treated.

CASE 2: SEBACEOUS CYST

CLINICAL DIAGNOSIS

1. The patient presents with a painless and slow growing swelling of skin of insidious onset.
2. It usually occurs on the scalp, face, neck, scrotum and trunk, and does not occur in the palm of hand and sole of foot.
3. It is smooth and hemispherical.
4. It is soft or firm, elastic and nontender.
5. There may be a black dot (punctum) on the top of the swelling (Figs 5 and 6).
6. It is mobile on deeper tissues but fixed to the skin at punctum.
7. It is not translucent.
8. Sometimes tooth paste-like yellowish white material may be expressed from it.
9. In hairy areas, the skin overlying the swelling tends to be bald.

VIVA VOCE

1. **What is a sebaceous cyst?**
   Two cysts are included under this heading: Epidermal cyst and tricholemmal cyst. None is derived from sebaceous glands.
2. **What is the origin of these cysts?**
   These cysts are derived from hair follicles.
3. **What is the site of origin of epidermal cyst?**
   It is considered to arise from the infundibular portion of a hair follicle.

4. **What is the site of origin of tricholemmal cyst?**
   It is derived from hair follicle epithelium.
5. **What are the sites of occurrence of epidermal cyst?**
   It can occur anywhere but the common sites are face, trunk, neck, extremities and scalp in that order.
6. **What are the sites of occurrence of tricholemmal cyst?**
   90 percent of cysts occur on the scalp.
7. **Why do they not occur in the palm or sole?**
   They do not occur in these areas as there are no hair follicles.
8. **How do the contents of an epidermal cyst look like?**
   - The contents of an epidermal cyst are pale, dirty looking, creamy and tooth paste-like. They may have an unpleasant smell.
   - The contents of a tricholemmal cyst may calcify which does not occur in an epidermal cyst.
9. **What is the lining of these cysts?**
   The epidermal cyst is lined by stratified squamous epithelium with a distinct granular layer. The tricholemmal cyst is lined by epithelial cells with palisading of the outer cell layer which surrounds the inner layers of pale swollen cells which undergo abrupt keratinization (Fig. 7).
10. **How does the lining of tricholemmal cyst differ from the lining of epidermal cyst?**
    It differs from the keratinization of lining cells of epidermal cyst which has an intervening granular cell layer which is not present in the lining of tricholemmal cyst.

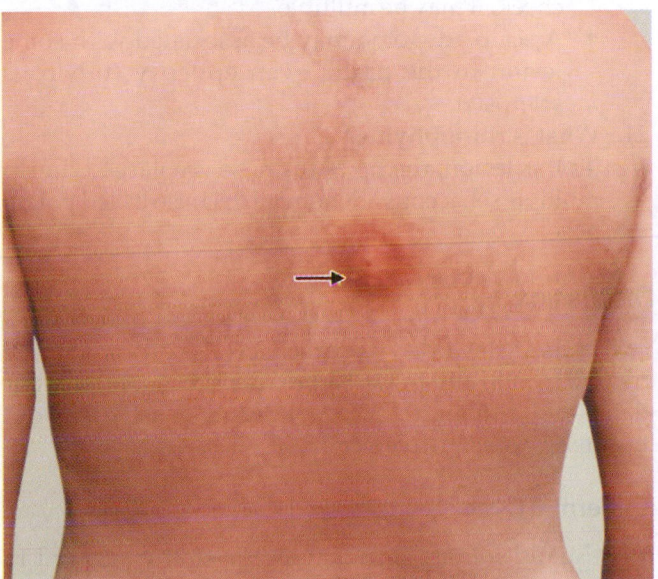

Fig. 5: Sebaceous cyst of back. Punctum is seen in the center

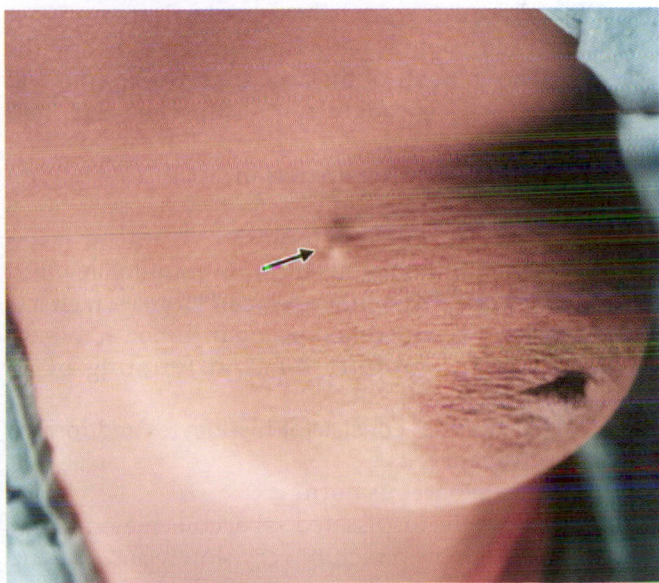

Fig. 6: A small sebaceous cyst of the breast with punctum

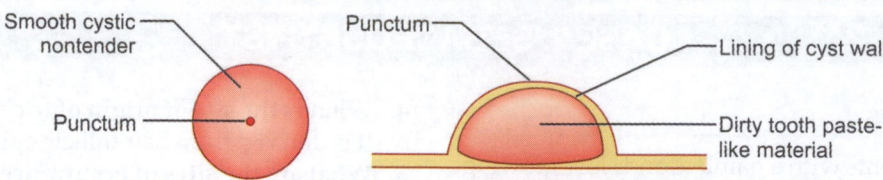

Fig. 7: Sebaceous cyst

11. **What are the complications?**
The complications include:
- Infection, suppuration
- Ulceration
- Calcification
- Cock's peculiar tumor
- Sebaceous horn (very rare)
- Basal cell carcinoma (very rare).

12. **What happens when the cyst gets infected?**
- The cyst enlarges and becomes painful with red overlying skin. The contents become semi-liquid and usually very fetid.
- Recurrent attacks of infection make the cyst wall adherent to surrounding subcutaneous tissue and hence a little difficult to excise.

13. **Which of these cysts calcify?**
The tricholemmal cyst tends to calcify which does not occur in an epidermal cyst.

14. **What is the cause of baldness of the skin overlying a cyst?**
It is due to interference in the blood supply of the skin overlying the cyst.

15. **How do you treat this lesion?**
It is treated by excision of the cyst either by incision-avulsion or dissection.

16. **What do you do in incision-avulsion?**
A small incision is made through the skin into the cyst. The contents of the cyst are squeezed out and the cyst wall is caught with a fine hemostat and avulsed completely.

17. **Can a cyst recur after operation?**
Yes, if it is not completely excised.

18. **What is Cock's peculiar tumor?**
- It is a granulomatous ulcer or granuloma which looks like a squamous cell carcinoma which it is not that is why called peculiar tumor. It follows infection, suppuration and bursting of an epidermal cyst.
- This "tumor" consists of histiocytes and foreign body giant cells.

19. **What is a sebaceous horn?**
Sometimes the inspissated sebaceous material may leak through the punctum very slowly and dries up in successive layers giving rise to a horny projection, called sebaceous horn (Fig. 8).

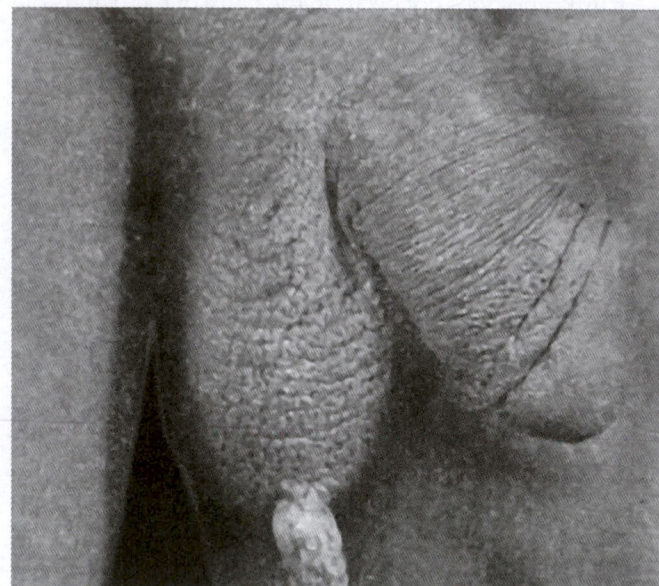

Fig. 8: Sebaceous horn of scrotum

20. **What is a sebaceous adenoma?**
- It is a benign tumor of sebaceous glands. The patient presents with a painless and slow growing solid swelling of scalp, forehead, nose or cheek. It may be multiple.
- A scalp adenoma may be associated with some lesion in the brain, even epilepsy (tuberous sclerosis).

21. **What is rhinophyma?**
In this lesion, the tip of the nose is enlarged due to multiple sebaceous adenomata. It is also called potato nose.

DISCUSSION

Two cysts are included under sebaceous cyst - epidermal cyst and tricholemmal cyst. None is derived from sebaceous glands and, although clinically indistinguishable they can be differentiated histologically.

Epidermal Cyst

It is usually solitary and may occur at any age and in almost any site but is most common on the face, trunk, neck, extremities and scalp, in that order. It is considered to arise from the infundibular portion of a hair follicle, or a traumatic inclusion.

The cyst can be of any size and presents as a hemispherical, smooth, firm to soft swelling which is attached to the skin. A black dot (punctum) is usually present on the top of the swelling which may be indentable with digital pressure, a feature which distinguishes it from a lipoma.

Multiple cysts occur in Gardner's syndrome in association with intestinal polyposis, desmoid tumors and osteomas.

Complications

- It may become infected with subsequent discharge of foul-smelling cheesy material.
- It may ulcerate and ulcer may look like a cancer when it is not cancer. Malignant change has been reported but very rare.

Histopathology

The cyst is filled with keratinous debris and is lined by stratified squamous epithelium with a distinct granular layer. The cyst may leak releasing keratinous material into the dermis resulting in a foreign body giant cell reaction.

An identical cyst occurs from traumatic implantation of epidermis (implantation or inclusion dermoid).

Treatment

The entire cyst is removed alongwith its contents.

Recurrence

It can reccur if even a small portion of its lining is left behind. Hence, the cyst should be removed intact with an ellipse of skin over the apex containing the punctum. To remove a cyst intact is a good technical exercise in making use of tissue planes and gentle handling of tissues.

- **Scrotal epidermal cyst:** Epidermal cysts are common in the scrotal skin. They are usually small, multiple, yellowish and hard (Fig. 9).
- **Meibomian cyst** is an epidermal cyst formed at the free edge of the eyelid. Chalazion is a chronic Meibomian cyst.

Tricholemmal cyst

This cyst is not as common as an epidermal cyst and in 90 percent patients, occurs on the scalp. It is often multiple, single being in about 30 percent of patients. There is a genetic predisposition with an autosomal mode of inheritance.

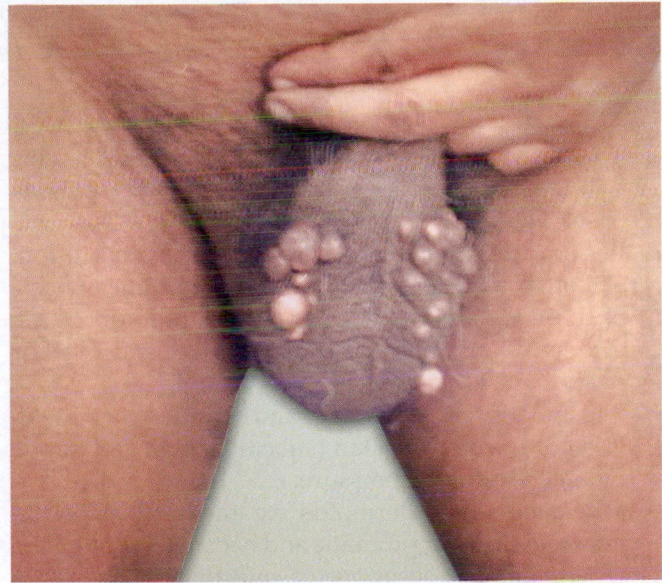

Fig. 9: Multiple epidermal cysts of scrotum

It is derived from the epidermis of the external root sheath of the hair follicle.

Histopathology

It is lined by epithelial cells with palisading of the outer cell layer which surrounds the inner layers of pale, swollen cells which undergo abrupt keratinization. This differs from the keratinization of lining cells of epidermal cyst which has an intervening granular cell layer, which is a normal component of epidermis, and supports the view that tricholemmal cyst is derived from hair follicle epithelium rather than epidermis.

The cyst contents may calcify which does not occur in an epidermal cyst. There may be proliferation of cyst epithelium sometimes, resembling that of a pilar tumor (proliferating tricholemmal cyst) and which may represent a transition between these two lesions.

Proliferating tricholemmal cyst or tumor: It is usually solitary and occurs on the scalp in 90 percent of patients. It may attain a very large size and ulcerate, and may resemble a squamous carcinoma both clinically and histologically. This lesion is called Cock's peculiar tumor. The proliferating tricholemmal cyst or tumor is benign, though it may recur after excision. It may undergo malignant change, grow rapidly and metastasize.

Treatment

The lesion should be excised completely.

CASE 3: DERMOID CYST

CLINICAL DIAGNOSIS

1. The patient is commonly a young person who presents with a painless, slow growing swelling of insidious onset (Fig. 10).
2. It is usually situated at the lines of embryonic fusion, e.g. outer and inner angles of orbit, midline of neck, back or abdomen, or at the site of union between ectoderm and another germinal layer, and testis or ovary.
3. It is smooth, soft, nontender and opaque.
4. It is not fixed to the skin (subcutaneous) and can be indented by digital pressure.
   (The deep-seated dermoids, e.g. mediastinal, pelvic, may remain asymptomatic and become symptomatic when some complication, e.g. infection occurs).

VIVA VOCE

1. **What is a dermoid cyst?**
   It is a cystic swelling lined by stratified squamous epithelium containing hair follicles and sebaceous and sweat glands in its wall. It contains dirty tooth paste like material, hair, teeth and other tissues (Figs 10 to 12).
2. **What are the types of dermoid cyst?**
   It is of three types—sequestration dermoid, tubulodermoid and implantation dermoid.

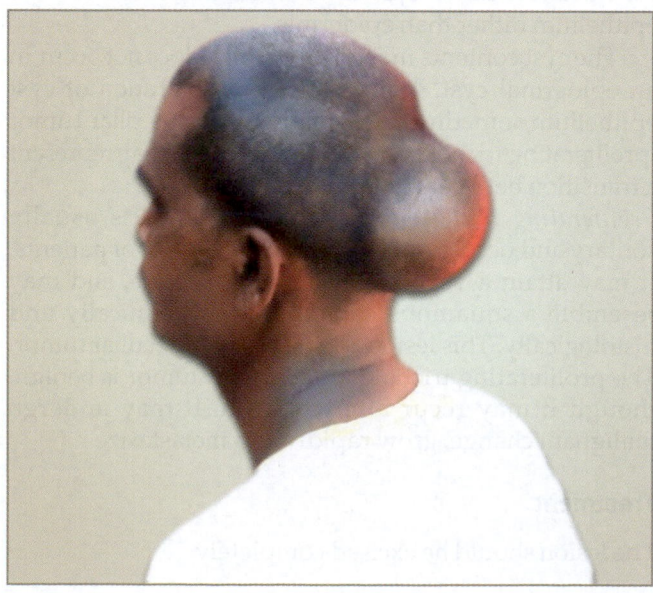

Fig. 10: Occipital dermoid cyst

3. **What is a sequestration dermoid?**
   A sequestration dermoid develops from ectodermal differentiation of multipotent cells pinched off at the time of closure of anterior neuropore. Hence, it occurs at the lines of embryonic fusion. It is the commonest type of dermoid.
4. **What is a tubulodermoid?**
   A tubulodermoid arises from fetal tubular structures or ducts, for example a thyroglossal cyst from thyroglossal tract. Other examples are branchial cyst, urachal cyst, vitellointestinal duct cyst.
5. **What is an implantation dermoid?**
   It arises from the fragments of dermis that are implanted in the tissues by punctures or cuts.
6. **What are the signs of an implantation dermoid?**
   It occurs in the palm of hand or a finger and rarely in the sole of foot. It is smooth, firm and nontender.
7. **What are the differences between an epidermoid (sebaceous) cyst and dermoid cyst?**
   The differences are given below:

Features	Epidermoid cyst	Dermoid cyst
Site	Can occur anywhere especially head, neck and trunk	Occurs at the sites of embryonic fusion, e.g. midline of body
Punctum	Usually present	No punctum
Fixity of skin	Fixed to skin at punctum	Not fixed to skin
Mobility	Mobile on deeper tissues	Fixed if it has an intracavitary extension
Indentation by finger pressure	Cannot be indented	Can be indented by finger pressure

8. **What are the investigations?**
   - In superficial dermoids, no investigation is needed except for routine investigations for operation.
   - If an intracavitary extension is suspected ultrasound, CT scan or MRI are required depending upon the site.
9. **What is an incidental dermoid?**
   It is the detection of an asymptomatic dermoid when the patient is being investigated for some other disease.
10. **What are the complications of a dermoid cyst?**
    The complications are infection, rupture and pressure symptoms on the neighboring structures.
11. **What are the signs of sublingual dermoid?**
    - A supramylohyoid cyst presents as opaque swelling in the floor of mouth lifting the tongue up.
    - An infrahyoid dermoid cyst presents as a swelling under the chin giving a double chin appearance as seen in the lateral view.

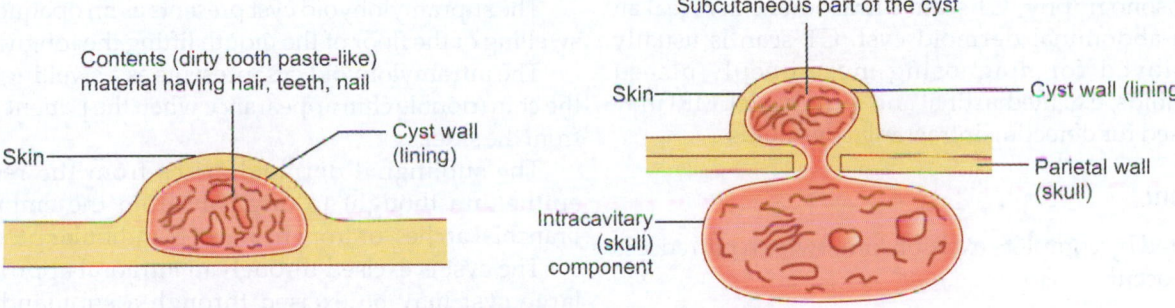

Fig. 11: Pathology of a dermoid cyst

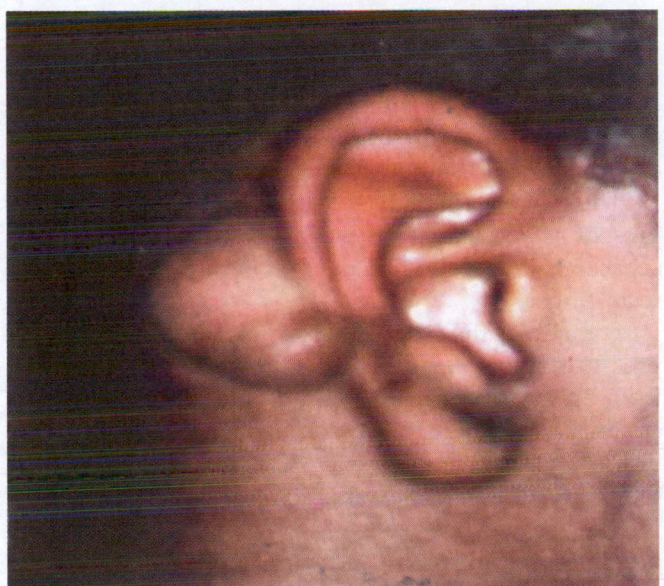

Fig. 12: Periauricular dermoid

12. How do you treat a sublingual dermoid cyst?
Most of the cysts can be excised by an intraoral approach. Large cysts can be excised by a submandibular incision.

13. What are the clinical presentations of a postanal dermoid?
- It may be asymptomatic and detected accidentally during digital rectal examination
- It may present as a postanal sinus which discharges offensive tooth paste like material.
- A large cyst may press the rectum causing its obstruction.

14. How do you treat it?
It can be excised by a postanal incision. The coccyx and lower sacrum may be excised for adequate exposure.

15. How do you treat dermoids of the head?
If there is no intracranial extension, excision is a simple operation. If intracranial extension is present, help of a neurosurgeon if it is required.

DISCUSSION

It is a cyst lined by stratified squamous epithelium containing hair follicles and sebaceous and sweat glands. The cyst cavity contains sebaceous material, hair, teeth and other tissues. It is of three types—sequestration dermoid, tubulodermoid and implantation dermoid.

Sequestration Dermoid

It develops from ectodermal differentiation of multipotent cells pinched off at the time of closure of anterior neuropore. Hence, it occurs at the lines of embryonic fusion, e.g. outer and inner angles of orbit (eyebrow), midline of neck, back or abdomen, or at the site of union between ectoderm and another germinal layer, e.g. pituitary fossa, floor of mouth, pharynx, esophagus and mediastinum. It may occur in the testis and ovary.

A superficially placed dermoid presents as a swelling more deeply placed than an epidermoid cyst (sebaceous cyst) and not attached to the skin. It is smooth, soft, nontender, opaque and may be indented by a finger.

A deeply placed dermoid is usually asymptomatic till some complication occurs. It is identified by ultrasound, CT scan or MRI.

Tubulodermoid

It arises from fetal tubular structures or ducts, for example, a thyroglossal cyst from thyroglossal tract.

Implantation Dermoid (post-traumatic cyst)

It occurs on the palm of hand or a finger and rarely on the sole of foot. It arises from the fragments of dermis that are implanted in the tissues by pricks or cuts. The cyst is smooth, firm and nontender. It grows rapidly. It is attached to the skin and contains cholesterol and fat. Its wall consists of fibrous tissue lined by squamous epithelium.

Investigations

- Plain radiography may show a heterogeneous soft tissue shadow.

- Ultrasonography/CT scan: Ultrasound can reveal an intra-abdominal dermoid cyst. CT scan is usually employed for diagnosing more deeply placed dermoids, e.g. mediastinal and intracranial. MRI may be used for detecting intracranial dermoids.

Treatment

It is treated by complete excision, otherwise recurrence is likely to occur.

External Angular Dermoid

This dermoid is sited at the line of fusion of frontal process with the maxillary process. There is a painless, slow growing swelling at the outer angle of the eyebrow. The bone underneath may be pitted or may have a depression (pressure atrophy). Rarely, it may have an intracranial connection which is confirmed by radiography and CT scan if indicated.

The cyst is excised completely which is curative. If there is an intracranial extension, help of a neurosurgeon may be sought.

Periauricular Dermoid

It is sited below and behind the pinna. It results from inclusion of epithelium when two adjacent auricular tubercles fuse during the development of pinna. It is smooth, soft, nontender and may be translucent. It should be excised.

Sublingual Dermoid

Sublingual area is one of the common site of a dermoid cyst which may be above or below the mylohyoid muscle of the floor of the mouth.

The supramylohyoid cyst presents as an opaque cystic swelling of the floor of the mouth lifting the tongue up.

The inframylohyoid cyst presents as a swelling below the chin (double chin appearance when the patient is seen from the side).

The sublingual dermoid arises from the residual epithelium thought to originate from the embryonic branchial arches, or from fusion of mandibular processes.

The cyst is excised through an intraoral approach. A large cyst may be excised through a submandibular incision.

Postanal Dermoid

It occurs in the space in front of lower part of sacrum and coccyx behind the rectum and anal canal. It is usually asymptomatic and may be discovered during digital rectal examination as a smooth, soft and nontender swelling.

The cyst may get infected and then it may rupture to present as a postanal sinus which discharges offensive sebaceous material when the cyst is compressed by the rectal finger.

Sometimes the cyst may grow to a large size to cause pressure on the rectum. This cyst has to be differentiated from an anterior sacral meningocele which occurs in children and is frequently associated with paralysis of the lower limbs and incontinence. It increases in size when the child cries while the dermoid remains the same.

The cyst can be seen by CT scan or MRI. If a sinus is present sinography may be done.

It should be excised. The excision of a large cyst is facilitated by the excision of coccyx. If a sinus is present it is excised with the coccyx.

CASE 4: CYSTIC HYGROMA

CLINICAL DIAGNOSIS

1. The patient is an infant or a child who presents with a slow growing swelling in the neck since birth (Figs 13 and 14).

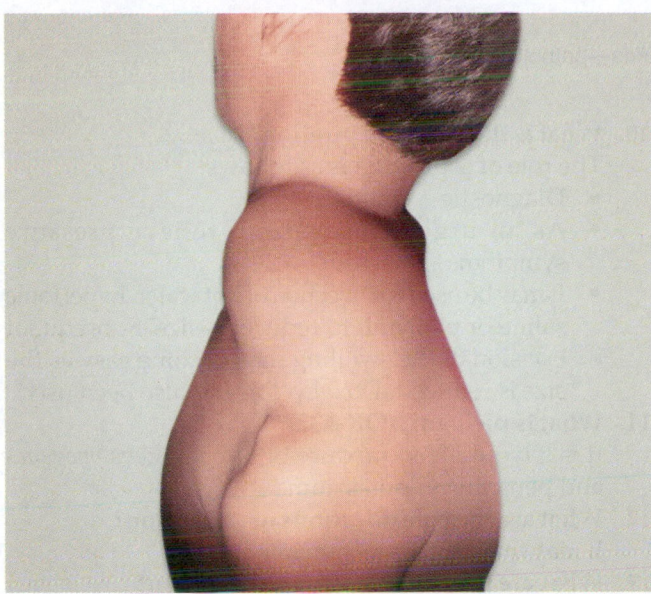

Fig. 13: Cystic hygroma left side of lower part of neck in an adolescent boy (*Courtesy:* Professor Ashish Wakhlu)

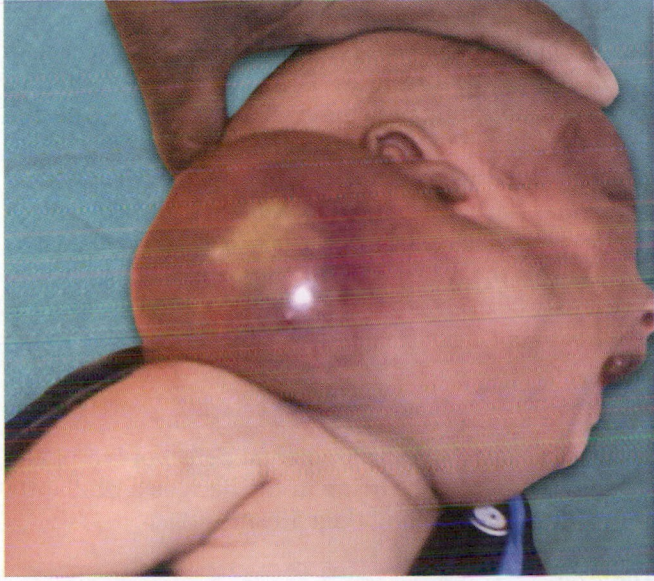

Fig. 14: Large cystic hygroma of neck (*Courtesy:* Professor Ashish Wakhlu)

2. It is usually present at the root of the neck in the posterior triangle deep to the sternomastoid (Fig. 15).
3. It is smooth or lobulated, soft, cystic, nontender and ill-defined.
4. It is brilliantly transilluminant.

VIVA VOCE

1. **What is cystic hygroma?**
   It is a congenital malformation of lymphatic channels containing a collection of lymphatic sacs.
2. **What is the cause of this condition?**
   It is due to sequestration of a portion of jugular lymph sac along with its lymphatic channels into the surrounding mesoderm. The secretion of the sequestrated lymph sac accumulates with time to produce a cystic hygroma.
3. **What are the sites of occurrence of a cystic hygroma?**
   The sites of occurrence are:
   - Root of the neck in the posterior triangle (commonest site)
   - Axilla and pectoral region
   - Inguinal region
   - Mediastinum
   - Tongue and buccal mucosa.
4. **What is the gross appearance of this lesion?**
   There is an irregular and lobulated swelling having multiple spaces and septa. Some of the septa are incomplete and thus many cysts intercommunicate with one another. The cysts are of variable size and the larger cysts are situated at the periphery and the smaller ones at the center. They are covered externally by a shell of lymphoid tissue (Fig. 15).
5. **What is the microscopic appearance?**
   The cysts are lined by columnar epithelium and are filled with clear and watery (lymph) or straw-colored fluid consisting of cholesterol crystals and lymphocytes. This fluid does not coagulate.
6. **What are the atypical presentations of a cystic hygroma?**
   The following are the atypical presentations of a cystic hygroma:
   - A large cystic hygroma may cause obstructed labor.
   - It may present as abscess in the neck if secondarily infected.
   - It may present with mediastinal syndrome, i.e. dyspnea, dysphagia, if it is situated in mediastinum.

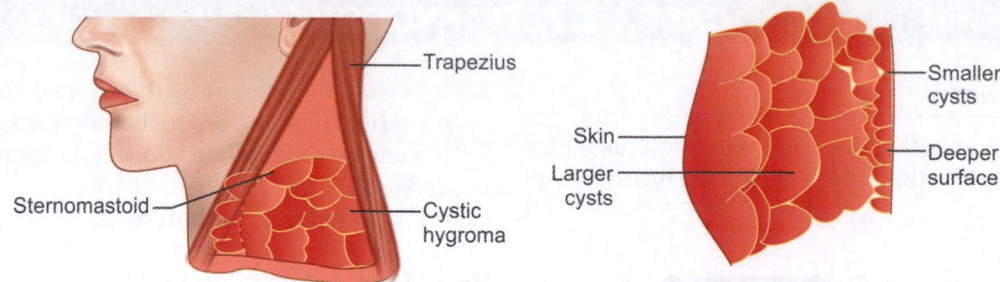

Fig. 15: Cystic hygroma—pathology

7. **What are the complications of this disease?**
   The complications are:
   - Recurrent infection
   - Hemorrhage
   - Respiratory distress due to sudden increase in size due to infection or hemorrhage.

8. **What are the investigations done in this swelling?**
   The investigations are:
   - X-ray chest to see for any evidence of mediastinal lesion (Fig. 16)
   - Aspiration with examination of fluid
   - Ultrasonography to delineate its extent and relationship with other structures. MRI gives better images.

9. **How do you treat this condition?**
   It is treated by excision. If there is no emergency, one can wait for 2 years as spontaneous recovery may occur.

10. **What is the role of aspiration?**
    The role of aspiration is as follows:
    - Diagnostic
    - As an urgent measure to relieve pressure symptoms
    - It may be used for injection of hot water, hypertonic saline or picibanil to reduce its size. Subsequent excision of the swelling may become easy as the size is reduced. Doxycycline has also been used.

11. **What is picibanil (OK-432)?**
    It is a lyophilized mixture of *Streptococcus pyogenes* and penicillin G potassium.

12. **What are the complications of aspiration?**
    It may introduce infection into it.

13. **What are the complications of excision?**
    The following complications can occur:
    - Hemorrhage
    - Lymphorrhea
    - Injury to spinal accessory nerve
    - Recurrence.

14. **What is the cause of lymphorrhea?**
    It is mainly due to division of many lymphatics communicating with the swelling. It may also be due to partial/incomplete excision of the lesion.

15. **How can the lymphorrhea harm the patient?**
    It may harm the patient by fluid and electrolyte loss leading to dehydration and electrolyte imbalance.

16. **What is the role of radiotherapy?**
    It may be used in a recurrent lesion or when surgical treatment is not feasible.

DISCUSSION

Cystic hygroma is a developmental defect of lymphatic vessels commonly occurring in the neck as a brilliantly transilluminant swelling (Figs 13 and 14).

Etiology

It occurs as a result of sequestration or obstruction of developing lymphatic vessels.

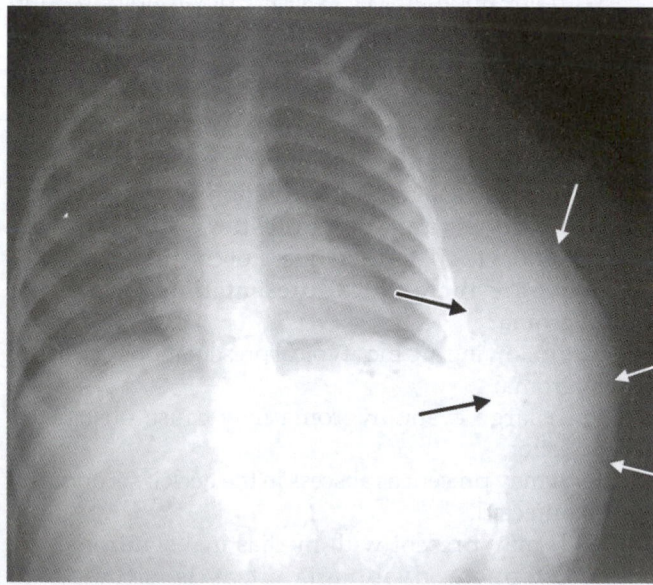

Fig. 16: Radiograph showing a left infra-axillary extra-thoracic soft tissue shadow of a cystic hygroma

Pathology

Although the lesion can occur anywhere, the common sites are in the posterior triangle of the neck (75%), axilla (20%), groin and mediastinum. It may involve parotid or submandibular salivary gland, tongue, cheek and floor of mouth. It may be bilateral. The lesion is usually multilocular lined by a single layer of epithelium with mosaic appearance and filled with lymph. Occasionally it is unilocular. Usually, there are many cysts 'infiltrating' the surrounding structures and distorting the local anatomy.

Clinical Features

The patient is a newborn baby or a young child who usually presents with a swelling in the lower part of posterior triangle of neck. The swelling may be apparent at birth or may appear and enlarge rapidly in the early weeks or months of life as the lymph accumulates; most of these present by the age of 2 years. It may be so large as to obstruct the labor.

The swelling is smooth or lobulated, soft, cystic, non-tender and ill-defined. It is brilliantly transilluminant. The behavior of this lesion in infancy is uncertain. It may expand rapidly and cause respiratory obstruction requiring urgent aspiration or even tracheostomy. It may get infected. The hygromas of neck may communicate behind the clavicle with an axillary or mediastinal hygroma, or rarely both.

Treatment

1. Surgical excision is the treatment of choice. Total extirpation may not be possible because of the extent of hygroma and its intimate relationship to adjacent nerves and blood vessels. Radical excision must not be done for this benign lesion. Conservative excision and de-roofing of the residual cyst is the recommended treatment. Repeated partial excision of residual hygroma may be required preserving all important structures in the vicinity. The complications of operation are:
   - Lymphorrhea resulting in dehydration
   - Seroma
   - Flap necrosis
   - Wound infection.
2. Injection of sclerosing agents like picibanil (OK-432) or bleomycin may be useful in a few patients. This therapy has not been widely used. It is not very effective as the lesion is multicystic. It is better if it is used in a unilocular lesion (which is rare). It may make subsequent surgery difficult due to fibrosis.

CASE 5: RANULA

CLINICAL DIAGNOSIS

1. The patient is usually a child or an adolescent person who presents with a painless and slow-growing swelling of floor of mouth.
2. It is situated on one side of frenulum linguae, or may occupy the whole floor if large (Fig. 17).
3. It is bluish in color.
4. It is cystic and nontender.
5. It is brilliantly transilluminant.
6. The submandibular salivary duct and ranine vein are crossing on its surface (Fig. 18).

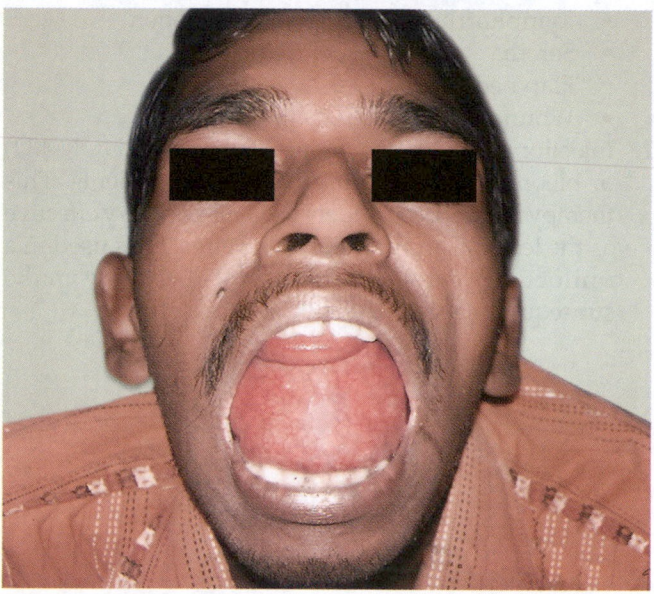

Fig. 17: Large ranula of floor of the mouth lifting the tongue up. It is so large that it has crossed midline
(*Courtesy:* Professor Sandeep Kumar)

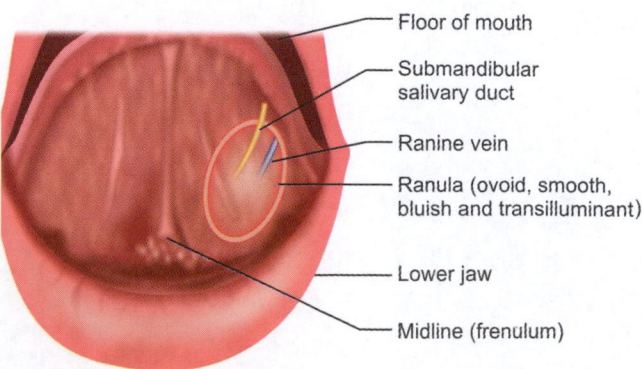

Fig. 18: Ranula

VIVA VOCE

1. **What is a ranula?**
   It is an extravasation cyst arising from a damaged sublingual gland.
2. **Why is it called ranula?**
   The term ranula is derived from the Latin word *Rana* that means a small frog; as this cyst is soft and bluish and looks like a frog's belly. That's why this name.
3. **What is the cause of this cyst?**
   It is due to extravasation of saliva from a damaged sublingual gland.
4. **What is its gross pathology?**
   A ranula is a spherical or ovoid cyst varying in size from 1 to 5 cm (diameter). It contains jelly-like material.
5. **What is the micropathology?**
   The wall of the cyst is composed of delicate capsule of fibrous tissue that is lined by a layer of macrophages.
6. **What are the types of ranula?**
   It is of two types:
   - Simple
   - Plunging.
7. **What is a simple ranula?**
   It is restricted to floor of mouth only.
8. **What is a plunging ranula?**
   This ranula has a cervical extension also. From floor of the mouth it passes (plunges) into the submandibular region of the neck.
9. **How does a plunging ranula develop?**
   This ranula develops when the leak occurs from the posterior part of sublingual gland that flows over the posterior border of mylohyoid down into the neck.
10. **What are the signs of a plunging ranula?**
    The signs are:
    - The patient presents with a painless and slow growing swelling in the floor of mouth as well as in the submandibular region near the angle of mandible.
    - The sublingual swelling is bluish, cystic and transilluminant.
    - The submandibular swelling is smooth, non-tender, soft and cystic.
    - Cross fluctuation is present between the oral and cervical swellings.
11. **What are the complications?**
    It may have the following complications:
    - Rupture and reformation
    - Infection
    - Repeated trauma
    - Difficulty in speech or swallowing (big ranula)

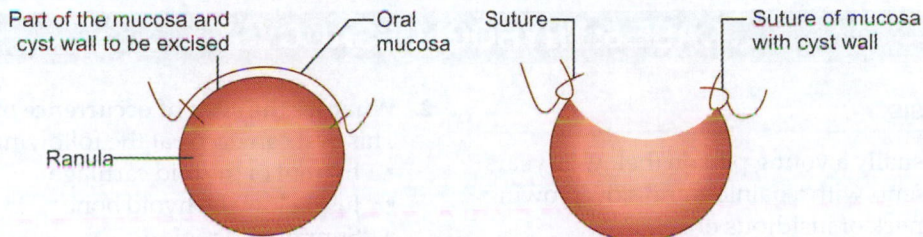

Fig. 19: Marsupialization of a large ranula

12. **How do you treat this condition?**
    The ranula is excised along with the sublingual salivary gland from which it is arising.
13. **What is marsupialization?**
    It is one of the methods of treatment of a large ranula. In this operation, the top of the cyst is excised and the cut edge of the cyst wall is stitched to the cut edge of the overlying mucosa. Thus the bottom of the ranula becomes part of the floor of the mouth (Fig. 19).
14. **How do you treat a plunging ranula?**
    Here the exploration of the neck is not required. The entire mass of sublingual gland on the side of the ranula is excised and a drain is passed from the wound down into the cavity of the neck.
15. **Does it need a cervical incision?**
    It is usually not required.
16. **What are the complications of operation?**
    The complications are:
    • Hemorrhage
    • Wound infection
    • Injury to Wharton's duct
    • Recurrence

DISCUSSION

Ranula is an extravasation cyst that arises from a damaged sublingual gland (Fig. 17). The word ranula is derived from Latin word *Rana* which means a small frog. This name is given to this swelling as it resembles the belly of a small frog. Hippocrates gave this name to this lesion.

Pathology

The extravasated saliva gets thickened and distends the floor of mouth resulting in this cyst. If the saliva leaks from the posterior part of sublingual gland it may flow over the posterior border of mylohyoid and down into the neck resulting in a plunging ranula. The size of the ranula is variable. It contains thick jelly-like material. The wall of this cyst consists of a delicate capsule of fibrous tissue and is lined by a layer of macrophages.

Clinical Features

The patient presents with a swelling in the floor of mouth which is bluish and translucent with prominent blood vessels running over its surface (Fig. 18).

Complications

1. Rupture and reformation
2. Infection
3. Repeated trauma
4. Difficulty in speech and swallowing (big ranula)

Treatment

The ranula is excised along with the sublingual gland from which it is arising. In a plunging ranula, the exploration of neck is not required. The entire mass of sublingual gland on the side of ranula is excised and a drain is passed from the wound down into the cavity in the neck.

Marsupialization: This operation is recommended for large cysts owing to multiple ramifications (Fig. 19). The major part of the cyst wall together with its overlying mucosa is excised. The cut edge of the cyst wall is sutured with the cut edge of the mucosa.

CASE 6: THYROGLOSSAL CYST

CLINICAL DIAGNOSIS

1. The patient is usually a young person (below 20 years of age) who presents with a painless and slow growing swelling in the neck of insidious onset.
2. It is situated just above or in front of thyroid cartilage slightly lateral to midline, usually to the left (Figs 20 and 21).
3. It is usually elongated with long axis vertically.
4. It moves up with swallowing and protrusion of tongue.
5. It is mobile from side to side but not vertically.
6. It is smooth, firm (tensely cystic), nontender and well defined.
7. It may be transilluminant.

VIVA VOCE

1. **What is a thyroglossal cyst?**
   It is a tubulodermoid arising from the remnants of thyroglossal duct (Fig. 22).

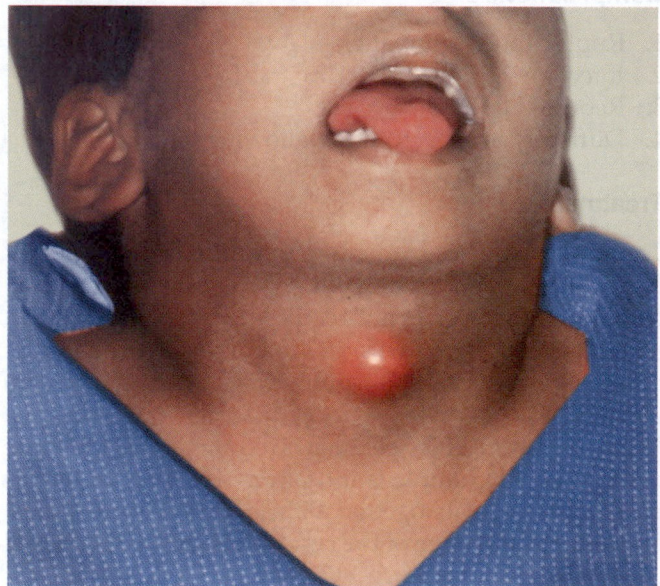

Fig. 20: Thyroglossal cyst (*Courtesy:* Professor Ashish Wakhlu)

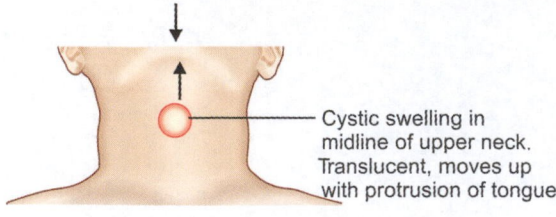

Cystic swelling in midline of upper neck. Translucent, moves up with protrusion of tongue

Fig. 21: Signs of thyroglossal cyst

2. **What are the sites of occurrence of this lesion?**
   This cyst can occur at the following sites:
   - In front of thyroid cartilage
   - Just below the hyoid bone
   - Suprahyoid region
   - Floor of mouth
   - In front of cricoid cartilage
   - In the substance of the tongue beneath the foramen cecum (Fig. 22).
3. **What is the commonest site?**
   Just below the hyoid bone.
4. **Which is the rarest site?**
   In the substance of the tongue.
5. **Why does it move up with deglutition?**
   Because it is attached to the hyoid bone by fibrous connective tissue.
6. **Why does it move up with protrusion of tongue?**
   It moves up with protrusion of tongue because it is attached to the tongue at foramen cecum by obliterated thyroglossal duct.
7. **What is the pathogenesis of this lesion?**
   This cyst develops from a part of thyroglossal duct which remains unobliterated and where secretions accumulate.
8. **What is the course of thyroglossal duct?**
   It starts at the foramen cecum of tongue and descends obliquely downwards and forwards through the genioglossi muscles up to the hyoid bone. At the level of hyoid bone it may descend in front, through or behind the hyoid bone.
   From there it descends up to the level of upper border of thyroid cartilage where it is attached to the thyroid gland.

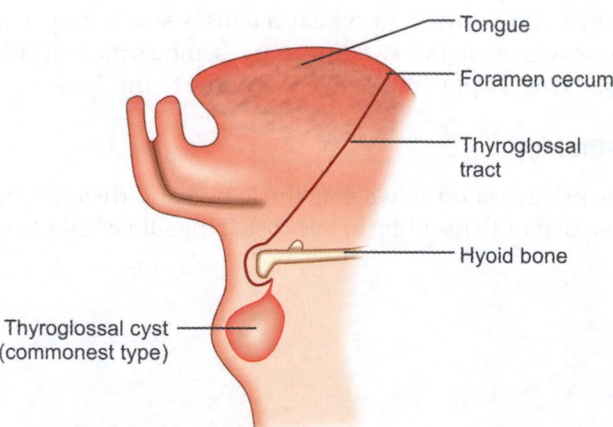

Tongue

Foramen cecum

Thyroglossal tract

Hyoid bone

Thyroglossal cyst (commonest type)

Fig. 22: Thyroglossal cyst and the thyroglossal tract on which it can occur anywhere

9. What is the fate of the thyroglossal duct?

Four things can occur to the thyroglossal duct:

- Complete disappearance except the lower part where it forms isthmus of thyroid and pyramidal lobe
- Disappearance of the part from foramen cecum to hyoid bone and persistence of the rest as levator glandulae thyroidae
- Development of ectopic thyroid tissue, e.g. lingual thyroid
- Persistence of lumen in a part with subsequent development of a thyroglossal cyst.

10. What is the pathology of this cyst?

It is an ovoid cyst of variable size. It contains thick transparent, jelly-like fluid in which cholesterol crystals may be present. It is lined by columnar, cuboidal or squamous epithelium and surrounded by a shell of lymphoid tissue. It may contain thyroid tissue.

11. What are the complications of this disease?

The complications are:

- Infection, abscess
- Rupture
- Thyroglossal fistula
- Malignancy (very rare)

12. How do you treat this condition?

Complete excision of the cyst with removal of every vestige of thyroglossal tract as far as possible up to the base of the tongue, is the treatment of choice. The body of the hyoid bone may obstruct complete excision of the tract, hence it should also be removed (Sistrunk's operation).

13. What are the complications of this operation?

The complications are:

- Wound infection
- Recurrence
- Fistula
- Perforation of larynx.

DISCUSSION

Thyroglossal cyst is a cystic swelling that occurs in thyroglossal duct remnants (Figs 20 and 22).

Pathogenesis

The thyroid gland develops from an evagination in the floor of the primitive pharynx between the first pair of pharyngeal pouches, during the fourth week of gestation. It is known as thyroglossal duct. It descends through the second branchial arch anlage, the hyoid bone, prior to its fusion in the midline. Because of this, the tract of a persistent thyroglossal duct usually extends through the body of hyoid bone.

Usually the thyroglossal duct disappears after the development of thyroid. If it persists it may form a cyst anywhere in its course.

Pathology

The cyst is usually small, ovoid and thin walled. It has got clear fluid usually filled under pressure. Thyroid follicles may be found in its walls in 30 to 40 percent of specimens.

Clinical Features

It can occur at any age but most common before age 20. The patient presents with a swelling of insidious onset in the neck in the midline just below the hyoid bone slightly to the left. It is firm, nontender and very well defined. It moves up with swallowing and protrusion of the tongue.

Differential Diagnosis

This lesion should be differentiated from an enlarged lymph node, dermoid cyst and enlarged delphian nodes containing metastasis.

Investigations

- Ultrasonography confirms the cystic nature of the swelling. It also detects the anatomic position of the thyroid.
- The cyst may be aspirated and the aspirate is sent for pathological examination, including the cytology.

Treatment

1. Acute infection: If there is acute infection it should be treated by local heat and antibiotics. If abscess forms it should be drained.
2. Quiescent phase: The cyst should be excised along with the duct. The midportion of the hyoid bone should be excised en-bloc with the thyroglossal tract to the base of the tongue (Sistrunk's operation).

CASE 7: BRANCHIAL CYST

CLINICAL DIAGNOSIS

1. The patient is a young person between 20 to 25 years who presents with a painless and slow growing swelling in the upper part of neck.
2. It is situated below the angle of mandible beneath the middle of sternomastoid and bulges along its anterior border (Figs 23 and 24).
3. It is ovoid, smooth, nontender, cystic and varies in size from 5 to 10 cm.
4. It has restricted mobility.
5. It is usually translucent.

VIVA VOCE

1. **What is a branchial cyst?**
   It is a cystic swelling of the upper part of neck arising from vestigial remnants of second branchial cleft (Figs 23 and 24).
2. **What does it contain?**
   It contains clear fluid or tooth paste like material. There are large number of cholesterol crystals in this fluid.
3. **What is the structure of its lining?**
   It is lined by squamous epithelium surrounded by a large amount of lymphoid tissue.
4. **What is the significance of this lymphoid tissue?**
   It indicates that the cyst probaby develops as a result of branchial epithelium becoming entrapped within a lymph node during development.

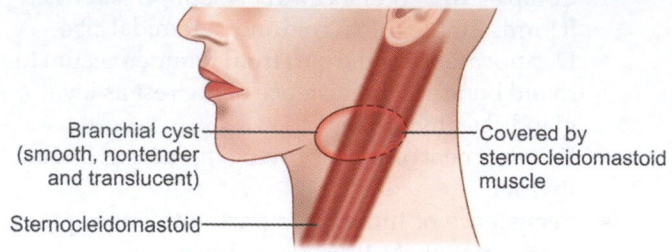

Fig. 24: Anatomical location of a branchial cyst

5. **What are its relations in the neck?**
   It usually lies superficial to the structures derived from second and third branchial arches, i.e. lesser cornu of hyoid, posterior belly of digastric, facial nerve and external carotid artery.
6. **What are the complications of this cyst?**
   The complications of this cyst are:
   - Recurrent infection, suppuration
   - Rupture
   - Fistula.
7. **What are the investigations?**
   The investigations are:
   - Ultrasound of cyst
   - Aspiration.
8. **What is the information given by an ultrasound scanning?**
   The information given by ultrasonography is given below:
   - It detects the cystic nature of the swelling.
   - It defines its extent and relations.
9. **What do you get on the examination of aspirate?**
   It reveals turbid fluid containing cholesterol crystals.
10. **How do you treat this condition?**
    It is treated by excision.
11. **What are the risks during operation?**
    The risks are:
    - Rupture of cyst resulting in difficulty in complete excision
    - Injury to cervical branch of facial, and spinal accessory and hypoglossal nerves
    - Perforation of pharynx.
12. **How do you prevent rupture of the cyst during excision?**
    After exposing the anterior wall of the cyst some of its content is aspirated so that its wall can be gently grasped in a suitable forceps.
13. **What do you remove in the operation?**
    Apart from the cyst, there may be a track passing through the fork of the carotids. It is also removed along with the cyst.

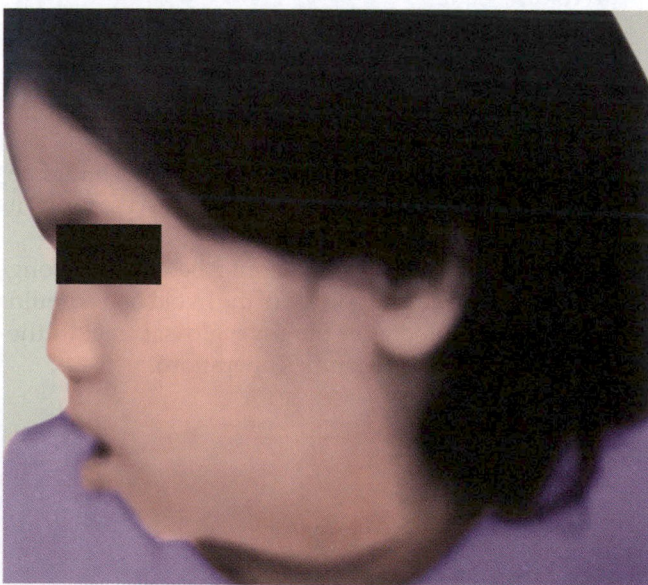

Fig. 23: Branchial cyst of left submandibular region

14. What are the cystic lesions containing cholesterol crystals?

The cholesterol crystal containing cystic lesions are:

- Branchial cyst
- Cystic hygroma
- Thyroglossal cyst
- Dental cyst
- Dentigerous cyst
- Old-standing hydrocele.

DISCUSSION

Branchial cyst is a cystic swelling of the upper neck of unknown etiology and lined by squamous epithelium.

Pathology

The cyst varies in size. It is thin-walled and contains turbid fluid or tooth paste like material full of cholesterol crystals. It is lined by squamous epithelium and surrounded by a layer of lymphadenoid tissue.

Origin

The tract of branchial origin (vestigial remnant of second branchial cleft) may form a complete fistula, or one end may be closed to form an internal or external sinus, or both ends may resorb, leaving an aggregate of cells that develops into a cyst.

Clinical Features

The patient is usually 20 to 25 years of age and presents with a painless and slow growing swelling of upper part of neck. The swelling is situated below the angle of mandible beneath the sternomastoid muscle and bulges along the anterior border of muscle. It is ovoid, smooth, nontender, cystic and varies in size from 5 to 10 cm. It has restricted mobility and may be translucent.

It is often soft in early stages that may make it difficult to palpate.

Complications

- Infection: If it is infected, it may look like a tuberculous abscess.
- If it ruptures, or is drained it results in a fistula.

Investigations

- Aspiration: The aspirated fluid contains cholesterol crystals.
- Ultrasonography: It reveals the cystic nature of the swelling. It helps in defining its extent and relationship with other structures of the neck.

Treatment

The treatment is surgical excision. The cyst wall is exposed by a skin crease incision in the neck and then the cyst is aspirated partially through a cannula. The wall of the cyst is grasped in a forceps and the cyst is dissected all round. In some cases, there is a track passing through the carotid fork up to the pharyngeal wall which is also excised by careful dissection. Care is taken to protect hypoglossal and spinal accessory nerves, as it passes superficial to the hypoglossal and glossopharyngeal nerves but deep to posterior belly of digastric muscle.

CASE 8: GANGLION CYST

CLINICAL DIAGNOSIS

1. The patient presents with a small hemispherical swelling at the dorsum of the wrist. It can occur on the volar aspect of wrist (Fig. 25).
2. It is a painless swelling of insidious onset. Slight discomfort may be there.
3. The swelling is smooth, tensely cystic and translucent.

VIVA VOCE

1. **What is a ganglion cyst?**
   It is a cystic swelling seen usually on the dorsum of the wrist. It develops due to herniation of the synovial lining of the joints or tendons in the surrounding tissue.
2. **What is the cause?**
   The cause is not known. Trauma to the wrist or hand may be responsible for the extrusion of synovium.
3. **What is the pathology of the cyst?**
   Cyst is usually small. Its wall is made of extruded synovium, and the cavity contains gelatinous translucent material.
4. **Can it produce pain?**
   It can be painful when it compresses the nerves in the vicinity.
5. **How will you confirm the diagnosis?**
   Usually no investigations are required. However, FNAC may be done to rule out a tumor.
6. **How will you differentiate a volar ganglion cyst from a brachial artery aneurysm?**
   The ganglion is not pulsatile while the brachial artery aneurysm has expansile pulsation.

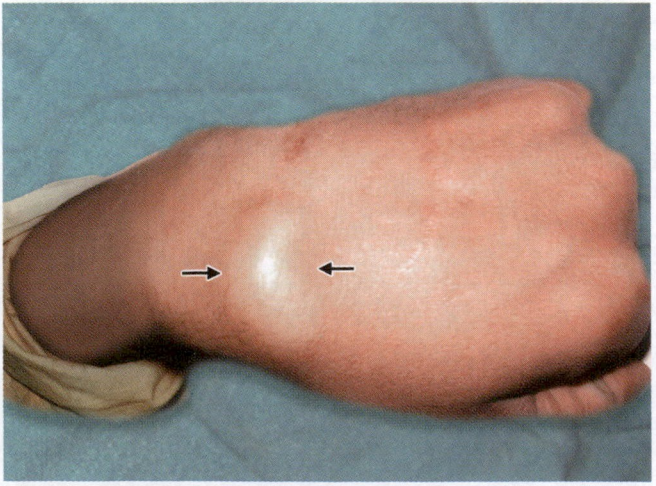

Fig. 25: Ganglion cyst of dorsum of hand
(*Courtesy:* Dr Uttam Grag)

7. **How do you treat it?**
   - It may disappear following needle aspiration or "sudden hit to rupture".
   - Surgical excision
8. **What is the technique of excision?**
   Under loupe magnification and a tourniquet the ganglion is excised completely including all attachments to the joint capsule and the underlying ligament or tendon.
9. **What is the postoperative care?**
   Prolonged splinting of the hand is required to prevent joint stiffness.
10. **What are the results of treatment?**
    Any method of treatment may be used, recurrence can occur.

DISCUSSION

A ganglion cyst is a small swelling containing gelatinous material. It develops by herniation of the synovial lining of the neighboring joints or tendons (tendon sheaths) into the surrounding soft tissue. Trauma to the wrist or hand may be responsible for the extrusion of synovium.

A ganglion cyst can originate from any joint of the hand but most commonly occurs on the dorsum of the wrist over the scapholunate ligament and the volar wrist near the radial artery. A ganglion cyst arising from a tendon is most common on the flexor sheath at the metacarpal head (A1 pulley).

The patient presents with a small hemispherical nodule that may be associated with some discomfort or pain (pressure on adjacent nerves). The swelling is smooth, nontender, cystic and translucent (Fig. 25). The diagnosis can be confirmed by needle aspiration. The viscous aspirate is sent for pathological examination.

A ganglion cyst may not be treated unless it is causing pain or functional impairment. The patient is given reassurance. It may resolve following needle aspiration or "hitting to rupture". The injection of empty sac with lidocaine and steroids may prevent recurrence but the majority recur.

Excision: It may be excised using a loupe magnification and a tourniquet. The ganglion is excised completely including all attachments to the joint capsule and the underlying ligament. Prolonged splinting of the hand is required to prevent stiffness.

Result: Any method of treatment may be used, recurrence can occur. This information must be given to the patient.

CASE 9: HYDROCEPHALUS

CLINICAL DIAGNOSIS

1. The patient is usually a child who presents with a rapid enlargement of head,
2. The scalp is stretched and thinned out, and veins are prominent and distended (Fig. 26).
3. The fontanelles are wide and tense.
4. The eyebrows overhang the roofs of the orbits.
5. The eyeballs are pushed downwards with exposure of sclera above, and the lower part of the corneas may be covered by lower eyelids (setting sun sign) (Fig. 26).

VIVA VOCE

1. **What is hydrocephalus?**
   It is increase in the intracranial pressure often associated with dilated ventricles of brain due to imbalance of CSF production and absorption.
2. **What is "setting sun sign"?**
   It is called "setting sun sign" as the eyeballs are pushed downwards and look like setting sun.
3. **What is the cause of this sign?**
   It is because of bulge of orbital plate downwards due to hydrocephalus and pressure on the eyeballs.
4. **How much CSF is produced daily?**
   Over 24 hours, a normal adult produces about 450 ml of CSF.
5. **What is the site of production of CSF?**
   CSF is mainly produced from the choroid plexus of lateral, third and fourth ventricles. A small amount of CSF is also derived from fluid that passes through the ependyma lining the ventricular walls.

6. **How is the CSF reabsorbed?**
   The CSF is reabsorbed into blood stream via the arachnoid villi projecting into sagittal and transverse venous sinuses.
7. **What is the genesis of hydrocephalus?**
   Normally the rate of ventricular CSF formation matches its absorption from the subarachnoid space. Thus, hydrocephalus can occur due to:
   - Reduction of absorption of CSF into blood stream
   - Obstruction to flow of CSF
   - Increased production (rare).
8. **What is noncommunicating or obstructive hydrocephalus?**
   When there is obstruction to the flow of CSF in the ventricular system or at the exit of the fourth ventricle, it is noncommunicating or obstructive hydrocephalus.
9. **What is communicating hydrocephalus?**
   If the distended ventricles communicate freely with the subarachnoid space, it is communicating hydrocephalus.
10. **What are the causes of communicating hydrocephalus?**
    The causes of communicating hydrocephalus are:
    - Intraventricular hemorrhage in premature infants
    - Subarachnoid hemorrhage, spontaneous or traumatic
    - Meningitis
    - Carcinomatous meningitis
    - High protein secretion into CSF by a tumor.
11. **What are the causes of obstructive hydrocephalus?**
    The causes of obstructive hydrocephalus are:
    - Neoplasms of third ventricle, e.g. colloid cyst, astrocytoma
    - Tumors causing distortion of third ventricle, e.g. pinealoma, craniopharyngioma, pituitary adenoma (giant)
    - Congenital aqueduct stenosis
    - Tumors of fourth ventricle, e.g. medulloblastoma, ependymoma
    - Tumors causing distortion of fourth ventricle, e.g. glioma of brainstem, acoustic neuroma, metastatic tumor
    - Congenital malformations of posterior fossa, e.g. meningomyelocele, Arnold-Chiari malformation, Dandy-Walker syndrome
    - Blood clots following subarachnoid hemorrhage.
12. **What are the signs of raised intracranial pressure?**
    The signs of raised ICP are papilledema, sixth nerve palsy, impaired upgaze, focal neurological deficit and

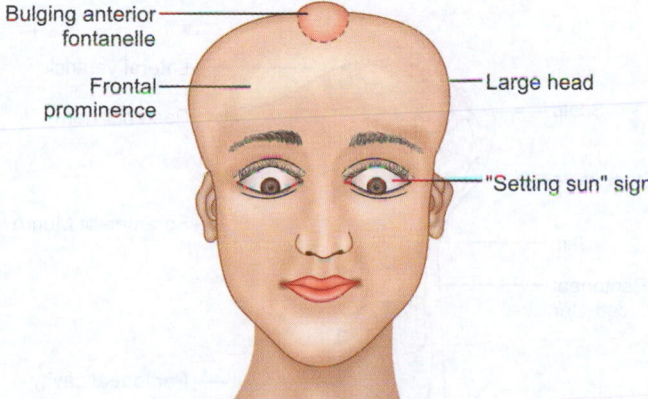

Bulging anterior fontanelle

Frontal prominence

Large head

"Setting sun" sign

Fig. 26: Signs of hydrocephalus

impaired conscious level. These are the signs in adults. In infants and children before the closure of sutures, it produces hydrocephalus.

13. What is carcinomatous meningitis?

It is an uncommon complication of cancer or leukemia in which there is invasion of subarachnoid space by malignant cells. Multiple cranial nerve palsies may occur with hydrocephalus.

14. What is Arnold-Chiari malformation?

It is an abnormality of the hindbrain in which, its commonly two-type forms, the cerebellum and medulla are found to lie partly below the level of foramen magnum. As a result of compression of outlet foramina of the fourth ventricle, or by virtue of associated stenosis of aqueduct of Sylvius obstructive hydrocephalus supervenes in 80 to 90 percent of patients. This malformation is commonly found in association with spina bifida or syringomyelia but diastematomyelia and various anomalies of brain may also occur.

15. What is Dandy-Walker syndrome?

It is characterized by the congenital absence of exit foramina of the fourth ventricle with marked dilatation of the entire ventricular system. The cerebellar hemispheres are widely separated and the vermis greatly thinned. The posterior fossa is large and the tentorium cerebelli is attached higher than normal. A pathognomonic radiographic feature is presence of high lateral sinuses.

16. What are the investigations?

The investigations are:
- Plain X-ray of skull
- CT scan of head
- Ultrasonography through patent fontenelle in infants
- MRI especially to see aqueduct stenosis, Arnold-Chiari malformation and syringomyelia.

17. What are the radiographic signs?

The X-ray signs are:
- Large skull with thinned out bones
- Wide separation of sutures
- Asymmetry of skull
- Pathological calcification
- Abnormal posterior fossa

18. What is the role of CT scanning?

It distinguishes between two main varieties of hydrocephalus and identifies the cause.

19. What is the role of lumbar puncture?

- In obstructive hydrocephalus it is not done as it is dangerous.
- In communicating hydrocephalus it helps in the diagnosis by measuring the opening pressure and

to drain some CSF to return the closing CSF pressure to normal.

- In normal pressure hydrocephalus CSF tap test and CSF infusion studies are done to confirm the diagnosis.

20. How do you treat hydrocephalus?

The essentials of treatment are:
- Removal of cause, e.g. a tumor or cyst should be excised.
- Shunting operation to drain CSF.

21. What will you do in a patient of acute hydrocephalus with severely raised intracranial pressure?

The patient is treated by tapping of lateral ventricles through posterior parietal or frontal holes and setting up external drainage (EVD).

22. What are the shunting procedures?

- Extracranial shunts: In these shunts the CSF is diverted from lateral ventricle into peritoneal or pleural cavity, or right atrium.
- Endoscopic third ventriculostomy (ETV): In this procedure, a hole is made in the floor of third ventricle for the CSF to drain into interpeduncular subarachnoid space.

23. What do you do in ventriculoperitoneal shunt?

In this procedure, the lateral ventricle (right frontal or occipital) is drained into the peritoneal cavity through a catheter having a shunt valve (Fig. 27).

24. What is the technique of shunting?

The catheter is inserted into lateral ventricle, and its other end is connected to a distal catheter that is passed subcutaneously down to be inserted into the peritoneal cavity (Fig. 27).

25. What is the action of this valve?

The valve opens when the CSF pressure exceeds the shunt valve pressure and the CSF then drains into the peritoneal cavity.

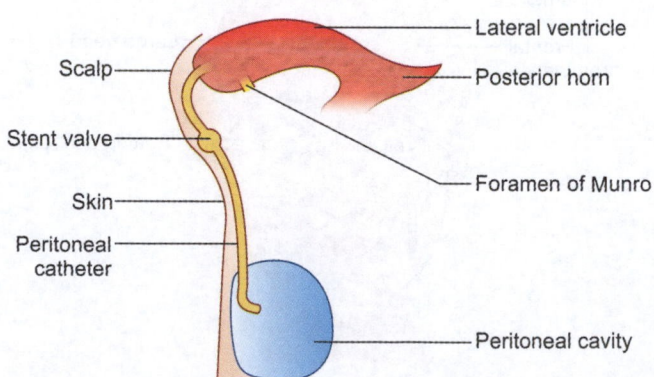

Fig. 27: Ventriculoperitoneal shunt

26. **What are the complications of ventriculoperitoneal shunt?**
    - The main complications are shunt obstruction and shunt infection and both are treated by revision of shunt.
    - Other complications are subdural hemorrhage, slit ventricle syndrome, seizures, CSF leak, stroke and intracerebral hemorrhage.
27. **What are the indications of endoscopic third ventriculostomy (ETV)?**
    Endoscopic third ventriculostomy (ETV) is employed to treat obstructive hydrocephalus with obstruction below the third ventricle, e.g. aqueduct stenosis or posterior fossa mass lesion.
28. **What is the technique of ETV?**
    A neuroendoscope is inserted into the frontal horn of the lateral ventricle and then through foramen of Munro into the third ventricle. A stoma is then made in the third ventricular floor between the mamillary bodies and the infundibular recess so that CSF from third ventricle can drain into interpeduncular subarachnoid space (Fig. 28).
29. **What are the advantages and results of this operation?**
    - The main advantage of this operation is that as no device (or foreign body) is inserted hence there is no risk of infection.
    - It has a success rate of more than 70 percent.
30. **What are the complications?**
    The ETV may block which may require a shunt for correction). Rare complications are basilar artery rupture and memory impairment due to injury to fornix.

DISCUSSION

This condition is characterized by raised intracranial pressure and often with dilated ventricular system due to disequilibrium between CSF production and absorption.

Ventricular enlargement can occur without hydrocephalus and even hydrocephalus can be there without ventriculomegaly.

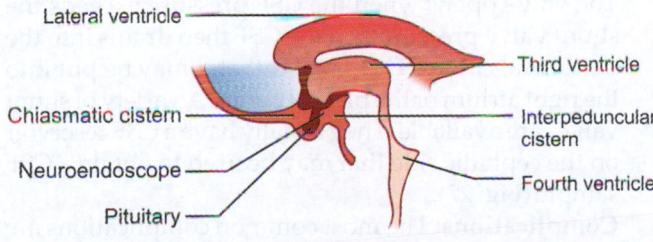

Fig. 28: Endoscopic third ventriculostomy (ETV)

CSF Physiology

The normal CSF volume in an adult is about 150 ml; about 450 ml of CSF is produced daily primarily by the choroid plexus of the ventricles. A small amount is derived from the fluid that passes through the ependyma of ventricular walls. The lateral ventricles communicate with the third ventricle via the foramina of Munro, and the aqueduct of Sylvius transmits CSF from the third to fourth ventricle from where it is transmitted by the midline foramen of Magendie and lateral foramina of Luschka to the subarachnoid space. The CSF is reabsorbed via the arachnoid villi projecting into the superior sagittal sinus. The reabsorption is pressure dependent. Normally there is a balance between CSF production and its absorption.

Etiology

Hydrocephalus is of two types: Obstructive and communicating:
- The obstructive hydrocephalus is due to some obstruction from the lateral ventricles to the fourth ventricle:
    - Lesions within the ventricle, e.g. colloid cyst of third ventricle
    - Lesions of the wall, e.g. congenital aqueduct stenosis
    - Lesions outside the ventricle but with a mass effect, especially posterior fossa mass lesions as the fourth ventricle is easily compressed.
- The communicating hydrocephalus is characterized by patent CSF pathways but there is impaired absorption as occurs following bleeding, CSF infection or raised CSF protein due to carcinomatous meningitis.

Clinical Features

1. Hydrocephalus in infancy
    - As the sutures separate the raised intracranial pressure is compensated. Hence headache, vomiting and papilledema are rare.
    - Lethargy and failure to thrive may be the only symptoms.
    - Increasing head circumference with prominent frontal bones (frontal bossing).
    - The eyes appear sunken and turned downwards. Hence, the upper sclera is exposed ("setting sun sign").
    - There may be bilateral abducent palsies.
    - Scalp veins are prominent.
    - The fontanelles bulge and sutures gape.
    - Other congenital anomalies such as spina bifida may be present.
    - Neurologic deficit occurs late.

2. Hydrocephalus in older children:
   - Disturbance in intellectual function, especially change in the ability at school.
   - Impairment of performance IQ.
   - Head enlargement may not be obvious.
   - Headache, vertigo, ataxia and loss of consciousness may be present.
   - Papilledema and disturbance of ocular movement, especially conjugate gaze are common.
   - Endocrine disturbances including sexual precocity, obesity and reduced skeletal growth may be present rarely.

3. Hydrocephalus in adults
   - Headache, drowsiness, altered mental state and ataxia.
   - Papilledema and disconjugate gaze are frequently observed.
   - Head enlargement cannot occur because of fusion of sutures.
   - Spontaneous CSF rhinorrhea may be present in tumors resulting in obstruction of third ventricle which then expands into the sella and erodes its floor.

4. Normal pressure hydrocephalus: It is a type of communicating hydrocephalus seen in elderly and characterized by ataxia, cognitive decline and urinary incontinence. If dementia predominates the diagnosis is missed. There is no headache and no papilledema. CT scan shows ventriculomegaly that is disproportionate to the degree of cortical atrophy. The CSF pressure is normal. It probably arises from impaired CSF absorption resulting in intermittent high pressures.

Investigations

- Lumbar puncture should not be done in obstructive hydrocephalus due to risk of tonsillar herniation.
- CT scan reveals ventriculomegaly. Chronic raised intracranial pressure in children may cause copper-beaten appearance of skull.
- MRI reveals better details of the causative lesions. It helps in the diagnosis of aqueduct stenosis (Fig. 29). A midline T2-weighted MRI helps in identifying the relationship of the floor of third ventricle, basilar artery and clivus. This information is important to see the suitability of the patient for third ventriculostomy.
- ICP monitoring may be done by putting a parenchymal probe into the frontal lobe through a drill hole.
- Lumbar puncture is done in communicating hydrocephalus to measure the opening pressure and to drain some CSF to return the closing CSF pressure to normal.

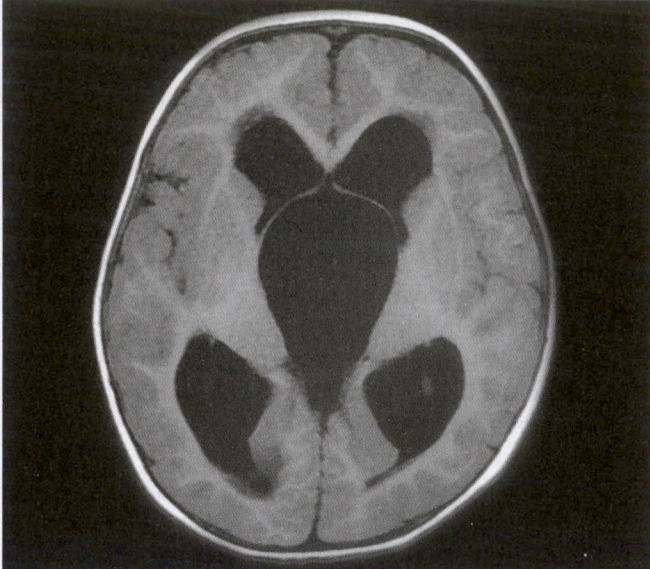

Fig. 29: MRI T1 image obstructive hydrocephalus due to aqueduct stenosis (*Courtesy:* Dr SS Sarkar of Sarkar Diagnostics)

- In normal pressure hydrocephalus, CSF tap test and CSF infusion studies are done.

Treatment

- **Removal of the cause**
  - Removal of the tumor and may be insertion of an external ventricular drain (EVD) to cover the early postoperative phase.
  - If the patient has impaired consciousness due to raised ICP, the hydrocephalus is treated with an EVD or ventriculoperitoneal shunt till recovery, and then the tumor is excised.
- **Ventriculoperitoneal shunt:** In this procedure, the lateral ventricle (right frontal or occipital) is drained into the peritoneal cavity through a catheter having a shunt valve. The catheter is inserted into the lateral ventricle and its other end is connected to valve under the scalp which is connected to a distal catheter that is passed subcutaneously down to be inserted into the peritoneal cavity.

  The valve opens when the CSF pressure exceeds the shunt valve pressure and the CSF then drains into the peritoneal cavity. The distal catheter may be put into the right atrium or the pleural cavity. A variety of shunt valves are available. They usually have a CSF reservoir on the cephalic side that may be used to obtain a CSF sample (Fig. 27).

  Complications: The most common complications are shunt blockage and infection. The obstruction can occur in the ventricular catheter, shunt valve or distal catheter. The causes of obstruction are choroid plexus adhesion, blood, cellular debris or misplaced distal catheter. The obstruction causes stasis that invites infection.

Shunt infection occurs in 1 to 7 percent of patients and is caused by cutaneous bacteria, most commonly by *Staphylococcus epidermidis*. Other organisms are *E coli* and hemolytic streptococci. The risk factors are: young children, open myelomeningocele, longer inserting time and excessive staff movement into and out of the operating room. The infection usually manifests within 6 weeks to 6 months. Treatment includes removal of shunt, external CSF drainage and antibiotics. After the infection is controlled a new shunt is inserted at a different site. Now antibiotic-impregnated catheters are available with a lesser chance of infection. A shunt may overdrain that may result in subdural hemorrhage or slit ventricle syndrome. Other complications are seizures, CSF leak, stroke and intracerebral hemorrhage.

- **Endoscopic third ventriculostomy (ETV):** This technique is employed to treat obstructive hydrocephalus with obstruction below the third ventricle, e.g. aqueduct stenosis or posterior fossa mass lesions.

A neuroendoscope is inserted into the frontal horn of the lateral ventricle and then through foramen of Munro into the third ventricle. A stoma is then made in the third ventricular floor between the mamillary bodies and the infundibular recess so that CSF from the third ventricle can drain into interpeduncular subarachnoid space. It has a success rate of more than 70 percent. The main advantage is that as no device is inserted so there is no risk of infection. The ETV may block which may require a shunt. Rare complications are basilar artery rupture and memory impairment due to injury to fornix (Fig. 28).

CASE 10: SPINAL MENINGOCELE

CLINICAL DIAGNOSIS

1. The patient is an infant who presents with a midline swelling in the lower back since birth.
2. It is hemispherical, cystic and brilliantly transilluminant (Fig. 30).
3. It becomes tense when the child cries.
4. Cross fluctuation may be present between the swelling and anterior fontanelle.
5. The overlying skin is thinned out but normal (it may be ulcerated in neglected cases).
6. There is no neurological deficit.

VIVA VOCE

1. **What is meningocele?**

   It is a congenital abnormality characterized by protrusion of meninges through a defect in the spinolaminar segment (or skull) containing cerebrospinal fluid (CSF) (Fig. 31).

2. **What is meningomyelocele?**

   It is a protrusion of meninges through a defect in the spinolaminar segment containing CSF and normally developed spinal cord or cauda equina that may be adherent to the posterior aspect of sac (Figs 30 and 31).

3. **What are the signs of meningomyelocele?**

   The signs of meningomyelocele are:

   - The patient is an infant who presents with a midline swelling in the lower back since birth.

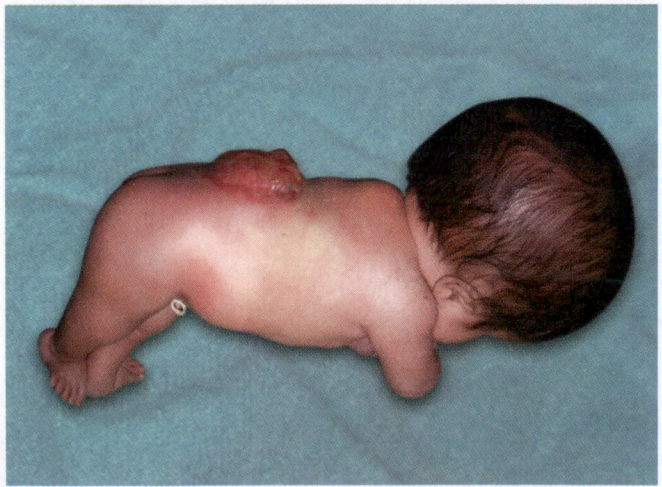

Fig. 30: Meningomyelocele with paralyzed lower limbs, deformed feet and hydrocephalus (*Courtesy:* Professor Ashish Wakhlu)

- It is hemispherical, cystic and translucent.
- It shows presence of cord and nerves inside by transillumination.
- Neurological deficit is present in the lower limbs. It is associated with incontinence (Fig 30).

4. **What is myelocele?**

   It is a congenital defect resulting from failure of closure of neural furrow characterized by the presence of an elliptical raw area in the midline of back discharging CSF from its upper end.

5. **What are the signs of myelocele?**

   The signs of myelocele are:

   - The patient is a newborn who presents with an elliptical raw surface in the midline of lower back.
   - It discharges CSF at the upper end.
   - Neurological deficit is present in the lower limbs with incontinence of urine and feces.
   - It is usually associated with talipes.

6. **What is syringomyelocele?**

   It is a congenital defect with protrusion of meninges through a spinolaminar defect containing dilated cord together with nerves arising from it.

7. **Which is the commonest type of spina bifida?**

   With the exception of spina bifida occulta, myelocele is the most common type of spina bifida.

8. **What is the fate of a myelocele?**

   Many cases of myelocele are stillborn. If the child is born alive, death ensues within a few days from infection of meninges and cord.

9. **How do you differentiate a meningocele from meningo-myelocele?**

   They are differentiated by the following features:

Differentiating features	Meningocele	Meningomyelocele
Translucency	Brilliantly transilluminant	Shadows of cord and nerves are visible
Depression on surface of the swelling	None	May have a depression due to adhesion of cord and nerves
Neurological deficit	None	Present; there may be extensive paralysis of legs with bladder and bowel involvement

10. **What is spina bifida?**

    It is a developmental defect characterized by failure of fusion of spinal arches in the intrauterine life (Fig. 31).

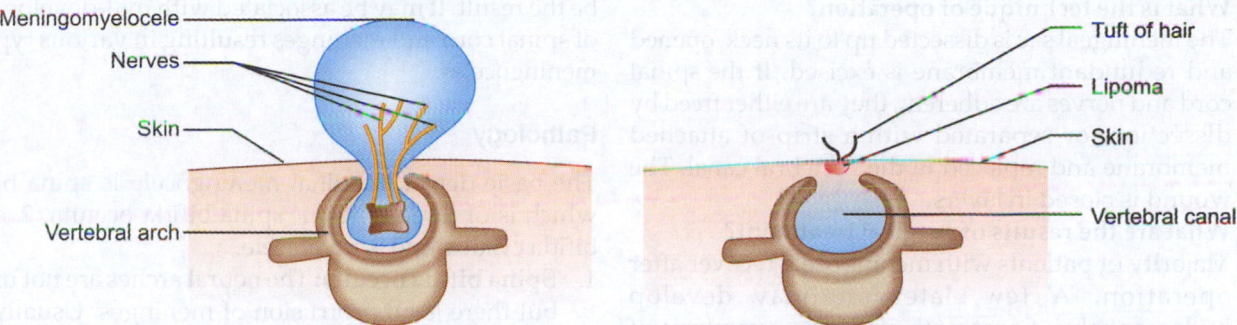

Fig. 31: Anatomy of spina bifida cystica (meningomyelocele) and spina bifida occulta

11. What are the types of spina bifida?
The spina bifida is of many types (Fig. 32):
- Spina bifida occulta
- Spina bifida cystica
  – Meningocele
  – Meningomyelocele
  – Syringomyelocele.
- Myelocele.

12. How is spina bifida related to meningocele?
Spina bifida is frequently associated with maldevelopment of spinal cord and meninges.

13. What is spina bifida occulta?
In this condition, the vertebral arches fail to unite but there is no protrusion of cord or membranes. Frequently only one vertebra is affected, most commonly in the lumbosacral region (Fig. 31).

14. What are the local signs of spina bifida occulta?
The local signs of spina bifida occulta are:
- A patch of hair
- Presence of a nevolipoma
- A dimple or depression in the skin
  There may not be any local sign.

15. Can spina bifida occulta affect any function of body or produce symptoms?
It may cause foot drop, nocturnal enuresis or backache as the child grows older or becomes an adult.

16. How does it produce these symptoms?
A fibrous band called membrana reunions connects the skin at the site of bifida to spinal theca. Growth of body causes the membrana to pull on the theca and nerve roots producing above symptoms.

17. What are the signs of meningocele affecting the skull?
The signs are:
- The patient is a newborn who presents with a swelling at the root of the nose or over the occipital bone since birth
- It is spherical, smooth and tensely cystic
- It is transilluminant and sometimes pedunculated
- It becomes tense when the child cries.

18. Do you know of a meningocele not affected by crying?
Sometimes the growth of skull may occlude the neck of meningocele sac and then the impulse on crying is lost.

19. What is encephalocele?
There is extrusion of a part of brain in the meningocele.

20. What is hydroencephalocele?
If an encephalocele contains part of a ventricle of brain, it is known as hydroencephalocele.

21. What are the specific signs of encephalocele and hydroencephalocele?
The specific signs are:
- The swellings may not be transilluminant.
- They have vascular pulsations.
- The patients are often stillborn or severely disabled.

22. How do you treat a meningocele?
It is treated by excision of sac.

23. What are the steps of excision?
After mobilizing the sac of meningocele up to the neck, it is opened and the redundant membrane is excised. The edges of the cut membrane are sutured over the cord, spinal muscles are approximated, and further reinforced with flaps of sheath from the erector spinae muscles.

24. When will you do the operation?
It is done as soon as the infant is deemed fit for operation. Often the operation is done within a few days of birth.

25. What is the risk of delay in operation?
The sac may grow out of proportion to the growth of the infant; the overlying skin may atrophy and ulcerate resulting in leakage of CSF and meningitis.

26. When do you treat a meningomyelocele?
If the neurological deficit is mild or moderate, operation may be done. In severe deficit, no operation is done.

27. How do you treat a meningomyelocele?
It is treated by excision of the sac, sparing and replacing spinal cord and nerves in the spinal canal.

28. **What is the technique of operation?**

The meningeal sac is dissected up to its neck, opened and redundant membrane is excised. If the spinal cord and nerves are adherent, they are either freed by dissection, or separated with a strip of attached membrane and replaced in the vertebral canal. The wound is closed in layers.

29. **What are the results of surgical treatment?**

Majority of patients with meningocele recover after operation. A few, later on, may develop hydrocephalus. Some patients having paralysis of one or both lower limbs may achieve some useful recovery.

30. **What is the cause of postoperative hydrocephalus?**

It is usually due to some associated congenital abnormalities at a higher level.

31. **What are the indications of operation in spina bifida occulta?**

It is indicated when neurological, urological or orthopedic symptoms progress or appear after infancy.

32. **What is the cause of neurological and/or urological symptoms in spina bifida occulta?**

The causes of symptoms are:
- Traction due to membrana reunions
- Compression of cord by intra- or extradural lipoma.

33. **What is distematomyelia?**

It is a condition in which the cord is split in midline by a bony spur that divides the vertebral canal beneath one lamina into two lateral compartments.

DISCUSSION

Spinal meningocele is a congenital anomaly characterized by protrusion of spinal theca with CSF through a defect in the vertebral arches. It occurs once in 300 live births.

Etiology

During the second week of intrauterine life, a longitudinal furrow develops on the dorsal surface of embryo by infolding of the epiblast. This is neural groove. The edges of this groove fuse with each other resulting in the formation of a tube. This epiblastic tube is separated from the surface by mesoblast that grows over it from both the sides. From this mesoblast vertebrae, spinal muscles, membranes, etc. are going to develop. In each segment bar of cartilage appears on both the sides of neural tube and fuse with each other to form vertebral arches during the fourth month. If these arches fail to fuse, spina bifida will

be the result. It may be associated with mal-development of spinal cord and meninges resulting in various types of meningoceles.

Pathology

The basic defect in spinal meningocele is spina bifida, which is of three types: 1. spina bifida occulta, 2. spina bifida cystica, and 3. myelocele.

1. **Spina bifida occulta:** The neural arches are not united but there is no protrusion of meninges. Usually one vertebra is affected most commonly in the lumbosacral region. At the site of bony deformity there may be a dimple, a tuft of hair or a lipoma. A fibrous band, membrana reunions, connecting the skin to the spinal theca is present. As the patient grows, this band pulls on the theca and nerve roots resulting in foot drop and nocturnal enuresis. This defect may be asymptomatic and may be diagnosed only when X-ray is done for some other reason (Fig. 31).

2. **Meningocele:** Here spina bifida is associated with protrusion of a sac of meninges containing CSF.

3. **Meningomyelocele:** The meningeal sac contains normally developed spinal cord or cauda equina. They may be adherent to the sac. The cord or nerves can be detected as dark shadows on transillumination (Figs 30 and 31).

4. **Syringomyelocele:** The central canal of the spinal cord is dilated and protruded along with the nerves arising from it into the meningeal sac. This lesion is very rare.

5. **Myelocele:** There is an elliptical raw area in the midline of the back discharging CSF from the upper end. It is due to arrest of development at the time of closure of neural furrow.

Clinical Features

Except spina bifida occulta, the myelocele is the commonest lesion. If the infant is born alive, death occurs within a few days from infection of meninges and cord. Gross talipes is present. Meningocele produces a brilliantly transilluminant swelling usually without any neurological deficit.

Meningomyelocele shows cord or nerves as dark shadows on transillumination. There may be a dimple on the protrusion due to adherent cord or nerves. It is usually associated with bilateral talipes and trophic changes. Later on, the patient may have paraplegia with incontinence.

Investigations

1. **Myelocele:** In this condition CT or MRI of the head and craniocervical region should be done to see for an

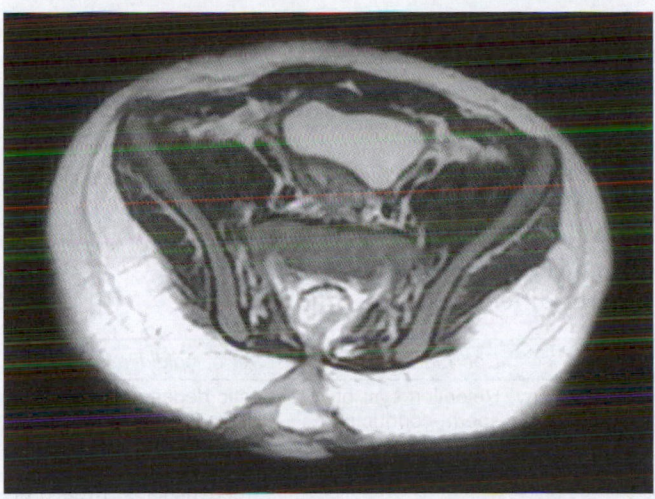

Fig. 32: MRI axial T2 image of open neural tube with meningocele (*Courtesy:* Dr SS Sarkar, Sarkar Diagnostics)

associated hydrocephalus, stenosis of aqueduct and Arnold-Chiari malformation.

2. **Spina bifida cystica:** In these defects ultrasonography or MRI may decide on the contents of the sac (Fig. 32).
3. **Spina bifida occulta:** Simple radiography and MRI can assess the degree of abnormality.

Treatment

The objective of surgical treatment is to restore the anatomical normality as far as possible by providing skin cover to the raw area (myelocele), excising the meningocele or excising and reconstituting the neural sac (meningomyelocele).

In meningomyelocele, the mass may be an extremely complicated structure and anatomical reconstitution may not be possible. The neurological deficit requires a multi-disciplinary approach in the management that includes a neurosurgeon, an urologist, an orthopedic surgeon and a pediatrician.

CASE 11: SPERMATOCELE

CLINICAL DIAGNOSIS

1. The patient is usually an adult who presents with a painless and slow growing nodule or swelling in the scrotum (Fig. 33).
2. It is situated above and behind the testis in the head of epididymis.
3. It is soft, smooth, non-tender and translucent.

VIVA VOCE

1. **What is spermatocele?**
   It is a retention cyst of epididymis of unknown etiology derived from some portion of the sperm conducting system of epididymis.
2. **Is this lesion unilateral or bilateral?**
   It is often bilateral.
3. **What is the time of occurrence of bilateral cysts?**
   They usually occur dys-synchronously.
4. **What is the morphology of this cyst?**
   It is an unilocular cyst of variable size usually small, filled with fluid resembling barley water containing spermatozoa.
5. **What is the most interesting clinical manifestation of this lesion?**
   Some of the patients imagine that they have three testicles, i.e. "some of these patients flatter themselves in thinking they are unduly provided" (Sir Robert Linton).
6. **What are the investigations done in this disease?**
   The cyst can be delineated by ultrasonography. Aspiration of the cyst may be done under ultrasound guidance.
7. **How do you treat a spermatocele?**
   A small cyst is left as such. A large cyst is treated by aspiration or excision.
8. **What is the technique of excision?**
   Through a scrotal incision, the thin coverings of the cyst are carefully peeled off, layer by layer. Then the residual attachments are divided and the cyst is excised.
9. **Will you like to excise a spermatocele in a young man?**
   It should be avoided in a young man before he has had children.
10. **Why?**
    The excision may impair epididymal function and sperm transport by postoperative fibrosis.

11. **Can this disease recur after excision?**
    Yes.
12. **How do you treat recurrence?**
    By epididymectomy.
13. **What are the differences between a spermatocele and cyst of epididymis?**
    The differences are as follows:

Feature	Spermatocele	Cyst of epididymis
Origin/etiology	Retention cyst of sperm-conducting system of epididymis	Cystic degeneration of: • Paradidymis (organ of Giraldes), or • Appendix of epididymis (pedunculated hydatid of Morgagni), or • Appendix of testis (sessile hydatid of Morgagni), or • Vas aberrans of Haller
Composition	Unilocular cyst	Aggregation of a number of cysts
Consistency	Soft, lax	Tense
Surface	Smooth	Feels like a bunch of grapes
Translucency	Translucent	Brilliantly transilluminant with fine tessellation (Chinese lantern appearance)
Aspirate	Barley water-like	Crystal clear
Treatment	Aspiration (can be completely aspirated) or excision	Excision (cannot be completely aspirated)

DISCUSSION

Spermatocele is a retention cyst of some portion of sperm conducting system of epididymis (Fig. 33).

Pathology

It is usually a small unilocular cyst that nearly always lies in the head of epididymis above and behind the upper

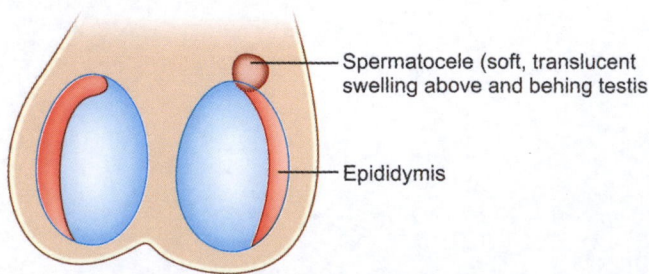

Fig. 33: Signs of a spermatocele

pole of testis. It has barley water-like fluid that contains spermatozoa.

Clinical Features

The patient presents with a painless and slow growing nodule or swelling in the scrotum. It is present above and behind the testis in the head of the epididymis. It is soft, smooth, non-tender and translucent.

Investigations

The cyst can be delineated by ultrasonography of the scrotum.

Treatment

If it is small it needs not to be treated. A large spermatocele is either treated by aspiration or excision.

Cysts of Epididymis

The cysts of the epididymis are quite common and are filled with crystal-clear fluid. They are multiple and bilateral and feel like a small bunch of grapes. These cysts are brilliantly transilluminant and separate from testis. They can be seen by ultrasonography.

If they are causing symptoms they may be excised but it may interfere with the transport of sperms from the testis.

Goiters

CLINICAL DIAGNOSIS

1. The patient is usually a child or an adolescent person between 12-20 years who presents with a painless and slow growing swelling of thyroid of insidious onset.
2. The whole of the thyroid is enlarged uniformly.
3. It is mild to moderate in size, smooth and soft (Fig. 1).
4. There is usually no other abnormality, e.g. pressure signs, signs of altered thyroid function or cervical lymph node enlargement.

VIVA VOCE

1. **What do you mean by a goiter?**
   - A goiter is a non-inflammatory and non-neoplastic swelling of thyroid.

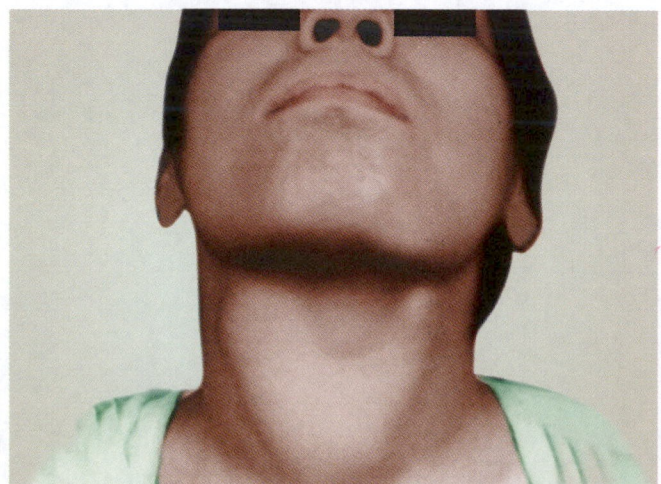

Fig. 1: Physiological goiter in a young female, 18 years of age. The swelling is generalized and smooth

- The term goiter is derived from the latin word Guttur, which means neck, as the goiter is one of the commonest swelling of the neck.
2. **What are the signs of a goiter?**
   The signs of a goiter are –
   - The patient presents with a painless slow growing swelling in the front of neck of insidious onset.
   - It moves up with swallowing.
   - It has the shape of thyroid.
   - It may be uniform (puberty or colloid goiter) or nodular (nodular goiter)
3. **What are the types of simple goiter?**
   The simple goiters are –
   1. Diffuse hyperplastic goiter which includes physiological, pubertal and pregnancy goiters
   2. Multinodular goiter
4. **What is a puberty goiter?**
   It is a diffuse hyperplastic goiter occurring at puberty when the metabolic demands are high.
5. **What is the cause of thyroid enlargement?**
   The enlargement is due to stimulation by pituitary, i.e. increased levels of circulating TSH.
6. **What is the cause of increased levels of TSH?**
   It is due to low levels of circulating thyroid hormone due to increased metabolic demands.
7. **What is the natural fate of a puberty goiter?**
   - If TSH stimulation stops early the goiter usually regresses.
   - If TSH stimulation continues for a longer period and then wanes away, it becomes a colloid goiter.
8. **What is a colloid goiter?**
   It is a late-stage of diffuse hyperplasia when many follicles are inactive and full with colloid.

9. **Can a puberty goiter recur?**
   It may recur later (but not as a puberty goiter) at the times of stress such as pregnancy and lactation.

10. **How do you treat a puberty goiter?**
    It is treated by giving L-thyroxine 0.15-0.2 mg per day for many months, and then slowly tapering it off to 0.1 mg per day which should be continued for many years.

11. **What are the results of treatment?**
    Usually the results are good as the goiter slowly disappears completely.

12. **Is there any indication for surgery?**
    In late cases there may be unsatisfactory or no response, hence surgery may be needed, especially if there is cosmetic problem or pressure symptoms.

13. **What do you do in such a case?**
    Partial thyroidectomy.

14. **What is advice to the patient at the time of discharge?**
    To continue L-thyroxine therapy for an unlimited period.

15. **What will happen if this instruction is not followed?**
    The goiter can recur.

DISCUSSION

Puberty goiter (diffuse hyperplastic goiter) is a simple goiter of thyroid usually occurring in teenagers mostly the girls, and characterized by mild diffuse enlargement of thyroid of insidious onset (Fig. 1).

Etiology

It usually occurs at puberty when the metabolic demands are high. There is diffuse hyperplasia of the thyroid in response to TSH stimulation. When the TSH stimulation ceases the goiter may regress, but may recur later at times of stress such as pregnancy and lactation.

The chances of goiter appearing at puberty are more in iodine-deficient areas when the patient is exposed to environmental goitrogens at the same time. Enzymatic deficiencies (dyshormonogenesis) may also be responsible.

In iodine-deficient areas the thyroid enlargement reflects a compensatory effort to trap iodide and produce sufficient hormone under conditions when the hormone production is relatively deficient.

The environmental goitrogens include cassava root, which contains a thiocynate, vegetables of Cruciferae family (e.g. brussels, sprouts, cabbage and cauliflower) and milk from regions where goitrogens are present in the grass.

Clinical Features

There is a mild, diffuse, uniform and soft enlargement of thyroid. It may become sufficiently enlarged to cause discomfort or even tracheal compression. Clinically the patient is euthyroid.

When the TSH stimulation wanes the goiter usually disappears. If it does not disappear it may become a colloid goiter with many inactive follicles full of colloid.

If the stimulation continues and is fluctuating, it results in a nodular goiter.

Investigations

Investigations are usually not required. The thyroid functions should be assessed to rule out subclinical thyrotoxicosis. The radiography of the chest and thoracic inlet shows tracheal compression or deviation, if present.

Ultrasound or CT scan may be required to see the extent and nature of the goiter, especially if it is causing tracheal compression.

Treatment

In endemic areas the incidence of goiter can be markedly reduced by the use of iodized salt.

The goitrogens are avoided.

The goiter may disappear if thyroxine is given in the dose of 0.15-0.2 mg daily early in the morning for a few months.

Partial thyroidectomy is very rarely required if the pressure symptoms are continued, or a large goiter is causing cosmetic problem.

CASE 2: NODULAR GOITER

CLINICAL DIAGNOSIS

1. The patient is usually a female between 25 to 40 years of age who presents with a painless and slow growing swelling of thyroid of insidious onset and long duration (many years).
2. The whole of the thyroid is enlarged.
3. It has one or more nodules which may be felt as elevations on its surface, some hard and some soft in consistency (Figs 2 and 3).
4. The nodules do not fluctuate or transilluminate, and are dull on percussion.
5. Pressure symptoms, dyspnea, dysphagia and stridor, may be present.

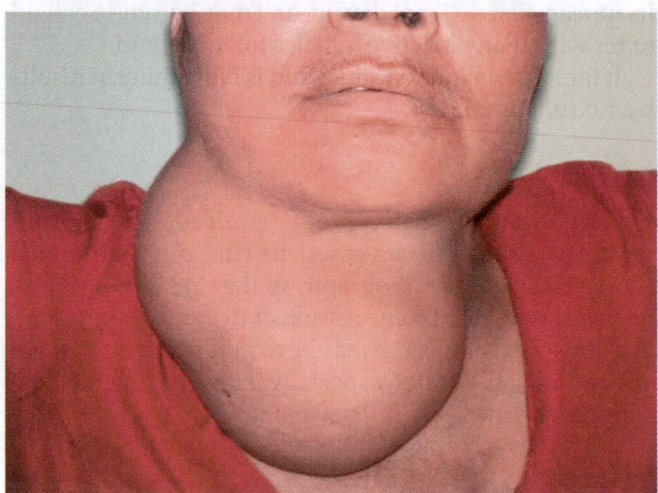

Fig. 2: Multinodular goiter (Courtesy: Professor Sandeep Kumar)

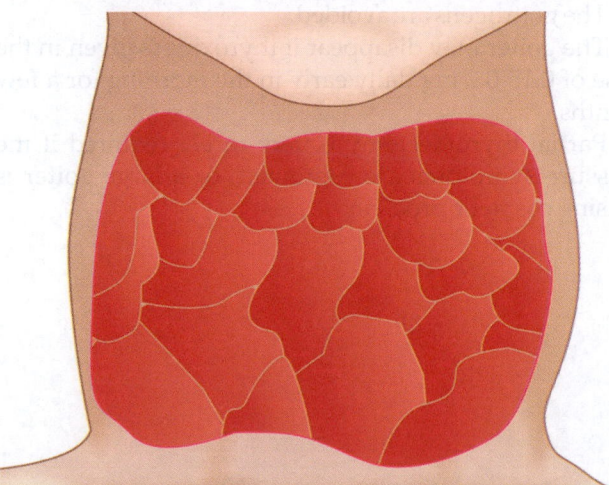

Fig. 3: Multinodular goiter

VIVA VOCE

1. **What is a nodular goiter?**
   It is a nonneoplastic and noninflammatory swelling of thyroid of varied etiology and characterized by one or more nodules in the thyroid (Figs 2 and 3).
2. **What is the cause of a nodular goiter?**
   The causes of a nodular goiter are many, i.e.
   1. Iodine deficiency in water and diet (endemic goiter) —commonest cause.
   2. Goitrogens in diet, some drugs.
   3. Genetic defects with defect in the enzyme system which is necessary for thyroxine synthesis (sporadic goiter).
3. **What is the normal daily requirement of iodine?**
   It is about 150-300 microgram.
4. **What are the causes of iodine deficiency?**
   The causes of iodine deficiency are—
   • Very low iodine content in water and food
   • Failure of intestinal absorption.
5. **What is the daily intake of iodine in endemic goiter area?**
   In endemic areas it is below 50 microgram per day.
6. **What do you mean by a goitrogen?**
   A goitrogen is a chemical or drug which produces a goiter when taken for some time.
7. **What are the examples of goitrogens?**
   The goitrogens are –
   • Vegetables of brassica family, e.g. cabbage, kale and rape which contain thiocyanate
   • Drugs – PAS, antithyroid drugs (thiocyanates, perchlorates, carbimazole, thiouracil compounds), resorcinol
   • Iodides in large quantities
8. **What is an iodide goiter?**
   A goiter produced by prolonged use of iodides in large quantities seen in asthmatics who have been taking proprietary preparations containing iodides over a prolonged period.
9. **What are the stages in goiter formation?**
   The stages in goiter formation are—
   • Persistent stimulation by TSH causes diffuse hyperplasia in which all lobules are composed of active follicles which may persist for a long time but is reversible if TSH stimulation ceases.
   • Subsequently due to fluctuating TSH level, a mixed pattern develops with areas of inactive lobules.
   • Active lobules become more vascular and hyperplastic until hemorrhage occurs causing

central necrosis and leaving only a surrounding rind of active follicles.

- Coalescence of necrotic lobules to form nodules filled either with iodine-free colloid or a mass of new but inactive follicles.
- Repeated cycles of above process result in a nodular goiter. Most nodules are inactive. Active follicles are present only in the internodular tissue (Fig. 3).

10. **Apart from TSH is the goitrogenesis related to some other growth factor?**
Apart from TSH there may be other thyroid growth factors responsible for growth and development of a nodular goiter. They include growth stimulating immunoglobulins (Studer). It is considered that chronic thyroid stimulation may affect particularly sensitive cells which are derived from growth prone cell clones. One of the hallmarks of such a nodular goiter is the heterogenecity of structure and function often between adjacent follicles of the same gland.

11. **How many nodules are present in a nodular goiter?**
Nodules are usually multiple. Sometimes only one macroscopic nodule is found but microscopic changes are present throughout the gland (Fig. 3).

12. **What is microanatomy of a nodule?**
Nodules may be colloid or cellular. Cystic degeneration and hemorrhage are common as is subsequent calcification.

13. **What is the time of appearance of a nodule?**
Nodules appear early in an endemic goiter and later (20 to 30 years of age) in a sporadic goiter, although the patient may not be aware of the goiter until the late forties or fifties.

14. **What do you mean by an endemic goiter?**
A goiter prevalent in the people of a district.

15. **What do you mean by a sporadic goiter?**
A goiter having haphazard occurrence in terms of geography.

16. **Why do the goiters occur more commonly in a female than a male?**
The cause for this fact is not known. It may be something to do with estrogen receptors which have been identified in normal thyroid tissue, and also in a nodular goiter.

17. **What investigations will you do in a nodular goiter?**
The possible investigations are—
- Hormone assay—TSH, T_3 and T_4
- Thyroid antibodies
- X-ray of neck
- Ultrasonography
- FNAC.

All the investigations are not done in every patient.

18. **What is the functional status of a nodular goiter?**
Usually the patient is euthyroid, subclinical mild hyperthyroidism may be present occasionally.

19. **Why do you estimate the titer of thyroid antibodies?**
It is done to differentiate it from Hashimoto's disease where antibodies are present.

20. **Why do you do a radiograph of neck?**
A radiograph of the neck is done to see—
- Soft tissue shadow of the goiter
- Calcification, if any
- Tracheal compression or deviation.

21. **What are the complications of a nodular goiter?**
The complications include -
- Tracheal obstruction
- Secondary thyrotoxicosis
- Carcinoma.

22. **What are the causes of tracheal obstruction in a nodular goiter?**
The causes of tracheal obstruction are -
- Compression in a lateral or anteroposterior plane
- Gross lateral displacement
- Hemorrhage into a nodule impacted in thoracic inlet (sudden or acute obstruction).

23. **What is the incidence of hyperthyroidism in this disease?**
The incidence is difficult to estimate but figures as high as 30 percent have been reported.

24. **What is the type of carcinoma that occurs in a nodular goiter?**
It is a follicular carcinoma.

25. **What is the incidence of malignant change?**
This complication is uncommon but an increased incidence has been reported from endemic areas.

26. **How do you treat a nodular goiter?**
If it is small and asymptomatic no treatment is required. If it is big and causing pressure on trachea it should be treated by subtotal thyroidectomy.

27. **What do you do in this operation?**
Most of the thyroid tissue including the nodules is excised and up to 8 grams of relatively normal tissue is preserved in each tracheoesophageal groove.

28. **Is there any medical treatment? Can this be treated by L-thyroxine or iodine?**
There is no medical treatment as the nodular goiter is irreversible. Hence L-thyroxine or iodine does not help. Sometimes, they may precipitate secondary thyrotoxicosis.

29. **Is there any indication for unilateral lobectomy?**
It is very rarely required and done when the disease is limited to one lateral lobe and the other lobe is normal or has minimal disease.

30. **Can this disease recur after operation?**
    Yes
31. **Why?**
    It is because of persistence of causative factors with continued TSH stimulation.
32. **How do you prevent recurrence?**
    It is prevented by giving 0.15-0.2 mg of L-thyroxine daily postoperatively until after the menopause.
33. **How do you treat recurrent goiter?**
    By radioiodine as the operation is difficult and hazardous.

DISCUSSION

Nodular goiter is a goitrous enlargement of thyroid having a single or multiple nodules (Fig. 2).

Pathology

The whole gland is enlarged and has multiple nodules. Occasionally, only one macroscopic nodule is present though microscopic alterations are present throughout the gland. The nodules may be colloid or cellular. Cystic degeneration, hemorrhage and calcification are common.

Pathogenesis—Due to iodine deficiency (or any other factor) there is impaired hormone production and release in circulation. It results in TSH stimulation which induces diffuse thyroid hyperplasia, followed by areas of focal hyperplasia with necrosis and hemorrhage. When this stimulus is continuous and/or repetitive, new areas of focal hyperplasia and degeneration including calcification may develop.

Clinical Features

- *Age*—Nodules appear early in an endemic and later (20-30 years) in a sporadic goiter.
- *Sex*—It is far more common in the female than in the male.
- The patient is euthyroid and presents with palpable and often visible nodules in the thyroid.
- They are smooth and usually firm.
- The goiter is painless and moves freely on swallowing. It may become painful if bleeding occurs in a nodule.

Investigations

- *Thyroid hormone estimation*—It is essential to rule out mild hyperthyroidism.
- *Thyroid antibodies*—The thyroid antibodies must be estimated to differentiate it from autoimmune thyroiditis.

- *Radiography of neck*—It may show calcification of goiter and compression or distortion of trachea.
- *FNAC*—It is very important, especially in a hard dominant painful nodule. For best results it is done under ultrasonographic guidance.
- Ultrasonography shows all the nodules, usually more than visible or palpable. A frequency probe may differentiate between a solid and cystic nodule.
- RAI uptake and scan usually reveal a patchy uptake with areas of increased uptake (hot nodules) and areas of decreased uptake (cold nodules).

Complications

Airway obstruction—The goiter may displace the trachea or compress it in a lateral or anteroposterior plane by retrosternal extension. Acute obstruction may occur following bleeding into a nodule incarcerated in thoracic inlet.

Secondary thyrotoxicosis—It may occur in about 30 percent of patients.

Malignancy—A nodular goiter may change into a follicular carcinoma. It is more likely to occur in endemic areas.

Calcification—A long-standing goiter may calcify and then the hardness of calcification may make it look like a carcinoma.

Etiology

- A nodular goiter may occur due to stimulation of thyroid by TSH, either from pituitary (rare), or in response to a low level of circulating thyroid hormone for a long time.
- The most important factor in endemic goiter is dietary deficiency of iodine.
- In a sporadic goiter defective hormone synthesis is most probable etiological factor.
- The follicular cell proliferation may also be due to other growth factors including immunoglobulins.
- The nodularity may be due to presence of clones of cells particularly sensitive to growth hormone.
- The goitrogens of some vegetables (cabbage, etc.) may be contributing to etiology.

Treatment

- The nodular change of a goiter cannot be reversed by any drug.
- Though nodular goiter is irreversible, more than 50 percent benign nodules regress in size over a period of 10 years (Kuma).

If there are no symptoms and the swelling is not very big and unsightly, operation is not indicated. The operation is indicated in the following situations –

- For cosmetic reasons
- Retrosternal extension with incipient or actual tracheal compression
- Presence of a dominant area of enlargement which may be malignant

During operation most of the bulk of gland is resected leaving up to 8 gm of relatively normal tissue in each remnant.

If one lobe is more significantly involved than the other, it should be totally excised. The less affected side should have subtotal resection (Dunhill procedure).

Recurrence: In many patients the etiological factors persist, therefore goiter can recur, especially in a young patient. Hence, the patient is given thyroxine (0.15-0.2 mg) to suppress TSH with the aim of preventing recurrence.

The postoperative recurrence has been treated by radioiodine which may reduce the size of goiter. Reoperation is difficult and hazardous.

Prophylaxis: Intake of iodized salt in endemic areas prevent the occurrence of a simple goiter.

CASE 3: SOLITARY THYROID NODULE

CLINICAL DIAGNOSIS

1. The patient presents with a painless slow growing solitary nodule in the neck of insidious onset.
2. It moves up with deglutition.
3. It is soft or firm and smooth.
4. It may be well or ill-defined.
5. The rest of the thyroid is usually not palpable (Figs 4 and 5).

VIVA VOCE

1. **What do you mean by a solitary nodule?**
   It is a circumscribed swelling in the thyroid which appears to be otherwise normal.

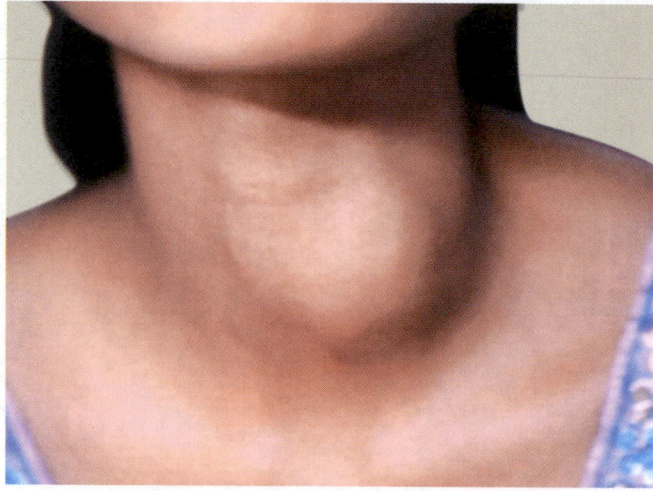

Fig. 4: Adenoma of left lobe of thyroid (solitary thyroid nodule)

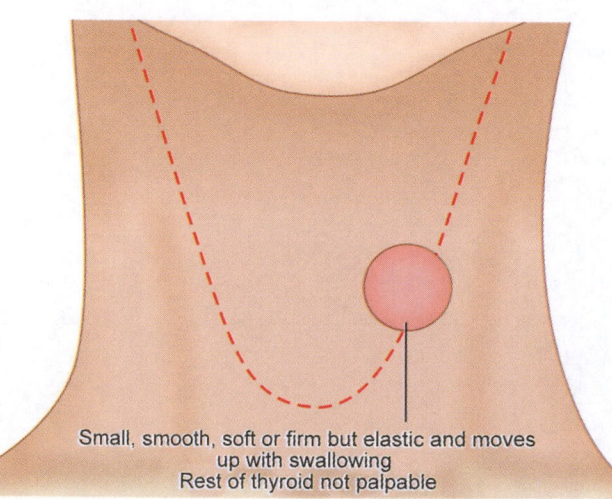

Small, smooth, soft or firm but elastic and moves up with swallowing
Rest of thyroid not palpable

Fig. 5: Solitary thyroid nodule

2. **What are the types of nodules?**
   The nodules are of two types -
   - Those in which there is a grave suspicion of malignancy.
   - Those which are probably benign.
3. **When do you clinically suspect malignancy?**
   Malignancy is more likely in the following nodules -
   - A nodule of recent onset
   - A nodule in a child
   - A nodule in a male
   - In patients with a history of head-neck radiation, family history of carcinoma of thyroid or another malignancy
   - If the nodule is large, adherent to trachea or strap muscles or associated with lymph node enlargement
4. **What do you do in first type of nodule?**
   It should be carefully investigated to rule out or confirm malignancy.
5. **What is the usual nature of second type of nodule?**
   50% are nodules of a multinodular goiter when exposed. Some are adenomas.
6. **What investigations are done to find the nature of nodule?**
   The possible investigations are –
   - Blood
   - Ultrasound examination
   - FNAC
   - Needle biopsy, excisional biopsy
   - Isotope scanning
7. **What is the incidence of malignancy in a solitary nodule?**
   About 10% of solitary nodules are carcinomas. It rises to about 40% in patients who have undergone previous cervical irradiation.
8. **What are the things you see in the blood?**
   The specific things to be seen in the blood are—
   1. Serum TSH and FT4
   2. Antithyroperoxidase antibodies and antithyroglobulin antibodies – very high levels are detected in Hashimoto's thyroiditis.
   3. Serum calcitonin is done in a suspicious patient of familial medullary carcinoma or MEN type 2.
9. **What is the role of ultrasonography?**
   - It is done to note the size of the nodule and to find if it is a part of multinodular goiter.
   - The nodule is more likely to be malignant if it has an irregular or indistinct margin, if it has heterogeneous nodule echogenicity, intranodular

vascular images, microcalcification, or a diameter more than 1 cm.

10. What is the role of radioiodine scan?

Radioiodine (^{123}I or ^{131}I) scan is of help if the patient has hyperthyroidism, otherwise it has very little diagnostic value because—

- The cold nodules have an increased risk of having cancer but most of the cold nodules are benign.
- Most of the hot nodules are benign but they may have cancer sometimes.

11. What is the role of CT scan?

It is done in a large nodule to find if there is tracheal compression, what is its extent, and whether it is extending into the mediastinum.

12. How will you confirm the diagnosis?

If there is suspicion of malignancy FNAC or needle biopsy is done. Larger nodules of one cm or more in size can be needle biopsied. Small nodules are aspirated or biopsied under ultrasonographic guidance.

13. What is the result of FNAC or needle biopsy of thyroid nodules?

In one study about 70% nodules were benign, 5% were malignant, 15% were not diagnosed and 10% were suspicious.

14. What will you do when the FNAC/FNAB report says it to be suspicious?

The suspicious nodules are excised.

15. What will you do with a cystic nodule?

It is aspirated dry and the aspirate is sent for cytology. A bloody aspirate has a higher chance of malignancy.

16. What are the results of FNAC/FNAB?

There are 4% false positive and 4% false negative rates.

17. What do you know of incidental thyroid nodules?

A thyroid nodule may be a coincidental finding during imaging studies – MRI, CT and ^{18}FDG-PET. The risk of malignancy is 17% in nodules detected on CT or MRI and 25-50% on ^{18}FDG-PET.

18. How will you treat a thyroid nodule?

The treatment depends upon the cause, and whether it is symptomatic or asymptomatic.

19. How will you treat an asymptomatic benign nodule?

- It may be kept under careful follow-up.
- A large benign nodule more than 2 cm in size with elevated serum TSH level may be treated with levothyroxine suppression (50 mcg daily starting dose).
- Ethanol injection may reduce its size.

20. How do you treat a symptomatic benign nodule?

- A toxic nodule may be treated by RAI (^{131}I)
- A nodule with indeterminate or suspicious cytology, compression symptoms or discomfort is treated by hemithyroidectomy.

21. How do you treat a malignant nodule?

Total thyroidectomy with hormonal replacement

DISCUSSION

Palpable thyroid nodules are very common. They are present in 4-7% of adult population in the regions of the world with sufficient intake of iodine. They are more common in iodine deficient areas. They are increasingly prevalent with age and more common in women than men.

On ultrasonography about 50% of solitary nodules are found to be a nodule of a multinodular goiter.

About 95% of thyroid nodules are benign, the causes include benign adenoma, colloid nodule, cyst, carcinoma or metastasis. The risk of a thyroid nodule being malignant is higher -

1. In patients with a history of head-neck radiation in the past.
2. In patients with family history of carcinoma of thyroid.
3. In patients with a history of another malignancy.
4. If the nodule is large, adherent to trachea or strap muscles or associated with lymph node enlargement.

Clinical Features

- Small nodules are mostly asymptomatic.
- Large nodules may cause cosmetic embarrassment, discomfort, hoarseness or dysphagia.
- Depending on their cause a thyroid nodule may be associated with hypothyroidism (Hashimoto's thyroiditis) or hyperthyroidism (toxic adenoma).

Investigations

- Serum TSH and FT4
- Antithyroperoxidase antibodies and antithyroglobulin antibodies – very high levels are found in Hashimoto's thyroiditis.
- Serum calcitonin in a suspicious patient of familial medullary carcinoma or MEN type-2.
- Ultrasound of the neck is done to measure the size of the nodule and to note if it is a part of a multi-nodular goiter. The nodule is more likely to be malignant if it has an irregular or indistinct margin, if it has heterogenous nodule echogenicity, intranodular vascular images, microcalcification, or a diameter more than 1 cm.
- Ultrasound is better than CT or MRI for its accuracy, ease of use and lower cost.
- RAI (^{123}I or ^{131}I) scan – This investigation is of help if the patient has hyperthyroidism, otherwise it has very little value because—
  1. Cold nodules have an increased risk of malignancy but most of them are benign.

2. Hot nodules are ordinarily benign but may sometimes be malignant.

- CT scan may be done in large thyroid nodules to find the extent of tracheal compression and extension into mediastinum.

- FNAC: If there is suspicion of malignancy FNAC or needle biopsy is done to confirm the diagnosis. Larger nodules (≥1 cm diameter) can be needle biopsied, small nodules are aspirated or biopsied under ultrasonographic guidance.

  In one study about 70% nodules were benign, 5% were malignant, 15% were nondiagnostic and 10%, were suspicious. The patients with malignant and suspicious nodules must undergo thyroid surgery.

  Cystic nodule are usually benign but the aspirate is examined cytologically. Bloody aspirate has a higher chance of malignancy.

  There are 4% false positive and equal false negative rates. Hence the patient with a negative result is kept under observation.

- Incidental thyroid nodules: A thyroid nodule may be a coincidental finding during imaging studies of the body for some other reason with an incidence—MRI 50%, CT 13% and ^{18}FDG–PET 2%. Such nodules are also investigated as outlined above. The risk of malignancy is 17% in nodules detected on CT or MRI and 25-50% on ^{18}FDG-PET.

TREATMENT

- Asymptomatic benign nodule:
  1. It may be kept under periodic monitoring.
  2. A large benign nodule more than 2 cm in size with elevated serum TSH level may be treated by levothyroxine suppression with a starting dose of 50 mcg daily. It prevents the nodule from enlarging. A few may shrink.
  3. Ethanol injection can be given in both solid and cystic nodules. Most nodules undergo partial shrinkage after injection.

- Symptomatic benign nodules:
  1. Removal of the cause, if any
  2. A toxic nodule may be treated by radioactive iodine (^{131}I). It shrinks at an average of 40% by 1 year and 59% by 2 years. It remains palpable and becomes firmer.
  3. Benign nodules with indeterminate or suspicious cytology, compression symptoms, discomfort or cosmetic embarrassment are treated by limited thyroid surgery depending upon the lesion.

- Symptomatic malignant nodules are treated by total thyroidectomy with thyroid hormone replacement.

CASE 4: RETROSTERNAL GOITER

CLINICAL DIAGNOSIS

1. The patient is usually a short-necked stocky male who presents with dry cough and dyspnea, especially nocturnal.
2. Engorged neck veins may be present over the upper part of chest.
3. A thyroid swelling may be present in the lower limit of which is not definable. It may not move up with deglutition (Fig. 6).
4. On elevating both the arms above the head the face may become congested and cyanosed.
5. The thyroid swelling may be appearing in the neck intermittently during coughing or sneezing.
6. The double deglutition sign may be positive.

VIVA VOCE

1. **What is retrosternal goiter?**
   It is a swelling of the thyroid which lies in the chest behind the sternum wholly or partially.
2. **What is double deglutition sign?**
   A patient of retrosternal goiter makes two efforts at swallowing a bolus. In first, the retrosternal goitre is pulled up or displaced to create space for the esophagus to open up; the second allows the bolus to pass down the thoracic inlet (PC Dubey).
3. **What is Pemberton's test?**
   The patient is asked to elevate both the arms above the head. If retrosternal goiter is present the patient's face becomes congested and cyanosed.

4. **What are the types of retrosternal goiter?**
   It is of three types (Figs 7 and 8)—
   1. Substernal type
   2. Plunging type
   3. Intrathoracic type.
5. **What is substernal type?**
   In this type the goiter in the neck is extending behind the sternum, i.e. the lower limit is not definable.
6. **What is a plunging goiter?**
   It is an intrathoracic goiter which appears intermittently in the neck during coughing or sneezing when the intrathoracic pressure is raised.
7. **What is an intrathoracic goiter?**
   The goiter is entirely intrathoracic and does not even come out during coughing or sneezing. It is detected only by investigations (CT scan).
8. **How does an intrathoracic goiter present?**
   The patient may present with signs of thyrotoxicosis without a goiter in the neck, or the patient may present with a past history of a goiter in the neck which has disappeared spontaneously.
9. **What is the genesis of a retrosternal goiter?**
   Most of these goiters arise from lower portion of thyroid. If the neck is short with strong pretracheal muscles, the negative intrathoracic pressure tends to pull the goiter into superior mediastinum.

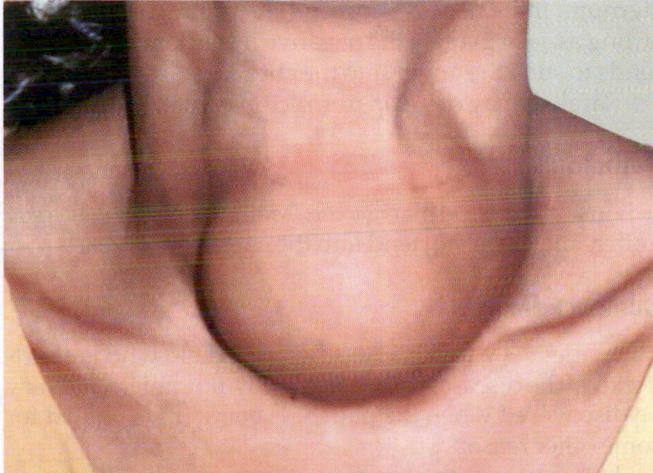

Fig. 6: Multinodular goiter with retrosternal extension (Courtesy: Professor Sandeep Kumar)

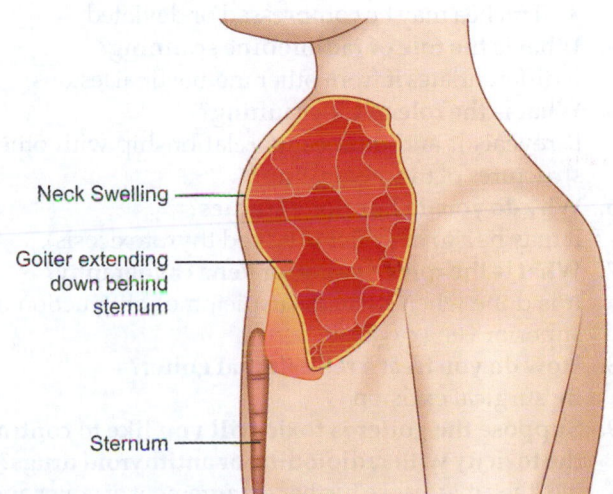

Fig. 7: Retrosternal goiter

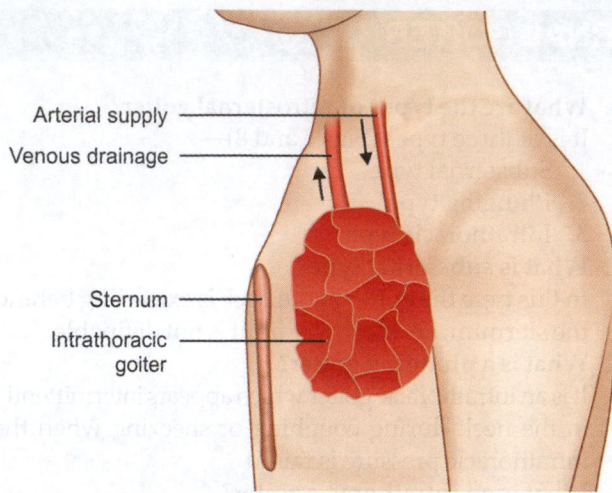

Fig. 8: Intrathoracic goiter

10. What is the pathology of this goiter?
It may be a simple, toxic or malignant goiter.

11. Can it cause recurrent nerve paralysis?
It may cause very rarely, especially if the goiter is malignant.

12. What are the investigations in this condition?
Usually the following investigations are done—
- X-ray of chest
- Isotope scanning of thyroid
- CT scanning
- Thyroid hormone estimation.

13. What are the radiographic signs?
The radiographic signs are—
1. A soft tissue shadow in superior mediastinum
2. The shadow may have calcification
3. Trachea may be compressed or deviated.

14. What is the role of radioiodine scanning?
It differentiates it from other mediastinal lesions.

15. What is the role of CT scanning?
It reveals it and defines its relationship with other structures of the mediastinum.

16. Why do you do hormone studies?
It may be a toxic goiter (masked thyrotoxicosis).

17. What is the role of superior vena cavography?
It is done when there is suspicion of obstruction of superior vena cava.

18. How do you treat a retrosternal goiter?
By surgical excision

19. Suppose the goiter is toxic will you like to control the toxicity with radioiodine or antithyroid drugs?
No, they may cause further enlargement of goiter and aggravate pressure symptoms.

20. How do you approach it for surgical excision?
It is usually done by cervical approach.

21. Will you not like to do median sternotomy?
It is rarely required.

22. What is the technique of excision?
The cervical part of goiter is first mobilized by ligation and division of superior thyroid vessels and middle thyroid veins. The retrosternal part can then be delivered out by traction and finger mobilization.

23. Will this final step not cause hemorrhage?
It does not cause hemorrhage as the goiter gets its blood supply from the neck vessels which have already been controlled.

24. What are the chances of recurrent nerve injury?
It should be identified if possible before delivery from chest as it is quite vulnerable to injury by traction and tearing.

25. If there is a large intrathoracic goiter which cannot be delivered, what will you do?
It can be removed by two methods—
- Doing a median sternotomy to provide better exposure
- Removing the goiter after fragmenting it into pieces.

26. What is the disadvantage of fragmentation?
A piece may be left over which may cause recurrence of the goiter.

DISCUSSION

Retrosternal goiter is a swelling of thyroid which is extending behind the sternum partially or completely.

Etiology

It is usually a nodular goiter the lower pole of which enlarges into the superior mediastinum behind the sternum. If the neck is short and the pretracheal muscles strong as seen in men, the negative intrathoracic pressure tends to suck the goiter into the chest.

Rarely it may develop from ectopic thyroid tissue.

Pathology

It is usually a nodular goiter. Malignant or even toxic goiters may rarely extend into the chest.

Clinical Features

The patient is usually a middle-aged male who is short-necked. The disease may be entirely symptomless and may be discovered when the patient is being investigated for some other reason.

In a symptomatic patient there may be following symptoms—

1. There may be dyspnea, particularly nocturnal. It may be associated with cough and stridor. Hence the patient may wrongly be diagnosed as asthma.
2. Dysphagia due to pressure on the esophagus

Due to extrinsic pressure on the veins (e.g. superior vena cava), the patient may present with engorgement of veins of the face, neck and upper chest wall.

Rarely the patient may present with symptoms and signs of recurrent laryngeal nerve palsy.

Investigations

- Radiography of the cervicothoracic junction reveals the soft tissue shadow of the goiter in the superior mediastinum. It may have calcification. The tracheal shadow may be compressed or deviated.
- CT scan shows the details of the goiter and its relationship with various structures of thoracic inlet.
- Flow-volume loop pulmonary function tests confirm the tracheal compression by showing deterioration in the flow.
- Thyroid function tests are done to find any evidence of thyrotoxicosis.
- FNAC is done under ultrasound or CT scan guidance to rule out malignancy, but one has to be very careful not to puncture a vessel.

Treatment

If a retrosternal goiter is associated with hyperfunction, the thyrotoxicosis must not be treated by radioiodine or antithyroid drugs, as they are likely to increase the size of the goiter.

The main aim of treatment is to relieve the pressure symptoms which can be done by doing excision of the goiter.

The goiter can be resected transcervically in most of the cases but it may be combined with median sternotomy, if necessary.

The goiter is mobilized by ligating and dividing the superior thyroid pedicle and the middle thyroid vein on both the sides, and then it is delivered from the chest by gentle pull. The risk of bleeding is not there as the goiter gets its vascular supply from the neck. The right recurrent nerve is identified and protected from avulsion during delivery. Most of the time the goiter comes out. It is resected and the wound closed around a drain.

Piecemeal excision - If the goiter cannot be delivered into the neck, it is broken into fragments and removed piecemeal. This should not be done if there is suspicion of malignancy. Further all the fragments of the goiter must be removed otherwise there is risk of recurrence.

It is better to avoid fragmentation, which can be done by a timely sternal split.

Hernias

CLINICAL DIAGNOSIS

1. The patient is usually an infant, a child or an adult who presents with an umbilical swelling (Fig. 1).
2. In an infant the swelling is present since birth or first few days after birth following neonatal sepsis.
3. In an adult, the swelling is of insidious onset and occurs due to significant ascites (Fig. 2).
4. The swelling becomes more prominent when the patient cries or strains.
5. It is reducible and a defect is palpable in the floor of umbilicus admitting the tip of a finger.

VIVA VOCE

1. **What is an umbilical hernia?**
   It is herniation of abdominal contents through the umbilical cicatrix (Figs 1 and 2).
2. **What is the difference between an umbilical and a paraumbilical hernia?**
   The umbilical hernia protrudes through the floor of umbilicus, while a paraumbilical hernia protrudes by the side of umbilicus usually in the upper part. Thus, in the first type the umbilicus is situated on the top of the swelling or lost in the swelling, while in the latter it is situated on the side of the protrusion.
3. **What are the types of an umbilical hernia?**
   It is of two types—
   • Umbilical hernia of infants and children (Fig. 1)
   • Umbilical hernia of adults (Fig. 2).
4. **What is the cause of an infantile hernia?**
   It is because of the weakness of umbilical cicatrix following neonatal sepsis.

5. **What is the cause of a hernia of an adult?**
   It is due to progressively increasing intra-abdominal pressure due to ascites (usually cirrhotic ascites) and stretching of umbilical cicatrix.
6. **What are the complications of this hernia?**
   The complications are –
   • In an umbilical hernia of infants and children obstruction and strangulation may occur, but are very rare below three years of age.
   • In an umbilical hernia of an adult incarceration and strangulation are common complications.
   • A fluid hernia of ascites may rupture with ascitic fluid leakage and risk of infection.

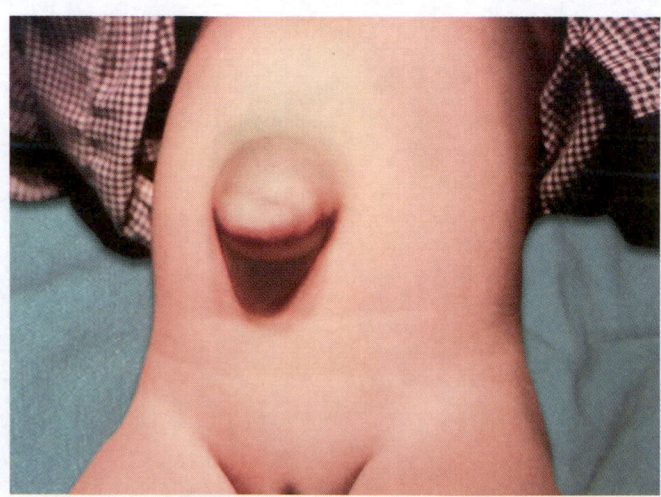

Fig. 1: A large umbilical hernia in a girl of 4 years

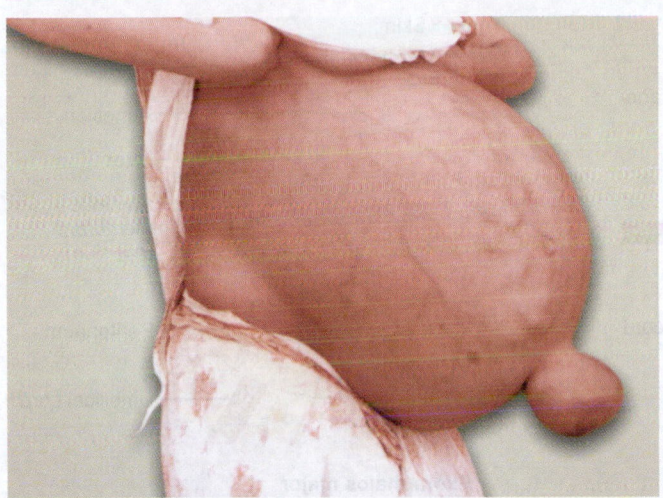

Fig. 2: Massive ascites of cirrhosis of liver with umbilical fluid hernia. Note the prominent veins is the abdominal wall indicative of portal venous obstruction

7. **How do you treat an umbilical hernia?**
   In infants, the umbilical ring reduces in size with passage of time and may close completely. Hence, one can wait up to 2 years or more. However, if the defect is more than 1.5 cm in diameter or the hernia is persisting at 2 years of age or more it is treated by an operation.
   In adults, all hernias are operated as early as possible.

8. **What is the technique of umbilical herniorrhaphy?**
   A small transverse curved incision is given below the umbilicus with convexity towards pubic symphysis. The skin flaps are dissected and the sac is identified and opened at neck. The sac is excised and the defect is closed by nonabsorbable sutures.

9. **Do you excise the umbilicus?**
   No, it is preserved for cosmetic reasons.

10. **How do you treat an umbilical hernia in an adult?**
    • The ascitic hernia of cirrhosis—The ascites should be controlled first by medical measures, and shunt if necessary and then the hernia is repaired.
    • The hernia is usually repaired utilizing a polypropylene mesh. The repair can be done by an open operation or laparoscopically.

11. **What are the advantages of laparoscopic approach?**
    The advantages are—lesser pain and early recovery.

12. **What is exomphalos?**
    It is a developmental defect due to failure of all or a part of midgut to return into the abdominal cavity in early fetal life, characterized by protruded abdominal contents at umbilicus, covered by a membrane consisting of an outer layer of amniotic membrane, middle layer of Wharton's jelly and an inner layer of peritoneum (Figs 3 and 4).

Discussion

It is the herniation of abdominal contents through the floor of a weak umbilical cicatrix. Depending upon the time of occurrence, it is of three types—umbilical hernia of infants and children, umbilical hernia of adults and exomphalos (omphalocele).

Umbilical Hernia of Infants and Children (Fig. 1)

A fascial defect at the umbilicus may be present at birth, especially in premature infants. The weakness of the umbilicus may be due to failure of the round ligament (obliterated umbilical vein) to cross the umbilical ring and partly from the absence of Richet fascia.

It is twice more common in the male children as compared to female children. It usually becomes obvious when the infant is several weeks old.

It is usually asymptomatic and the child is brought with the complaint of an umbilical swelling which increases when the child cries. The crying may cause pain making the infant to cry more. It is spherical but may assume a conical or tubular shape as it grows in size.

Complications—Obstruction and strangulation may occur but very rare below three years of age.

Treatment—Normally after birth the umbilical ring progressively diminishes in size and eventually closes. Thus, the fascial defects less than 1 cm in size close spontaneously in 95 percent of patients by 5 years of age.

The indications for operation are fascial defects larger than 1.5 cm in diameter, hernia persisting at 2 years of age or more, or if incarcerated.

Umbilical herniorrhaphy—A small curved incision with concavity upwards is made immediately below the umbilicus, which is dissected upwards. The neck of the sac is cleared all round and the sac opened at the neck. The contents are reduced and the sac is excised or inverted into the abdomen. The defect in the linea alba is closed by nonabsorbable sutures.

Umbilical Hernia of Adults (Fig. 2)

It is due to gradual yielding of the cicatricial tissue which closes the ring due to persistently raised intra-abdominal pressure. The predisposing factors are ascites, obesity, large intra-abdominal tumors and multiple pregnancies with prolonged labor. Cirrhotic ascites is the commonest cause.

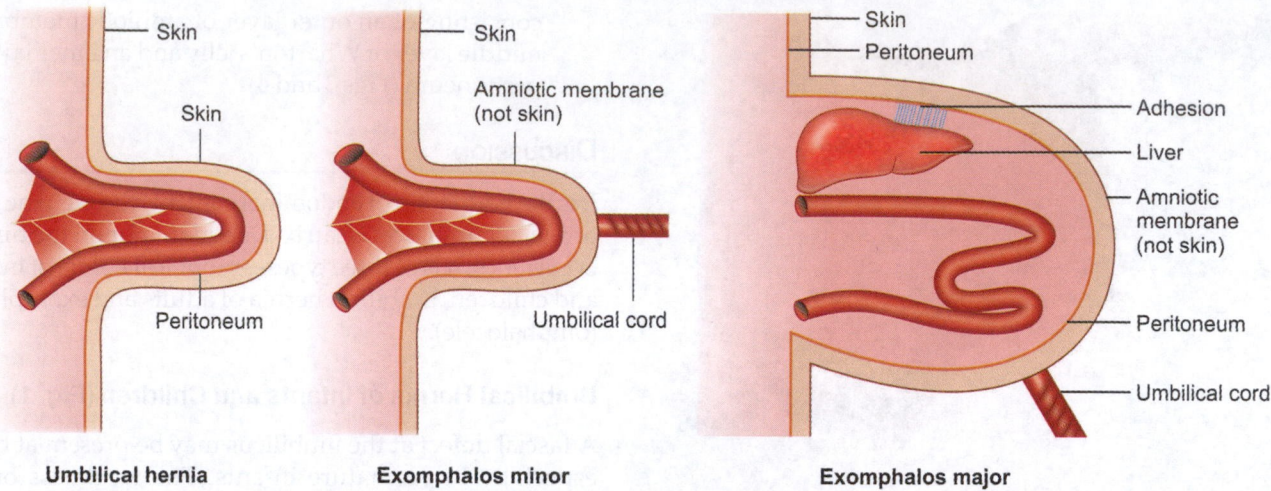

Fig. 3: Anatomy of umbilical hernia and exomphalos

The hernia sac may have multiple loculations, and it usually contains ascitic fluid, or omentum. Small and large bowel may be present.

As the ring is usually tight, the patient may have pain on coughing or straining. A large hernia may produce a dragging or aching sensation.

Incarceration and strangulation are common complications. A fluid hernia of ascites may rupture with ascitic fluid leakage.

Treatment—In cirrhotic patients, the ascites should be controlled by medical measures or shunt if necessary. The nutritional status must be improved.

The hernia is usually repaired utilizing a polypropylene mesh. The repair can be done by an open operation or laparoscopically.

Prognosis—The prognosis depends on the size of hernia, age and the nature of the predisposing disease. In good-risk patients, the results are good with a low rate of recurrence.

Exomphalos (Omphalocele) (Figs 3 and 4)

It is a developmental defect which occurs due to the failure of all or a part of midgut to return into the abdominal cavity in early fetal life characterized by protruded abdominal contents at umbilicus, covered by a membrane consisting of an outer layer of amniotic membrane, middle layer of Wharton's jelly and an inner layer of peritoneum.

It occurs once in 5000 live births. A large exomphalos may rupture during delivery. It may be associated with other abnormalities in 30 to 70 percent of cases, e.g. chromosomal anomalies (trisomy 13, 18, 21), congenital heart disease and Beckwith–Wiedemann syndrome,

Depending upon the size of the defect the exomphalos is of two types – exomphalos minor and exomphalos major.

a. **Exomphalos minor**—It is also called herniation of the umbilical cord. Here the fascial defect is less than 4 cm. The protrusion is small and the umbilical cord is attached to its summit. It may have a single loop of small bowel which may be ligated and transected accidentally resulting in an umbilico-enteric fistula.

Treatment—The attached umbilical cord is gradually twisted to reduce the contents into the abdomen, and retained by strapping at least for 2 weeks. The exomphalos disappears as the sac is obliterated.

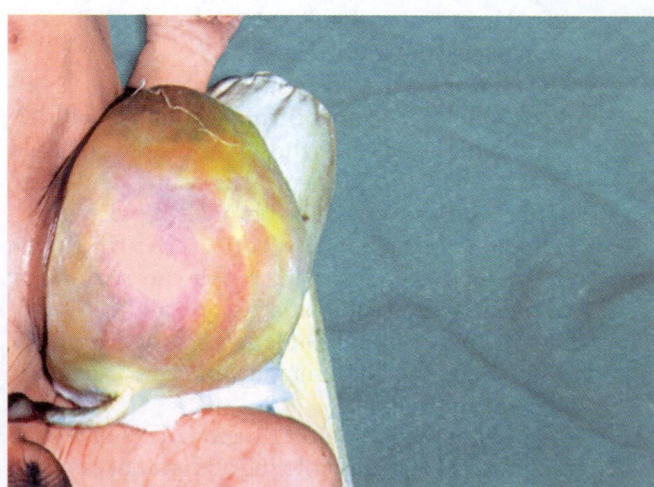

Fig. 4: Exomphalos major (*Courtesy:* Professor Ashish Wakhlu)

b. **Exomphalos major (Fig. 4)**—The fascial defect is more than 4 cm, but it is usually more than 10 cm. The sac is large and contains small and large bowel and nearly always a portion of liver. The umbilical cord is attached to the inferior aspect of the swelling. The liver has dense adhesions to the sac.

Treatment—To avoid the complications of rupture and infection, the problem must be treated within the first few hours of birth. There are four methods of treatment –

1. **Nonoperative treatment**—It is usually indicated in poor risk infants with a gigantic intact sac. The sac is painted daily with a desiccating antiseptic which leads to formation of an eschar with inflammatory reaction. It gradually reduces the swelling to a ventral hernia which is repaired subsequently.

2. **Skin flap closure**—Flaps of skin are made on either side by undermining the subcutaneous tissue and brought together over the sac. Relaxing incisions are given in both loins to facilitate closure. The abdominal distension is prevented by nasogastric suction for a few days.

   After a few months or years when the hernia is being repaired, one would be surprised to find that the peritoneum and muscles can be easily brought together for closure.

3. **Staged closure**—Silastic sheeting sutured to the fascial edges or a preformed one-piece silo with a collapsible ring at its base. The silo is progressively compressed to return the contents of sac into the abdomen, to bring the edges of linea alba together by stretching the abdominal wall muscles. This usually happens in 5 to 7 days when the defect can be closed, The intra-abdominal pressure created by the silo should not be more than 20 cm H_2O to prevent impairment of venous return from the bowel and kidneys.

4. **Primary closure**—The sac is trimmed away from the skin. The bowel is completely emptied through a nasogastric tube. The abdominal wall is stretched in quadrants which increases the capacity of abdomen. The abdominal contents are then replaced and the fascial layer is closed usually under some tension.

Prognosis – The minor defect has a good prognosis. The exomphalos major has significant mortality from wound dehiscence and wound infection, and associated anomalies.

CASE 2: PARAUMBILICAL HERNIA

CLINICAL DIAGNOSIS

1. The patient is usually a middle-aged multiparous obese female who presents with a swelling in the umbilical region of insidious onset.
2. The swelling protrudes by the side of umbilicus (Figs 5 and 6).
3. It is globular or pyriform in shape.
4. It is soft and nontender (if reducible), or may be tense and tender (if irreducible).
5. The umbilicus is stretched out or displaced.

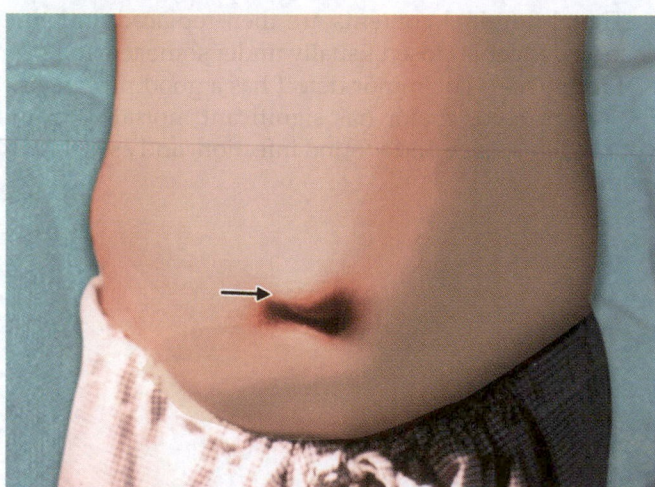

Fig. 5: Small paraumbilical hernia

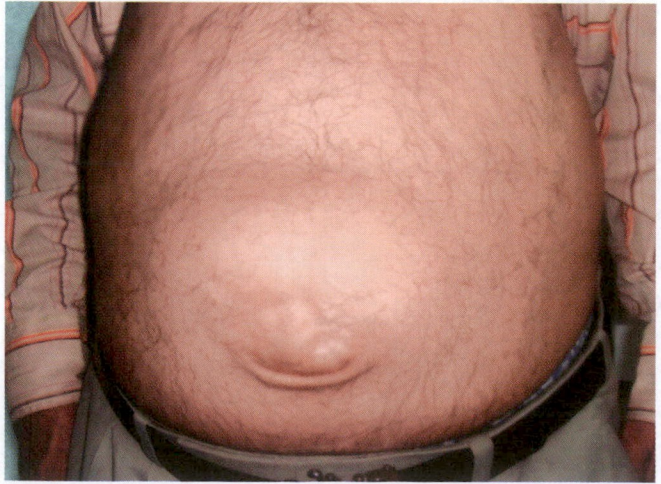

Fig. 6: A para-umbilical hernia of moderate size bulging from upper edge of umbilicus

VIVA VOCE

1. **What is a paraumbilical hernia?**
   It is a protrusion of abdominal contents by the side of umbilicus (not through umbilicus).
2. **What is the cause of this hernia?**
   This hernia is always acquired and results from repeated or persistent stretching of abdominal wall at umbilicus due to obesity, repeated pregnancy, chronic cough or chronic straining.
3. **What are the contents of the sac?**
   The sac usually contains omentum, and may contain small bowel and transverse colon.
4. **What is Richter's hernia?**
   It is the protrusion of a part of circumference of bowel.
5. **What is the peculiarity of Richter's hernia?**
   This hernia can strangulate without intestinal obstruction.
6. **What are the complications of this hernia?**
   The complications are –
   • Irreducibility
   • Intestinal obstruction
   • Incarceration
   • Strangulation
   • Ulceration of overlying skin
   • Intertrigo.
7. **What are the causes of irreducibility?**
   The irreducibility is due to:
   • Progressive enlargement of contents of hernia
   • Adhesions between the sac and contents
   • Inter-content adhesions.
8. **What is incarcerated hernia?**
   The term incarcerated hernia is used as an alternative to obstructed hernia, but actually it indicates that a portion of colon is the content of hernia and is blocked with feces.
9. **How do you clinically recognize an incarcerated hernia?**
   The hernia has a doughy feel and the inspissated feces can be indented.
10. **What is intertrigo?**
    It is the erythema or dermatitis of contiguous cutaneous or mucocutaneous surfaces.
11. **What is the risk of intertrigo?**
    It may cause wound infection if not adequately treated before operation.
12. **How do you treat a paraumbilical hernia?**
    The essentials of the treatment are:
    • Reduction of body weight

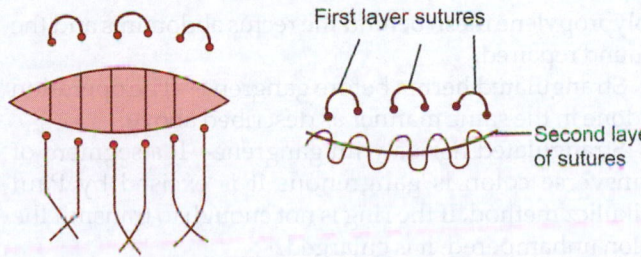

First layer sutures

Second layer of sutures

- 3-5 stitches of unabsorbable material depending upon size of defect
- Away from the edge in upper flap and near the edge in lower flap
- Upper flap overlaps the lower flap and covers the suture knots of first layer

Fig. 7: Mayo's double breasting operation for a paraumbilical hernia

- Control of any other contributory factor such as chronic cough and chronic constipation
- Control of skin infection
- Surgical repair of hernia.

13. How do you repair the hernia?

The hernia can be repaired by:

1. Overlapping or double breasting the flaps of anterior rectus sheath either from above and below (Mayo) (Fig. 7) or from side to side (Wells) and suturing them with interrupted unabsorbable sutures, or
2. Polypropylene mesh hernioplasty, where a patch of mesh is sutured in the weakness deep to the rectus sheath (inlay graft).

14. Where do you open the sac of hernia?

It is opened at the neck.

15. Why?

To avoid injury to the contents as they are frequently adherent at the fundus of the sac.

16. What do you do to the omentum?

It may be reduced, but usually the prolapsed part is excised.

17. What are the dangers of omentectomy?

The dangers (complications) of omentectomy are—

- Hemorrhage
- Injury to transverse colon.

DISCUSSION

Paraumbilical hernia is a protrusion of abdominal contents through the linea alba just above, or sometimes just below the umbilicus (Fig. 6)

Increasing obesity with flabbiness of the abdominal muscles, and repeated pregnancy are the main etiological factors.

Pathology

As the sac comes out of the defect it gradually enlarges and becomes rounded or oval in shape with a tendency to sag downwards. Thus, this hernia may grow to a large size.

The neck of the sac is narrow as compared to the size of sac and volume of contents consisting of greater omentum, small intestine and a portion of transverse colon. In long-standing cases, the sac may become loculated due to adherence of omentum to its findus.

Clinical Features

Age—Usually between 35 and 50 years of age.
Sex—It is 5 times more common in females than males.
Body build—The patient is usually obese with flabby abdominal muscles.
Symptoms—The patient presents with an abdominal protrusion which soon becomes irreducible because of omental adhesions inside the sac.

A large hernia may cause local dragging pain because of its weight.

Gastrointestinal symptoms may occur and are probably due to pull on the stomach or transverse colon. Often there are transient attacks of intestinal colic because of subacute intestinal obstruction.

Complications

- Irreducibility
- Intestinal obstruction, incarceration
- Strangulation—It is because of the pressure of narrow neck and fibrous edge of the linea alba. Gangrene occurs early, hence early operation is recommended. It is important to note that in large hernias the presence of loculi may result in a strangulated knuckle of bowel in one part of otherwise soft and nontender hernia.
- Rupture
- Intertrigo and trophic ulceration of fundus.

Treatment

All the patients should be operated as early as possible as delay may invite complications. In asymptomatic obese persons, one can wait until weight has been reduced. This hernia is usually treated by Mayo's operation or polypropylene mesh hernioplasty.

Mayo's operation (William James Mayo, 1901)—A transverse elliptical incision is made around umbilicus enclosing the protrusion and the sac is dissected upto the neck. The sac is opened at the neck and the contents are examined. The excess adherent omentum is removed with the sac. The peritoneum is closed at the neck. Transverse cuts of 2.5 cm or more are made on both sides of the umbilical ring to make two flaps of aponeurosis to allow an overlap of 5 to 7.5 cm. The flaps are overlapped with the help of 3 to 5 mattress sutures of fine unabsorbable material (e.g. prolene 2/0) as the row of stitches is tied. The edge of overlapping upper flap is stitched lower down to the rectus sheath and midline aponeurosis. The wound may be drained by a suction drain at each angle of the wound if required (Fig. 2).

In obese patients the above procedure may be combined with lipectomy by designing the incision to include a larger area of fat laden abdominal wall in excision.

Paraumbilical polypropylene mesh hernioplasty—If the hernial fascial defect is more than 4 cm or the hernia is recurrent type, the defect is repaired by putting a polypropylene mesh behind the rectus abdominis and the wound repaired.

Strangulated hernia before gangrene—The operation is done in the same manner as described above.

Strangulated hernia with gangrene—If a segment of transverse colon is gangrenous it is excised by Paul Mikulicz method. If the ring is not enough to transmit the colon unhampered, it is enlarged.

The small intestine must be thoroughly checked as a small gangrenous loop may slip back when the constriction is being released. If it escapes the postoperative abdominal pain may be taken as postoperative discomfort till the patient deteriorates to die in a few days.

CASE 3: EPIGASTRIC HERNIA (FATTY HERNIA OF LINEA ALBA)

CLINICAL DIAGNOSIS

i. *Asymptomatic*—The patient has no symptoms and the hernia is discovered during routine abdominal examination.

ii. *Symptomatic*
1. The patient is usually an adult, commonly a male who has an average build or mild obesity and presents with an epigastric nodule or pain or both, of insidious onset (Figs 8 and 9).
2. The nodule or swelling is situated in the epigastrium or supraumbilical region in midline.
3. It is firm but elastic (may feel like a lipoma).
4. It may be reducible or irreducible (or partially reducible).
5. If reducible completely, the defect in the linea alba is palpable as a depression with a sharp edge.
6. The cough impulse is present (if reducible).
7. The patient may have pain suggestive of acid peptic or gall bladder disease.

VIVA VOCE

1. **What is an epigastric hernia?**
   It is the protrusion of extraperitoneal fat through a defect in the linea alba any where between xiphoid process and umbilicus, usually midway between these structures.
2. **What is the cause of this condition?**
   It is usually due to a localized defect (hole) in linea alba.

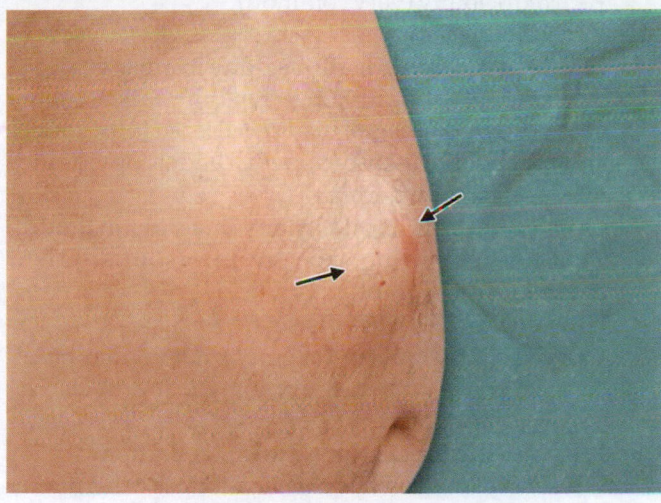

Fig. 8: Recurrent epigastric hernia

3. **What are the contents of this hernia?**
   In early stage, it contains extraperitoneal fat only without any well formed sac, but this fat is attached to the underlying peritoneum (Fig. 9).
   As the disease advances the extruded extraperitoneal fat grows bigger and drags a pouch of peritoneum after it. The sac is usually empty or may contain omentum and small bowel occasionally.
4. **Why is the sac commonly empty?**
   The mouth of the sac is very narrow and does not permit herniation of abdominal organs.

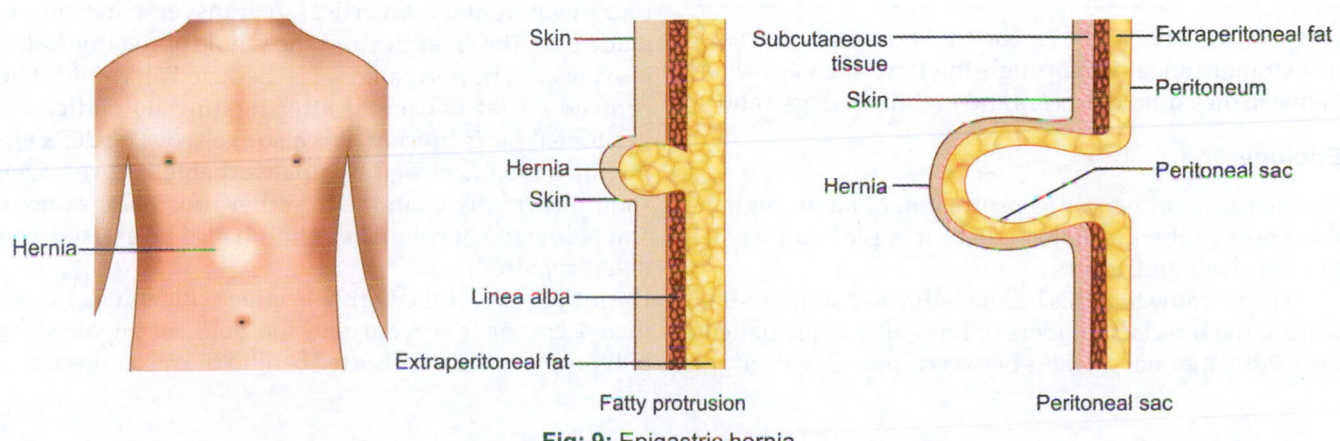

Fatty protrusion — Peritoneal sac

Fig: 9: Epigastric hernia

5. **What are the complications of this hernia?**
   The complications are:
   • Irreducibility (very common)
   • Strangulation.

6. **What are the investigations done in such a case?**
   Apart from routine investigations, the patient should be investigated for gall bladder disease (ultrasound) and acid peptic disease (upper GI endoscopy) as they may coexist with hernia.

7. **Can you see this hernia by any imaging method?**
   This hernia can be seen by ultrasound, CT or tangential radiography.

8. **How do you treat this disease?**
   If the hernia is small and asymptomatic it may be left as such. If it is large or symptomatic it is treated by herniorrhaphy.

9. **What are the precautions during operation?**
   The whole linea alba is checked for other hernias as multiple protrusions are not uncommon.

10. **What is the prognosis?**
    It has a 10 to 20 percent recurrence rate which is very high.

11. **Why?**
    It is partly due to failure to recognize and repair other small defects.

12. **What is diastasis recti?**
    It is a diffuse widening and attenuation of linea alba without a fascial defect which presents as a fusiform linear bulge between the two rectus abdominis muscles.

13. **How will you treat this condition?**
    As there is no risk of incarceration, it does not need any treatment. If one tries to repair it, the chances of recurrence are very high.

DISCUSSION

Fatty hernia of linea alba (epigastric hernia) is a protrusion of extraperitoneal fat through the linea alba anywhere between the xiphoid process and umbilicus (Figs 8 and 9).

Etiology

This hernia commences as protrusion of fat through the weakness in the linea alba where it is pierced by small blood vessels and nerves.

It is probable that this hernia is due to a sudden strain tearing the interlacing fibers of linea alba as the patients are mostly manual workers between 30 to 45 years of age.

Pathology

The hernia is frequently the size of a pea consisting of extraperitoneal fat only. If the protrusion grows it drags a pouch of peritoneum after it to become a true hernia. The hernia sac is usually empty as the mouth of the hernia is too small to permit a portion of abdominal viscus to enter it. If it grows it may contain omentum and rarely a part of small bowel (Fig. 9).

Clinical Features

1. *Asymptomatic*—This hernia may be entirely symptomless and may be discovered as a small lipoma-like swelling in the midline of upper abdomen on routine clinical examination. Often more than one hernia is present.

2. *Symptomatic*
   a. Local pain—There may be local pain which is worse on physical exertion, associated with local tenderness. It may be due to fatty contents becoming nipped sufficiently to produce partial strangulation. It may be associated with bloating, nausea and vomiting.
   b. Referred pain—The patient may not complain anything about the hernia but has pain suggestive of acid peptic or gall bladder disease.

Treatment

• If the hernia is asymptomatic and small no treatment is necessary.
• If hernia is symptomatic or large it is treated by an operation.

Herniorrhaphy—The site of the hernia should be marked on the skin before giving anesthesia as it may be difficult to locate the defect if the protrusion retracts into the abdomen. A vertical or transverse incision is made over the swelling and the whole of the linea alba is exposed. The herniated fat is dissected all round. The protruding fat is excised after ligating its pedicle. If peritoneal sac is present, it is also excised. The defect in the linea alba is closed by unabsorbable sutures. One should carefully examine for other protrusions above and below the hernia. They should also be excised and defect repaired.

Hernioplasty—If the hernia is large with a defect more than 4 cm, or it is recurrent, the defect is repaired by polypropylene mesh inserted behind the recti muscles.

CASE 4: FEMORAL HERNIA

CLINICAL DIAGNOSIS

1. The patient is usually a middle-aged or elderly female who presents with a swelling on the inner side of inguinofemoral region, over the saphenous opening just below the inguinal ligament (Fig. 10A).
2. It is hemispherical, smooth and soft.
3. It is reducible partially or completely.
4. If it is reducible a defect can be felt at the root of the thigh. If it is occluded by pressure, the hernia does not protrude on coughing or straining.
5. Sometimes the patient may present with signs of intestinal obstruction and an un-noticed femoral hernia.

VIVA VOCE

1. **What is a femoral hernia?**
   It is the protrusion of extraperitoneal fat and peritoneum with or without abdominal contents through the femoral canal. The sac passes through the femoral ring and enters the femoral canal.
2. **What is femoral canal?**
   It is the medial-most compartment of the femoral sheath. It is about 1.25 cm long, and 1.25 cm wide at base that is directed upwards.
3. **What is femoral sheath?**
   It is a funnel-shaped fascial prolongation around the femoral vessels below the medial half of inguinal ligament. The anterior wall of the sheath is made by fascia transversalis and the posterior by fascia iliaca (Fig. 10B).
4. **What are the compartments of femoral sheath?**
   The femoral sheath has three compartments separated by fibrous septae:

1. The lateral compartment contains the femoral artery and femoral branch of genitofemoral nerve.
2. The intermediate compartment contains the femoral vein.
3. The medial compartment is known as femoral canal and contains some fibrofatty tissue and lymphatic tissue (Cloquet's node).

5. **What is femoral ring?**
   It is the mouth of the femoral canal and lies at its base. The hernia enters the canal through femoral ring. It is closed above by septum crurale.
6. **What are the boundaries of femoral ring?**
   The boundaries of femoral ring are:
   - Anterior—Inguinal ligament
   - Posterior—Pectineal line of horizontal ramus of pubis, pectineal ligament (Cooper's)
   - Medial—Crescentic edge of lacunar (Gimbernat's) ligament
   - Lateral—Fibrous septum separating the canal from femoral vein.
7. **Is the ring open in normal circumstances?**
   No. It is closed above by septum crurale, a condensation of extraperitoneal tissue pierced by lymphatics.
8. **What is the cause of this hernia?**
   The etiological factors are:
   1. It is an acquired hernia.
   2. It occurs in the females, and is due to wider pelvis.
   3. Repeated pregnancy with raised intra-abdominal pressure may be an initiating factor.
9. **What is the course of a femoral hernia?**
   The femoral hernia has a tortuous course having three movements in a serial manner:

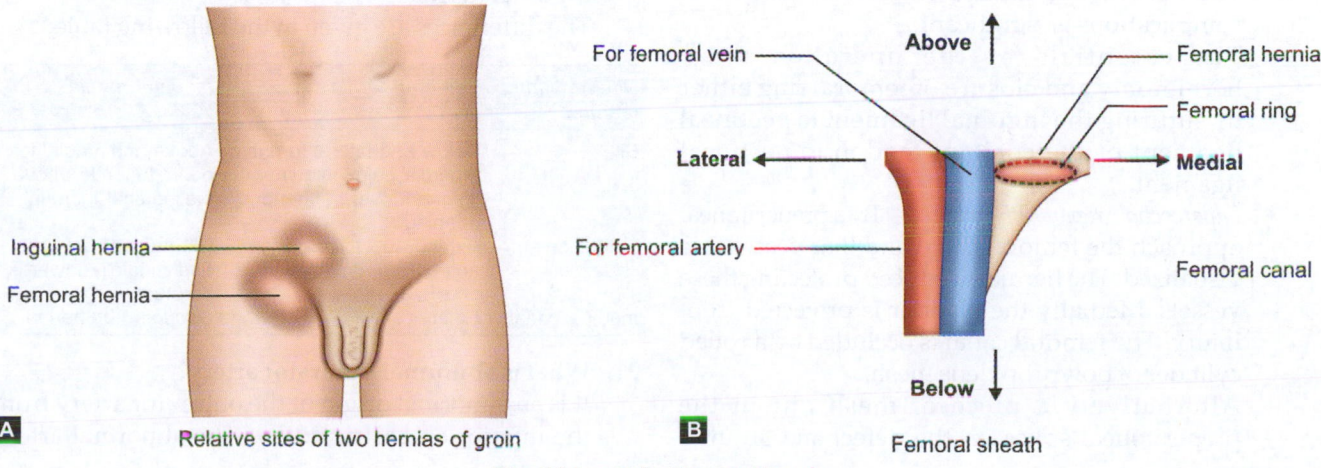

A Relative sites of two hernias of groin

Inguinal hernia
Femoral hernia

For femoral vein
Above
Femoral hernia
Femoral ring
Lateral
Medial
For femoral artery
Femoral canal
Below
B
Femoral sheath

Fig. 10A and B: Femoral hernia

- *Vertical descent*—The hernia sac enters through the femoral ring and descends vertically down into the femoral canal upto the lower border of fossa ovalis where it lies in close relation to long saphenous vein. Due to attachment of Scarpa's fascia to fascia lata at lower border, the sac cannot pass down the thigh.
- *Forward movement*—As the sac cannot pass down it courses forward and gets enlarged.
- *Upward movement*—As the sac enlarges further it courses upward and thus the distal part of the sac overlies the inguinal ligament and occupies the inguinal region.

10. What are the coverings of the sac?

The coverings of the sac from outside in are:
1. Skin
2. Superficial fascia
3. Cribriform fascia
4. Fascia transversalis
5. Extraperitoneal fat

11. What are the contents of the sac?

The sac may contain the following structures:
- Omentum
- Small bowel
- A part of circumference of bowel (Richter's hernia).

12. What are the complications of a femoral hernia?

The complications are:
1. Irreducibility
2. Intestinal obstruction
3. Strangulation.

13. What is the incidence of these complications as compared to an inguinal hernia?

These complications are more common in a femoral hernia than in an inguinal hernia.

14. How do you treat a femoral hernia?

- The treatment is always surgical as the risk of complications is significant.
- The essentials of the operation are—herniotomy and closure of femoral ring either by suturing the inguinal ligament to pectineal ligament or the conjoint tendon to pectineal ligament.
- *Laparoscopic repair (TEP repair)*—By a preperitoneal approach the femoral canal and iliac vessels are visualized. The hernia is reduced protecting these vessels. Medially the bladder is protected from injury. The femoral canal is occluded by a rolled cylinder of polypropylene mesh.

Alternatively a piece of mesh put in the preperitoneal space on the defect and sutured inferiorly to the iliopectineal line, inferomedially to Cooper's ligament and superomedially to the rectus sheath. The wound is closed.

15. Will you like to use a truss?

A truss is useless as it cannot control a femoral hernia.

16. What are the approaches for surgery?

There are three surgical approaches: Low or subinguinal (Lockwood's), inguinal (Lotheissen's), and high or suprainguinal (McEvedy's)

17. What are the advantages and disadvantages of Lockwood's approach?

- The advantages are:
  1. Direct approach to sac
  2. Speedy and simple
  3. Suitable for small and uncomplicated hernias
- The disadvantages of this approach are:
  1. Resection of gangrenous bowel is difficult, hence not suitable for a strangulated hernia.
  2. The repair of femoral ring is difficult.

18. What are the advantages and disadvantages of Lotheissen's approach?

- Advantage—It is easy to deal with gangrenous bowel.
- Disadvantage—The posterior wall of inguinal canal becomes weak.

19. What are the advantages and disadvantages of McEvedy's approach?

- The advantages are:
  1. Gangrenous bowel can be resected easily.
  2. The repair of femoral ring is easy.
- The disadvantages are:
  1. The access to the fundus of the sac is difficult. Hence excision of sac poses some difficulty.
  2. If infection of the wound occurs, an incisional hernia may develop.

20. How do you differentiate a femoral hernia from an inguinal hernia?

The differences are given in the following table:

Differentiating features	Femoral hernia	Inguinal hernia
Site	Below and lateral to pubic tubercle below inguinal ligament over saphenous opening	Above and medial to pubic tubercle above the inguinal ligament
Extension	Extends up towards the anterior abdominal wall	Extends downwards and medially towards scrotum
Inguinal canal	Empty	Occupied by hernia

21. What is abnormal obturator artery?

It is an abnormal origin of the obturator artery from the inferior epigastric artery. The abnormal artery descends closely related to the posterior surface of Gimbernat's ligament.

22. **What is the significance of this artery?**
    This artery may be lacerated during the division of Gimbernat's ligament to release the strangulation.

DISCUSSION

Femoral hernia is the protrusion of abdominal contents through the femoral canal which is the medial-most compartment of femoral sheath. It is the third most common hernia after inguinal and incisional hernias and accounts for 20 percent of hernias in females and 5 percent in males.

Etiology

This hernia is more common in females who have borne children than in nulliparas. The broader female pelvis predisposes to this hernia.

Pathology

The hernia comes down upto the saphenous opening and then comes into the loose areolar tissue of the thigh. While it is in the femoral canal it is narrow, but outside the saphenous opening it expands, sometimes considerably and may extend above the inguinal ligament. Thus, a fully developed hernia is retort-shaped.

Because of the tortuous course and rigid and narrow surroundings of the femoral canal this hernia soon becomes irreducible and likely to strangulate.

Clinical Features

Age and sex—The male to female ratio is 1:2. The female patients are usually elderly while the males are usually 30 to 45 years of age. It is rare before puberty.

Side—The right-sided hernia is twice more common than the left. It is bilateral in 20 percent of cases.

Symptoms—The hernia is so small that it often goes unnoticed by the patient till it strangulates. Sometimes, there may be dragging pain. Rarely, the patient may come with a large swelling.

Signs—There is an ovoid swelling just below the medial part of inguinal ligament and pubic tubercle. It has cough impulse if reducible.

Differential diagnosis – It should be done from the following diseases:

1. *Inguinal hernia:* The femoral hernia lies below and lateral to the pubic tubercle while the inguinal hernia lies above and medial to it. An inguinal hernia is more easily reducible than a femoral hernia.

2. *Saphena varix:* Saphena varix is a cystic and reducible swelling placed along the course of saphenous vein. It disappears on lying down unlike a femoral hernia. Tapping the vein distally may produce a fluid thrill over the varix.

3. *Enlarged femoral lymph node:* If other femoral lymph nodes are enlarged, the diagnosis is simple but if it is Cloquet's lymph node alone the diagnosis is difficult in the absence of a septic focus.

4. *Psoas abscess:* It is often associated with an iliac abscess with cross fluctuation. The diagnosis is confirmed by examination and radiography of spine.

Treatment

All femoral hernias should be operated without any delay due to a very high risk of strangulation. The operation consists of reduction of the contents and excision of sac above neck. Repair is carried out by closing the femoral ring by suture of the inguinal ligament or the conjoint tendon to the Cooper's ligament. This may be done by an approach from below the inguinal ligament (Lockwood), through the inguinal canal (Lotheissen) or by an extraperitoneal approach from above (McEvedy).

Strangulation of a femoral hernia is very common especially of the Richter's type. The commonest constricting agent is the neck of the sac itself. The strangulation is released by division of the neck of the sac medially by carefully dividing the Gimbernat's ligament. An abnormal obturator artery may run along the free margin of this ligament and may be injured during division.

Low operation (Lockwood)—A groin crease incision is given and the sac is dissected upto neck, the contents are reduced, the neck of the sac is pulled down, ligated as high as possible and divided. The femoral ring is now closed by suturing the inguinal ligament to the iliopectineal line using 3 unabsorbable sutures. The disadvantages of this method are – (1) maximum chance of damage to an abnormal obturator artery, and (2) limited exposure to deal with gangrenous bowel.

Or, the ring can be occluded by a rolled sheet of polypropylene mesh and fixing it by nonabsorbable sutures passed medially, superiorly and inferiorly.

High (McEvedy) operation—A vertical incision is given on the hernia which is continued upwards above the inguinal ligament. The sac is dissected out and the external inguinal ring is identified and an incision 2.5 cm above the ring and parallel to the outer border of rectus muscle is given and deepened to expose the extraperitoneal space. The hernia sac entering the femoral canal is found by gauze dissection in this plane. If the sac is small and empty it can be pulled up, opened and excised. If it is large the fundus is opened and the contents are reduced before the sac is pulled from above. The femoral ring is closed by suturing the conjoint tendon to iliopectineal ligament by nonabsorbable sutures. The advantages of this approach are – (1) If resection of bowel is required it can be done easily (2) an excellent view of iliopectineal ligament is obtained for repair, and (3) the origin of abnormal obturator artery is protected. The disadvantage of this procedure is that if infection occurs an incisional hernia can occur. Other method of repair is to stitch a piece of polypropylene mesh over the femoral ring.

Inguinal (Lotheissen) operation—The inguinal canal is opened and the transversalis fascia is incised medial to inferior epigastric artery. The peritoneum is exposed and opened to see if any intraperitoneal structure is entering the femoral sac. The sac is emptied of its contents and cut edges of the peritoneum are held with hemostats and the sac is dissected and withdrawn from the femoral canal. The sac is now excised and the conjoint tendon is sutured to the iliopectineal line to form a shutter. The external iliac-femoral vein is protected with the forefinger and unabsorbable sutures are passed through the periosteum and Cooper's ligament overlying the iliopectineal line. Now the sutures are passed from within outwards through the conjoint tendon and tied, thus approximating the conjoint tendon and iliopectineal line. The wound is closed.

Laparoscopic repair (TEP repair)—By a preperitoneal approach the femoral canal and iliac vessels are visualized. The hernia is reduced protecting these vessels. Medially the bladder is protected from injury. The femoral canal is occluded by a rolled cylinder of polypropylene mesh.

Alternatively a piece of mesh is put in the preperitoneal space on the defect and sutured inferiorly to the iliopectineal line, inferomedially to Cooper's ligament and superomedially to the rectus sheath. The wound is now closed.

Infections

CASE 1: TUBERCULOUS COLD ABSCESS

CLINICAL DIAGNOSIS

1. The patient is usually a young person who presents with a painless slow growing swelling of insidious onset.
2. The swelling is usually present in the neck, chest (Fig. 1), axilla, paravertebral region or groin.
3. It is hemispherical, soft, smooth and nontender.
4. The edge is soft and may not be well defined.
5. It is usually fluctuant.
6. There may be clinical signs of tuberculosis of lymph nodes, bones or joints.

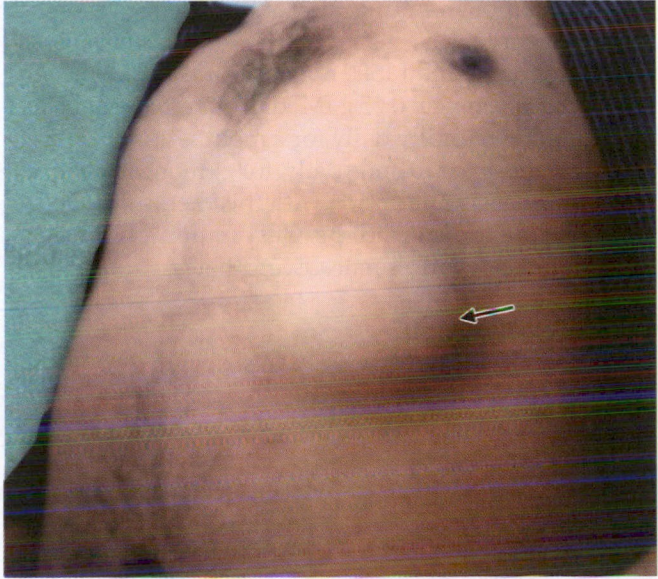

Fig. 1: Cold abscess of left costal margin

VIVA VOCE

1. **What is a cold abscess?**
   It is a localized collection of pus without signs of acute inflammation.
2. **What is the cause of this type of abscess?**
   The usual cause of a cold abscess is tuberculosis of lymph nodes, bones or joints. Tuberculosis of other organs and tissues can also result in a cold abscess formation. Rare causes of a cold abscess are:
   1. Nodular leprosy with degeneration.
   2. Actinomycotic abscess.
   3. Gumma with degeneration.
3. **Why is a cold abscess painless?**
   A cold abscess is painless because:
   • It does not have signs of acute inflammation.
   • It is a low tension abscess.
4. **What is the source of pus in a cold abscess?**
   The caseous necrotic tissue when liquefies produces pus.
5. **What do you know about tracking of pus in a cold abscess?**
   In cold abscesses, the pus may present quite far off from its site of formation. This is usually seen in cold abscesses occurring due to tuberculosis of vertebral column. The pus tracks down along the fascial planes or course of nerves coming out from the affected region. For example—
   • In upper cervical region, the pus may pass forwards and present as a posterior midline swelling in the pharynx (chronic retropharyngeal abscess). It may track downwards behind the

prevertebral fascia and carotid sheath to reach the posterior triangle behind the posterior border of sternomastoid.

The pus may track down in the neck from lymph nodes deep to the cervical fascia and may form a collar-stud abscess.

- The pus may follow the posterior primary divisions of spinal nerves and present as a paravertebral abscess.

6. **What is collar-stud abscess?**

It is a bilocular abscess with an intervening narrow communication. One loculus of the abscess is deep to deep fascia and at a higher level, the other one is just beneath the skin at a lower level.

7. **What are clinical types of collar-stud abscess?**

A collar-stud abscess is seen in two clinical situations:

1. Tuberculous cervical lymphadenitis – There is formation of a cold abscess deep to deep fascia. As the time passes the pus erodes through the deep fascia and comes to lie under the skin usually at a lower level than the main loculus.

2. Pyogenic collar-stud abscess of the palm of hand – In this situation the superficial loculus lies superficial to palmar fascia and the deep loculus is deep to it with a narrow communication connecting the two.

8. **What are the investigations done in this lesion?**

The investigation are:

- Blood—TLC, DLC, ESR and hemoglobin
- Tuberculin test
- X-ray of chest, vertebral column or any other bone/joint where there is suspicion of primary disease
- Sputum smear if the patient is having productive cough
- Lymph node biopsy if possible
- Examination of aspirate for tuberculous infection
  All these investigations are not required in every case.

9. **Why do you radiograph the chest?**

Because chest X-ray may show primary complex with enlarged mediastinal lymph nodes or any other sign of tuberculosis (Fig. 2).

10. **What are the radiographic signs of vertebral column tuberculosis?**

The X-ray signs are—osteoporosis, reduction in the intervertebral disc space, destruction of vertebra and increased paravertebral shadow.

11. **What are the findings on the bacteriological examination of aspirate?**

- A smear stained by Ziehl-Neelsen method may reveal acid fast bacilli.
- Ordinary culture is usually sterile.

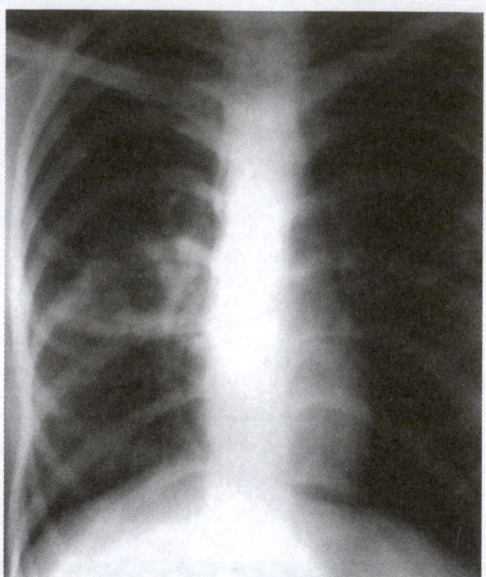

Fig. 2: X-ray of chest showing a tuberculous cavity in the middle zone of right lung

- A culture done on Lowenstein-Jensen medium may show tubercle bacilli.
- DNA and RNA amplification for tuberculosis which gives results within a few hours.

12. **How do you treat a cold abscess?**

The essentials of the treatment are:

- A full course of antituberculous drugs
- Treatment of the source of abscess.

13. **What is schedule of antituberculous drugs?**

It is as follows:

- Isoniazid 300 mg daily orally for 9 months
- Rifampicin 450 mg daily orally on empty stomach for 9 months
- Pyrazinamide 1500 mg daily orally for 2 months
- Streptomycin 0.75 g IMI daily or ethambutol 800-1000 mg orally daily for 2 months
- Pyridoxine 10 mg daily for 9 months. A small abscess may subside with this therapy alone.

14. **What are the indications of aspiration?**

It is indicated in a small abscess that can be aspirated completely.

15. **How do you do it?**

Aspiration is done with a large needle through the healthy skin by antigravity valvular method.

16. **What is evacuation?**

In this method the abscess is opened, the pus and all necrotic material is removed and the wound is closed around a drain.

17. **What are the indications of evacuation?**

Any cold abscess can be evacuated but it is ideal for a large abscess.

18. How do you treat the source of pus?

The common sources of a cold abscess are lymph nodes, bones and joints, hence their disease should be treated as outlined below:

1. *Tuberculous lymph node disease*—If it is not responding to antituberculous drugs the diseased nodes may be excised.
2. *Bone and joint tuberculosis*—The affected bone or joint is immobilized. Fusion may be required in selected cases.

DISCUSSION

Cold abscess is an abscess of comparatively slow development with little evidence of inflammation. It is one of the commonest surgical manifestation of tuberculosis. The pus in cold abscess usually collects in and around the organs or part having the original focus of disease. In many patients however, the pus gravitates down or migrates along the anatomical passages or nerves and presents far away from the source of pus.

Clinical Features

A tuberculous cold abscess can occur at any age, both male and female, but it commonly occurs in young persons. Clinically, it may present in 3 manners—

- The cold abscess is the only symptom.
- The cold abscess is associated with other symptoms of the causative lesion.
- The cold abscess is asymptomatic and discovered on clinical examination, investigations or exploration.

The patient presents with a painless and slow growing swelling of insidious onset at any of the following sites.

- *Neck*—Lateral aspect, posterior triangle, front of neck, back of neck
- *Chest*—Front, lateral wall, back
- *Abdomen*—Subcostal margin (Fig. 1), back, iliac region (iliopsoas abscess)
- Inguinal region
- Multiple sites.

The swelling is smooth, soft, nontender, fluctuant and not transilluminant.

Pathology

A cold abscess commonly follows osteo-articular or lymph node tuberculosis. The caseation and liquefaction of infected tissues lead to formation of pus which may accumulate in the tissues, migrate or rupture.

Investigations

1. Needle aspiration—It confirms the presence of pus which may be sent for bacteriological examination,

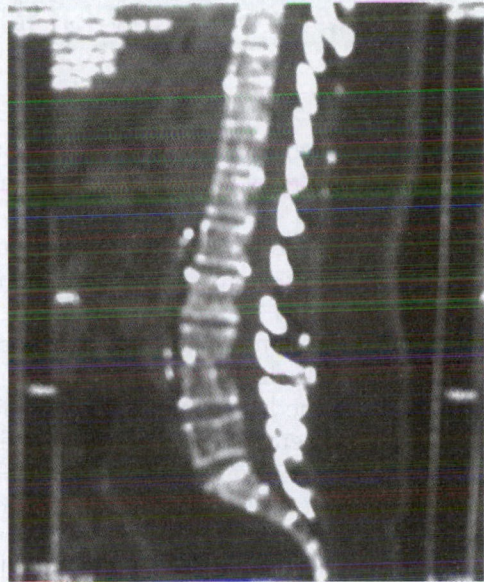

Fig. 3: CT scan of lower spine (lateral view) showing tuberculosis of L3 and L4. The intervertebral disc space is obliterated. This patient had a left psoas abscess

including culture for mycobacteria and DNA and RNA amplification for tuberculosis.

2. Radiography of chest or suspected bone or joint to find any evidence of tuberculosis (Fig. 2).
3. Ultrasound examination, especially for the diagnosis of a deep seated abscess such as iliopsoas abscess. CT scan may be done (Fig. 3).

TREATMENT

The advent of antituberculous drugs have revolutionized the treatment as any type of surgical treatment can be done with excellent results. A small cold abscess may disappear with chemotherapy alone. However, a majority or cold abscesses require surgical intervention. If the surgical treatment is combined with chemotherapy, the healing is rapid with curtailment of morbidity, which is nearly half of that of conservative treatment. The usual operative treatment is evacuation where the abscess is opened, the pus is mopped away, and all the solid necrotic tissue is excised followed by closure of the wound around a drain. Rarely, a sinus may form following surgical treatment the causes of which are:

- Persistent debris
- Secondary infection
- Infection by resistant mycobacteria
- Presence of a foreign body.

The sinus heals rapidly after the elimination of the causative factor.

CASE 2: FILARIAL ELEPHANTIASIS OF SCROTUM

CLINICAL DIAGNOSIS

1. The patient is usually an adult who presents with gradual and, or recurrent progressive enlargement of scrotum.
2. In early stage, the scrotal swelling pits on pressure (lymphedema). Later on, it presents with nonpitting edema (fibredema).
3. The whole of the scrotum is enlarged. It may be massive enlargement (scrotum like a water melon).
4. The skin is thickened, rough, rugose and may be fissured and hyperkeratotic and resembles the skin of a bitter gourd. This change is maximum at the bottom and minimum at the neck of scrotum (Figs 4 and 5).
5. The hair may be lost.
6. It may not be possible to palpate the testes, epididymis and the lower end of spermatic cords.
7. A hydrocele is usually present but fluctuation and transillumination are difficult to elicit due to thickened skin.
8. The penis is usually buried in the anterior wall of scrotum and the prepuce is stretched out. The penis may remain outside scrotum and may be elephantoid.
9. A history of filarial fever may be present.

VIVA VOCE

1. What is filarial fever?

It is a periodic fever which comes up suddenly with rigor. The temperature is often high (103-104°F) which continues for 3 to 5 days and comes down by crisis with profuse sweating. It may be associated with any of the acute manifestation of filariasis, e.g. funiculitis, lymphangitis, lymph adenitis, cellulitis, etc.

2. What are the clinical manifestations of lymphatic filariasis?

The clinical manifestations of lymphatic filariasis are–

i. Common manifestations
  a. Predominantly inflammatory
    1. Filarial fever.
    2. Epididymo-orchitis.
    3. Funiculitis.
    4. Lymphadenitis.
    5. Abscess.
  b. Predominantly obstructive
    1. Hydrocele.
    2. Elephantiasis.
    3. Chyluria.
ii. Uncommon manifestations
  a. Predominantly inflammatory
    1. Lymphangitis
    2. Cellulitis (Fig. 5)
    3. Ulceration
    4. Gangrene
    5. Pericarditis
    6. Cystitis
    7. Thrombophlebitis
    8. Peritonitis
    9. Synovitis
    10. Arthritis

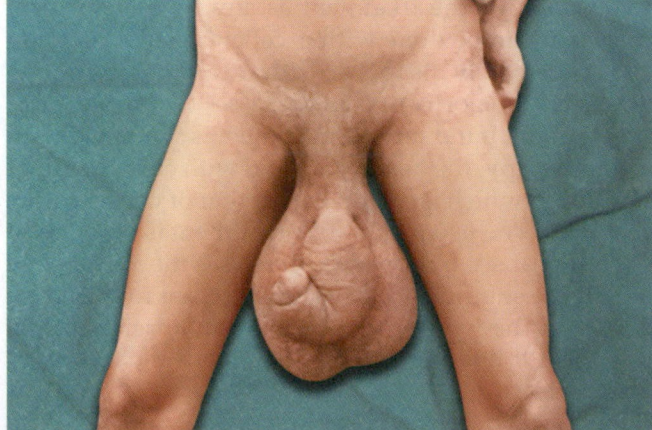

Fig: 4: Filarial elephantiasis of scrotum and penis—The penis is not buried in the scrotum in this patient but is also involved in the elephantoid process and has become curved like a Ram's horn (Ram-horn penis)

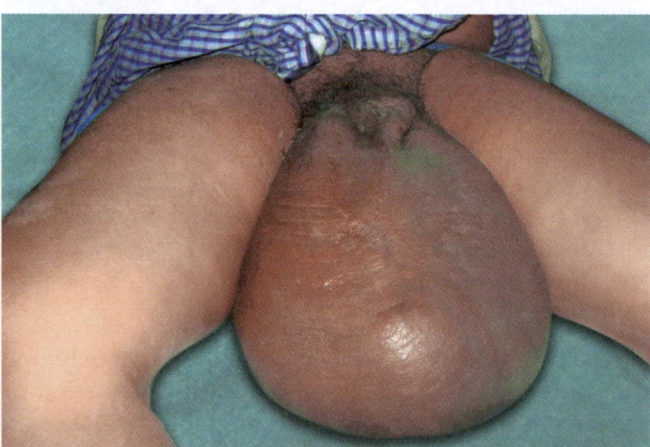

Fig. 5: Chronic filarial lymphedema of scrotum with cellulitis of skin, more marked on the right side. (*Courtesy:* Professor Sandeep Kumar)

11. Myositis
12. Salpingo-oophoritis.
   b. Predominantly obstructive
   1. Lymph-varix
   2. Lymph adenovarix
   3. Lymph scrotum
   4. Lymphorrhea
   5. Lymphuria
   6. Chylous ascites, chylous diarrhea, chylothorax, chylous arthritis, chylous pericardial effusion.

3. What is the cause of this condition?
It is caused by a parasite, Wuchereria bancrofti which is a nematode transmitted to human beings by mosquito bite (culex fatigans).

4. How many hosts does this parasite have?
This parasite passes its life cycle in two hosts man and mosquito. The man is the definitive and the mosquito is intermediate host.

5. What is the pathogenesis of elephantiasis?
Filarial infection causes adenolymphatic obstruction following which the lymph accumulates in the scrotum resulting in lymphedema. Each attack of filarial infection adds protein rich exudate to the edema fluid, which provides suitable environment for the luxurious growth of fibroblasts (fibredema) (Fig. 6).

6. What are the sites of elephantiasis in the body?
The sites are—lower limb, scrotum, penis, vulva, breast and upper limb.

7. Why are the lower limb, scrotum and penis the common sites of elephantiasis?
The commonest site of localization (and death) of adult worm is the adenolymphatic system of ilio-inguinal region, hence these are the sites of adeno-lymphatic obstruction.
Further, these areas are dependent parts of the body hence lymphedema is most manifest in these areas.

8. What is the mechanism of burial of penis into the scrotum?
As the scrotum enlarges it borrows skin from the penis, thus the penis is gradually buried into the scrotum (Fig. 7).

9. What are the investigations?
The investigations are:
- Blood for eosinophilia
- Midnight thick blood film for microfilaria
- Serologic tests include bentonite flocculation, indirect hemagglutination, ELISA and indirect fluorescent antibody tests.

10. How do you treat this lesion?
The essentials of treatment are:
1. Prevention of further mosquito bite.

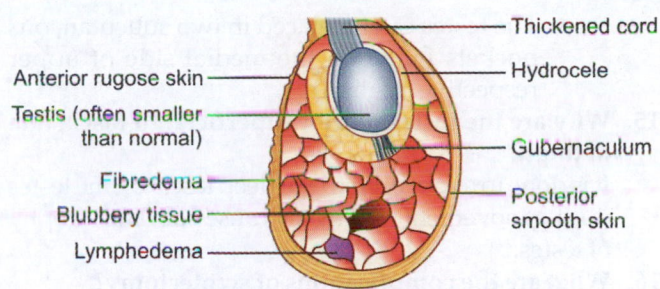

Fig. 6: Pathology of elephantiasis of scrotum

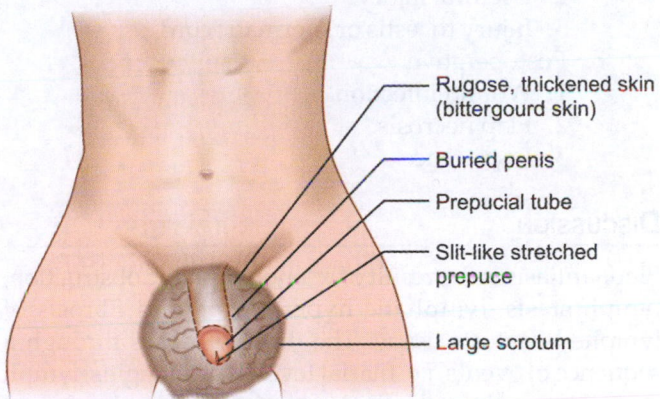

Fig. 7: Filarial elephantiasis of scrotum with penis buried completely in the anterior wall of scrotum

2. Diethylcarbamazine 100 mg thrice daily after food for 3 to 4 weeks.
3. Antibiotic therapy to control secondary infection.
4. Subtotal or total excision of scrotum.

11. What are the complications of diethylcarbamazine?
As such it is a very safe and effective drug. Some times the patient may have symptoms of allergy caused by dead microfilarial worms. Hence, an antihistaminic drug may be given alongwith diethylcarbamazine.

12. How do you prevent the allergic reaction?
The treatment should begin with a lower dosage with escalation over the first 4 days of treatment.

13. What is the newer antifilarial drug?
Ivermectin (400 mcg/kg orally) single dose may be as effective as a full course of diethylcarbamazine.

14. How do you deal with exposed testes?
1. In subtotal excision of scrotum, the testes can be covered by reconstructing the scrotum by stitching together the remnants of scrotum.
2. In total scrotectomy any of the following procedures may be employed:
   - A new scrotum can be reconstructed from skin flaps obtained from thigh or abdominal wall.

- The testes can be placed in two subcutaneous pockets made on the medial side of upper respective thighs.

15. **Why are the testes placed superficial to fascia lata of thigh?**

It is done to avoid pressure of deep fascia on the testes during movement which may cause pain and atrophy of testes.

16. **What are the complications of scrotectomy?**

The complications are:

a. Intraoperative
   1. Hemorrhage.
   2. Urethral injury.
   3. Injury to testis or spermatic cord.
b. Postoperative
   1. Wound infection.
   2. Flap necrosis.
   3. Recurrence.

DISCUSSION

Elephantiasis is the result of adenolymphatic obstruction, lymph stasis, lymphatic hypertension and fibrosis of lymphedematous tissue. The disease passes through a sequence of events, i.e. filarial fever, lymphangitis, lymph stagnation and finally elephantiasis. In the early stage of disease after an attack of adenolymphangitis the part becomes swollen due to lymphedema which pits on pressure. When the attack subsides the swelling is reduced to some extent but the status quo ante is seldom attained. With subsequent attacks, the swelling increases further and becomes more firm due to overgrowth of connective tissue. The static and protein-rich lymph provides a suitable medium for the luxurious growth of fibroblasts. Ultimately a firm and nonyielding swelling is produced which does not pit on pressure. The overlying skin gets thickened, rough and dry (elephantiasis). The surface of the skin becomes rugose with warty growths. Secondary infection and trauma may cause cellulitis, suppuration, ulceration and gangrene.

Filarial elephantiasis of scrotum is due to ilioinguinal adenolymphatic obstruction caused by filarial infection. It is the selective blockage of scrotal drainage which results in this type of elephantiasis.

Pathology

On section, the hypertrophied skin forms the outermost layer, then there is dense fibrous layer, deep to this layer there is a layer of gelatinous lymph clogged mass known as blubbery tissue of variable thickness. The tunica vaginalis has a variable amount of serous fluid (Fig. 6).

The lower pole of testis is anchored to the botton of scrotum by hypertrophied gubernaculum testis. The testis may be normal or atrophied (Fig. 7).

Clinical Features

Scrotal elephantiasis is one of the common manifestation of filariasis. Owing to dependent position of scrotum and quite lax subcutaneous connective tissue a lot of fluid can accumulate resulting in a very large swelling which may be the size of a large water melon or even bigger. Later, the skin starts becoming thickened first in the most dependent part of the scrotum which then extends upwards. It involves mostly the anterior rugose skin.

The enlarging scrotum gradually engulfs the penis completely and then its orifice is indicated on the anterior wall of scrotum by the hypertrophied prepuce, whence a long channel goes upwards to meet the glans penis (Fig. 7).

Investigations

1. Blood for eosinophilia.
2. Parasitological—Night blood smear may be positive for microfilaria, especially if the patient had an acute attack recently.
3. Immunological assay for filarial antibodies and antigens.
4. Lymphography—It does not have much clinical value.

Treatment—Further mosquito bite must be prevented.

Diethylcarbamazine 100 mg thrice daily for 3 to 4 weeks is the most effective usual drug.

A course of antibioitics to control secondary infection is usually required.

In moderate or severe elephantiasis usually surgical help is required in the form of partial or complete excision of scrotum with scrotal reconstruction which is done by residual scrotal skin or from a flap obtained from abdominal wall or thigh.

CASE 3: FILARIAL ELEPHANTIASIS OF PENIS

CLINICAL DIAGNOSIS

1. The patient is an adult who presents with swelling of the skin of penis of insidious onset.
2. The swelling is maximum near the tip and gradually becoming less near its base (Fig. 8).
3. The skin of the penis is thickened, rough, dry and may pit on pressure.
4. The prepuce cannot be retracted and glans penis cannot be seen (filarial phimosis) (Fig. 9).
5. The penis may be deformed to assume the shape of a ram's-horn (ram horn penis) (Fig. 5.8).
6. There may be a history of recurrent attacks of fever with rigor, every attack adding to the penile swelling.

VIVA VOCE

1. **What is elephantiasis?**
   It is the enlargement of any part due to chronic lymphedema caused by adenolymphatic obstruction and characterized by elephantoid thickening of skin.
2. **What are the causes of chronic lymphedema of penis?**
   The causes of lymphedema of penis are:
   - Filarial adenolymphangitis of inguinal lymphatic system
   - Tuberculous inguinal lymphadenitis
   - Lymphogranuloma inguinale

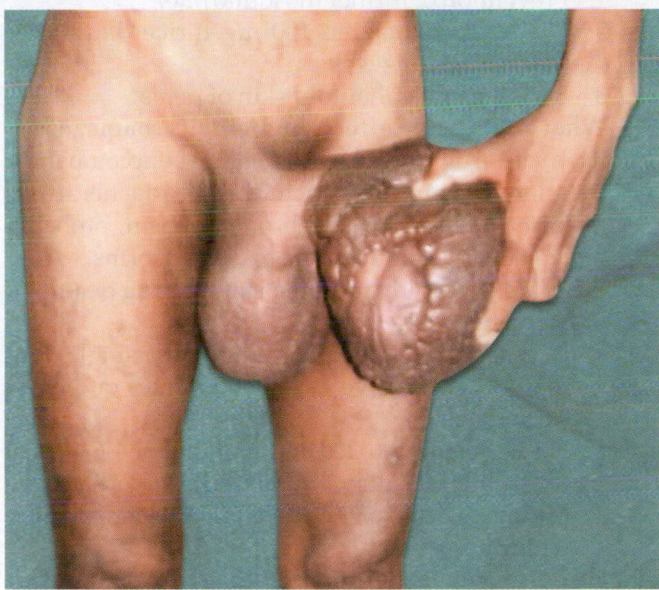

Fig. 9: Filarial elephantiasis of penis
(*Courtesy:* Professor Sandeep Kumar)

   - Following block dissection or irradiation of inguinal nodes.
3. **What are the causes of inability to retract the prepuce?**
   The causes of inability to retract prepuce are:
   - Phimosis
   - Subprepucial adhesions
   - Penile elephantiasis
   - Diabetic posthitis
   - Prepucial carcinoma.
4. **How does elephantiasis cause inability to retract prepuce?**
   Because of chronic lymphedema and fibredema the prepuce loses its elasticity and stretchability, hence cannot be retracted.
5. **What are the investigations done to prove its filarial etiology?**
   The investigations are:
   1. Blood for eosinophilia
   2. *Parasitologic*—Night blood smear (thick) is examined on three occasions for microfilariae. It is usually negative unless the patient has a bout of fresh infection.
   3. *Immunologic*—They are usually positive and include bentonite flocculation, indirect hemagglutination, ELISA, and indirect fluorescent antibody test.

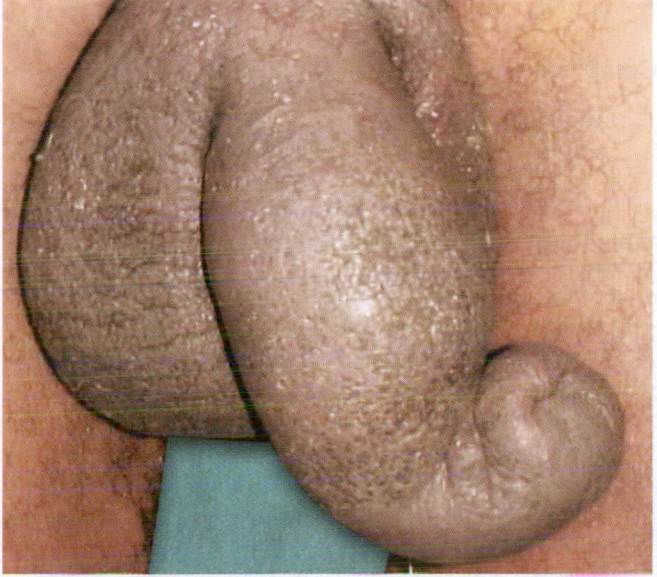

Fig. 8: Filarial elephantiasis of penis—Ram horn penis
(*Courtesy:* Professor Sandeep Kumar)

6. **How do you treat this condition?**
   The essentials of treatment are:
   1. Prevention of further mosquito bite.
   2. Diethylcarbamazine 100 mg thrice daily after meals for 3 to 4 weeks.
   3. Excision of elephantoid skin of penis.

7. **What are the side effects of diethylcarbamazine?**
   It is a safe drug, but it may sometimes be accompanied by allergic symptoms including headache, fever, malaise hypotension and bronchospasm, probably due to release of antigens from dying worms.

8. **What are newer advancements in the drug treatment of filariasis?**
   - Ivermectin (400 mcg/kg orally) in a single dose may be as effective as longer courses of diethyl carbamazine
   - Doxycycline (100-200 mg/d orally for 4-6 weeks) kills obligate intracellular Wolbachia bacteria, leading to death of the adult filarial worms. Hence, it may be given.

9. **How do you provide skin cover to penis after excision of elephantoid skin?**
   Usually the inner layer of prepuce is healthy and unaffected, hence it should be preserved. It is everted on the penis to provide a cover after excision (Fig. 10), if this not possible skin grafts obtained from thigh may be used.

10. **Can you treat this condition by lymphangioplasty?**
    They have been tried but failed to give any satisfactory results.

11. **What is the role of compression therapy ?**
    In an early case, it gives satisfactory relief. Benzopyrones may be combined with it for better results.

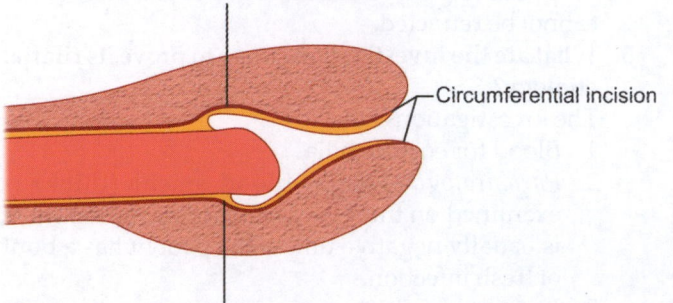

Plane of separation of two layers
(the inner layer is everted to cover raw
penis after excision of outer layer)

—Circumferential incision

Plane of separation of two layers
(everted to cover raw penis)

Fig. 10: Excision of elephantoid tissue of penile elephantiasis

DISCUSSION

The penis may be affected alongwith the scrotal disease or independently. The penile skin is swollen due to lymphedema and later on thickened. It may be enormously swollen, thickened and distorted due to unequal contraction of hypertrophied fibrous tissue and fascia around the penis resulting in a ram horn penis (Figs 8 and 9).

Except for swelling the patient does not have any other symptom. The prepuce cannot be retracted (filarial phimosis). The sexual dysfunction is invariably present.

Types of Elephantiasis of Penis

1. **Straight hypertrophied penis** - There is elephantiasis of penile skin without distortion or burial of penis (Fig. 9).
2. **Ram horn penis** - It is due to unequal accumulation of elephantoid tissue resulting in distortion of prepuce resembling a ram's horn. The length of prepuce is increased and it cannot be retracted to expose the glans (filarial phimosis). In the prepucial sac dirty blackish and inspissated smegma or epithelial debris accumulates (Fig. 8).
3. **Embedded penis** with penile elephantoid skin becoming a part of scrotum—As the scrotum enlarges in filariasis due to elephantiasis and/or hydrocele it borrows the penile skin gradually burying the entire penis in the anterior elephantoid wall of scrotum.

Investigations

- Blood for eosinophilia
- Night blood smear for microfilaria
- Serologic tests for filarial infection.

Complications

1. Phimosis.
2. Cellulitis, gangrene.
3. Ulceration.

Treatment

- Further mosquito bite must be prevented.
- Diethylcarbamazine 100 mg thrice daily for 21 to 30 days.
- Excision of elephantoid tissue cures this condition. A racket incision is made whose handle is a vertical midline incision along the dorsum of penis and the blade of racket encircles the root of penis. The handle ends in a circumferential incision around the prepuce. The skin of the penis, all elephantoid tissue and outer layer of prepuce are excised. The raw area is covered by turning back the inner layer of prepuce or partial thickness skin grafts (Fig. 10).

CASE 4: BREAST ABSCESS

CLINICAL DIAGNOSIS

1. The patient is usually a young woman who has recently given birth to a baby and presents with pain and swelling of the breast.
2. The breast is red, hot and tender (Fig. 11).
3. These signs are usually localized to a segment of the breast.
4. Fever and toxemia may be present depending upon the severity of disease.
5. The axillary lymph nodes of the same side may be enlarged and tender.

VIVA VOCE

1. **What is a breast abscess?**
   It is a localized collection of pus in the breast.
2. **What is the etiology of this condition?**
   The causative organism is *Staphylococcus aureus* which enters the breast tissue from a sore or cracked nipple. Stasis in the lactiferous ducts due to epithelial debris invites infection.
3. **What about the fluctuation as a sign of pus?**
   It is a late sign of the disease. One must not wait for fluctuation to recognize this disease.

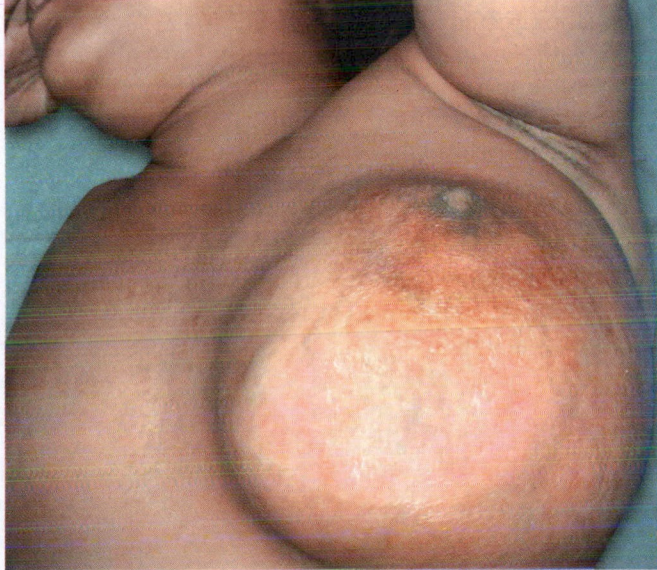

Fig. 11: A large breast abscess pointing on the skin and about to rupture (*Courtesy:* Professor Sandeep Kumar)

4. **How will you confirm the presence of pus?**
   It can be confirmed by ultrasonography and needle aspiration.
5. **How do you treat this condition?**
   If the duration is short the patient may be given antibiotic (flucloxacillin or amoxiclav), analgeic and hot fomentation.
   If there is no relief within 48 hours the pus must be removed.
6. **How will you remove the pus?**
   - The traditional method of removal of pus is surgical drainage.
   - Now the pus is being removed by repeated needle aspiration, may be under the guidance of ultrasound.
7. **What is the technique of open drainage?**
   - It is usually done under general anesthesia, but it can be done under local anestheisa if an analgesic cream e.g. EMLA which contains lidocaine is applied locally half an hour before the operation.
   - A radial incision is given on the top of the abscess, the abscess cavity is opened, all the loculi are broken and the pus and necrotic tissue is removed and the wound is dressed.
8. **What is the cosmetic method of drainage?**
   - The abscess is drained by a circumareolar incision.
   - A counter drainage tube may be required to be inserted in the abscess cavity.
9. **What is an antibioma?**
   If an acute abscess is treated with antibiotics without drainage the abscess is encapsulated by a thick fibrous wall. The patient has a painless, firm mass in the breast which looks like a carcinoma.
10. **What is subareolar abscess?**
    It is a small furuncle-like abscess of the areola which occurs due to infection of Montgomery tubercles. It is treated by excision of affected tubercle.
11. **What is a retromammary abscess?**
    It is not a true breast abscess as the pus collects behind the breast usually due to tuberculosis of ribs. The patient presents with a breast swelling.
    It is treated by antituberculous drugs and removal of pus by aspiration or evacuation.

DISCUSSION

It is the formation of pus in the breast. Depending upon the collection of pus in relation to breast parenchyma the

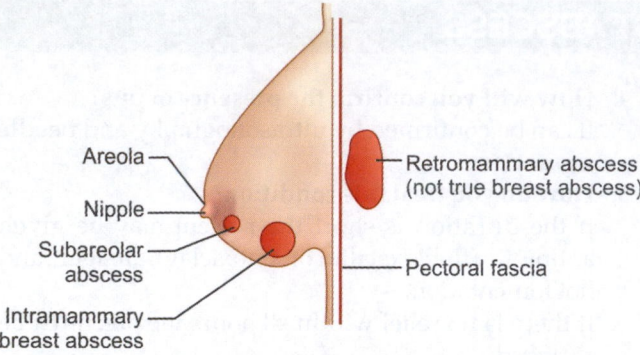

Fig. 12: Side view of the breast showing various types of breast abscesses

breast abscesses are of three types - intramammary, retromammary and subareolar (Fig. 12).

Intramammary Breast Abscess

Acute breast abscess is a common problem which follows bacterial mastitis which is associated with lactation in most of the patients.

It is mostly caused by *Staphylococcus aureus* which may enter the breast from a sore or cracked nipple. It may be due to stasis as the lactiferous ducts may be blocked by epithelial debris or plugs. Hence, breast abscess is very common in a female with retracted nipple. After the bacteria enter the lactiferous sinus they cause curdling of the milk and then the bacteria multiply within the clot, invade the tissues and cause tissue necrosis.

Clinical Features

The patient has recently delivered a baby and develops pain and swelling in the breast, Usually a segment of the breast presents with signs of acute inflammation. Initially, it is due to cellulitis followed by localization and abscess formation.

The blood will show polymorphonuclear leukocytosis. The pus can be seen by ultrasonography.

Treatment

1. Early inflammation may be treated with an antibiotic, e.g. flucloxacillin or co-amoxiclav, breast support, local heat and analgesics. The breast feeding should continue if the patient can do it.
2. *Drainage*—If the infection is not resolved within 48 hours, the abscess is drained under general anesthesia. All the loculi are broken and the cavity is cleaned and dressed.
3. It can be done under local anesthesia if an analgesic cream, e.g. EMLA which contains lidocaine is applied locally 30 minutes before operation. The incision employed is a direct radial incision or a cosmetic circumareolar incision.
4. *Aspiration*—Now the abscess can be treated by minimal invasion, by repeated needle aspiration under antibiotic cover. The aspiration can be done under ultrasonographic guidance.
   - *Chronic abscess or antibioma*—If an acute abscess is treated with antibiotics without removal of pus, the abscess becomes encapsulated by a thick fibrous wall. The patient presents with a painless firm mass which cannot be differentiated from carcinoma clinically. One differentiating feature is that the swelling is stationary.
   - *Subareolar abscess*—The patient presents with a furuncle-like abscess on the areola. It is due to infection of Montgomery tubercles. The patient is usually a young or middle aged women who is not lactating. If it is treated by incision it recurs, hence the affected tubercle is excised.
   - *Tuberculous abscess*—Tuberculous abscess in relation to the breast is of two types retromammary abscess and intramammary abscess. The former occurs behind the breast due to tuberculosis of ribs or sternum. It is quite common.
   Intramammary tuberculous abscess is due to tuberculosis of breast. It is an uncommon problem. The patient is given antituberculous drugs and the pus may be removed by repeated needle aspiration or evacuation.

CASE 5: ACUTE PARONYCHIA

CLINICAL DIAGNOSIS

1. The patient presents with pain and swelling in a digit of the hand.
2. The nail fold is swollen, red, hot, tense and tender.
3. The pus may be visible in the swelling (Fig. 13).

VIVA VOCE

1. **What is paronychia?**
   It is acute inflammation of the nail fold with pus formation due to infection by *Staphylococcus aureus*.
2. **How do the bacteria enter the nail-fold?**
   They enter the nail-fold directly through a puncture or injury during nail-paring.
3. **What is the extent of infection?**
   From the nail-fold the infection may spread to the base of the nail (eponychia), or pus may form under the nail (subungual abscess).
4. **How do you treat this condition?**
   The pus is drained by a longitudinal incision on the necrotic skin and the abscess cavity is deroofed. If the pus has gone under the nail it should be removed from there also. If necessary the part of the nail overlying the abscess is excised.
5. **What is chronic paronychia?**
   It is a chronic infection of nail folds including the nails, usually seen in persons whose hands are frequently immersed in water, e.g. dishwashers.
6. **What is the nature of infection?**
   It is usually a mixed bacterial infection. It may be caused by fungi.

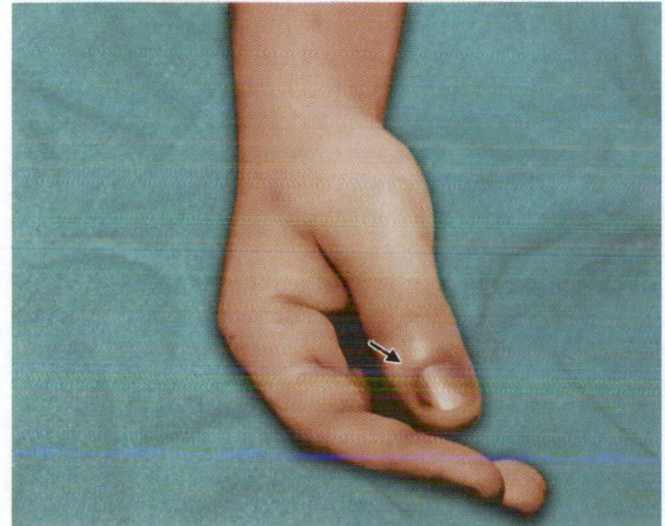

Fig. 13: Paronychia of thumb

7. **How do you treat it?**
   - It is treated by controlling infection by local antibacterial or antifungal creams.
   - Gloves may be worn to keep the cream in position.
   - The hands must be kept dry.
   - The pus pockets are opened and necrotic tissue, if any is excised.
8. **How does the chronic paronychia related to acute disease?**
   The chronic paronychia has nothing to do with acute disease.

DISCUSSION

Acute paronychia is the formation of pus in the nail fold and is characterized by acute pain and swelling.

Etiology

It is usually caused by *Staphylococcus aureus* which enters the nail fold by inappropriate nail trimming or a puncture. The infection is subcuticular as it is situated entirely within the dermis.

Clinical Features

There is pain and swelling of the nail fold. It becomes red, tense and tender. The pus may be visible under the skin.

Treatment

It is drained by a longitudinal incision and the cavity is deroofed. Frequently the pus goes under the nail which must be removed with or without excision of outer part of the nail.

Chronic paronychia (perionychia) is the chronic infection of the nail folds as well as the nail. It usually affects all the nails.

It is nothing to do with acute paronychia. The infection may be mixed bacterial or fungal. It is usually seen in persons whose hands are frequently immersed in water.

The nail folds are swollen and chronically inflamed. The nails may be thickened and discolored. There may be subungual discharge.

The discharge and scrapings are sent for culture, especially fungal culture.

Treatment – The hand is kept dry. Local anti-fungal creams are applied and the hand may be kept in a glove to keep the cream applied. Surgical help may be required in removing pus and necrotic tissue.

12. **What is imiquimod and how do you use it?**

It is a local interferon inducer. A 5 percent cream is applied once daily on alternate days per week for 8 to 12 weeks.

13. **What are the advantages and disadvantages of imiquimod?**
    - It is a treatment of choice in female patients.
    - It is an expensive drug.

14. **What are the indications of surgery?**

If the local medical treatment has failed and the lesions are large or pedunculated surgical treatment is indicated.

15. **What is the technique of excision?**

Under general or local anesthesia the individual wart is excised with scissors, and the residual and the base of the lesion is treated with electrocautery.

16. **Is there any risk during this procedure?**

The smoke of electrocoagulation contains viable organisms, hence must be thoroughly evacuated.

17. **What are the indications of laser therapy?**

It is indicated in recurrent warts.

18. **What are the results of CO_2 laser therapy?**

It is an effective method of treatment but the recurrence rate is slightly more.

19. **What is the role of cryotherapy?**

It also destroys the warts by two freeze-thaw cycles given every 2 to 4 weeks for several visits. It is the first line surgical treatment.

20. **What are the disadvantages of cryotherapy?**

Scarring and permanent depigmentation in pigmented persons.

21. **Do you know of intralesional injection therapy?**

Yes, intralesional injection of interferon-alfa have been used with good results.

22. **How do you treat intraurethral lesions?**

The urethral warts are first seen and localized by urethroscopy and then treated by intraurethral fulguration, CO_2 laser, or injection of interferon-alfa.

23. **Can this disease recur, if so what are the causes of recurrence?**

This disease can recur as this virus is autoinoculable and has an incubation period that can be as long as one year. Both these factors account for many treatment failures.

24. **How do you prevent recurrence?**
    - After successful treatment, the patient is seen weekly to treat any recurrence as soon as it appears.
    - The patient should observe sexual hygiene and discretion.

25. **How do you prevent occurrence of this disease?**
    - Administration of vaccine
    - Examination of sexual partners
    - By observing sexual hygiene and discretion.

DISCUSSION

Condylomata acuminata are warty lesions caused by human papillomaviruses (HPVs) occurring on the penis, scrotum, urethra, vulva, vagina, cervix, perineum, perianal region and anal canal (Figs 14 and 15).

Etiology

It is caused by various types of human papillomaviruses which are transmitted by sexual intercourse, including homosexuality. Immunosuppression, especially in transplant recepients and HIV patients, and pregnancy favor their growth. HPV infection, apart from these lesions also causes intraepithelial neoplasia (carcinoma in situ) and squamous cell carcinoma, which may affect anus, vulva and cervix.

There are more than 80 subtypes of HPV, but the subtypes 16,18, 31, 33 are associated with more risk of progression to dysplasia and malignancy.

Clinical Features

The disease may be asymptomatic, or the patient may have pruritus, discharge, bleeding or pain.

- **Anal disease**—The early anal warts are separate pinkish-white warts near the anal verge and may be on the anoderm within the distal anal canal upto 2 cm above the dentate line. Later on, they enlarge and coalesce to produce larger condylomata. These lesions are seen in 25 percent of homosexual men. Rarely, they may produce giant condylomata (Buschke-Lowenstein tumor) which may obstruct the anal opening.
- **The penile warts** occur commonly under the prepuce in the coronal sulcus, but they can occur anywhere including urethra.
- **In females they** occur most commonly on the vulva, but may line the vagina, and can occur on the cervix. The vaginal lesions may show diffuse hypertrophy or a cobblestone appearance. Fissures may be present at the fourchette.

Investigations

- Biopsy—It is done in large and suspicious lesions as it will also reveal dysplasia, if present.
- Tests for venereal diseases, e.g. syphilis, AIDS are done as they may be associated with these warts.

- Aceto-whitening—If acetic acid (4%) is applied to the lesion it turns white with prominent papillae. The vaginal and cervical lesions can be seen by colposcopy after pretreatment with acetic acid.

Complications

- Condylomata acuminata may be associated with anal intraepithelial neoplasia (AIN) and squamous cell carcinoma of the anus. In a women, there may be vulvar intraepithelial neoplasia (VIN), cervical intra-epithelial neoplasia (CIN) and cancers.
- Large genital warts in a woman may obstruct the vagina.

Treatment

There is no treatment which can guarantee a remission or prevent recurrence. Hence, there are many methods of treatment.

- *Podophyllum resin* (podofilox) is applied by the patient twice daily for 3 consecutive days a week for cycles of 4 to 6 weeks. After one 4-week cycle, 50 percent of patients are wart-free but recurrence occurs in 60 percent of patients at 6 weeks. Thus, many cycles of treatment are needed.

  In the hospital or office each wart can be painted protecting normal skin very 2 to 3 weeks with 25 percent podophyllum resin (podophyllin) in compound tincture of benzoin. It is the treatment of choice in men. It cannot be applied in the anal canal.

- *Imiquimod*—It is a local interferon inducer having moderate activity in clearing external genital warts, A 5 percent cream is applied once daily on 3 alternate days per week. The response comes at 8 to 12 weeks (in 44-69% of patients) better in women. 13 percent of patients have recurrences in the short term. It is the treatment of choice in women. It is an expensive drug.

- *Surgical excision*—Snip biopsy (scissors) excision followed by light electrocautery is good especially for patients with pedunculated or large lesions.
- *Laser therapy*—CO_2 laser destroys the warts and leaves open wounds which heal by granulation tissue over 4 to 6 weeks.
- *Cryotherapy*—Liquid nitrogen is applied to obtain a thaw time of 20 to 45 seconds. Two freeze-thaw cycles are given every 2 to 4 weeks for several visits. It causes scarring and depigmentation.
- *Anal disease*—Small external perianal warts are treated by topical application of podophyllum resion, imiquimod cream or podofilox 0.5 percent gel.

  Anal canal lesions need topical application of bichloroacetic acid, cryotherapy or electrocautery.

  Refractory or large warts may be treated by local injection of interferon-alfa beneath the lesions or surgical excision.

- *Vulvar disease* is treated by podophyllum resin 10-25% in tincture of benzoin (not to be used during pregnancy), or 80 to 90 percent trichloroacetic acid or bichloroacetic acid applied with care to protect skin. The pain of acetic acid application can be reduced by sodium bicarbonate paste. Podophyllum in washed after 2 to 4 hours. Podofilox 0.5 percent gel or imiquimod 5 percent cream can be used by the patient.
- *Vaginal condylomata* are treated with cryotherapy with liquid nitrogen, trichloroacetic acid or podophyllum resin.

  Extensive disease is treated with CO_2 laser.

Prevention

- Administration of a vaccine against genital HPV types
- Examination of sexual partners
- Condom does not prevent HPV transmission but it may help in accelerated regression of associated lesions.

Miscellaneous Swellings

CASE 1: GYNECOMASTIA

CLINICAL DIAGNOSIS

1. The patient is an adolescent or adult male who presents with gradual enlargement of one or both breasts.
2. The enlargement of the breast may be diffuse, soft and nontender (fatty gynecomastia) (Figs 1 and 2).
3. It may be firm, granular and somewhat tender (glandular gynecomastia).
4. There may be a tender discoid swelling 2 to 3 cm diameter under the areola (pubertal gynecomastia).

VIVA VOCE

1. **What is gynecomastia?**
   It is the presence of a female-like breast in a male.
2. **What is the harm in having gynecomastia?**
   - Except for psychological embarrassment gynecomastia is of no cosequence in most of the patients, where the cause is not known (idiopathic gynecomastia)
   - In symptomatic gynecomastia, the harm depends upon the cause of gynecomastia.
3. **What are the causes of gynecomastia?**
   The causes of gynecomastia are:
   - Indiopathic, where the cause is not known
   - Physiologic
     1. Puberty
     2. Old age.
   - Systemic diseases
     1. Chronic liver disease
     2. Chronic renal disease
     3. Refeeding after starvation.

- Endocrine disorders
  1. Androgen resistance syndromes.
  2. Hyperprolactinemia.
  3. Hyperthyroidism.
  4. Klinefelter's syndrome.
  5. Male hypogonadism.
- Tumors: Adrenal tumors, bronchogenic carcinoma, testicular tumors
- Drugs (partial list): Cimetidine, estrogen, spironolactone, chorionic gonadotropins, digitalis, diazepam, isoniazid, methyl dopa, calcium channel blockers, phenothiazines,

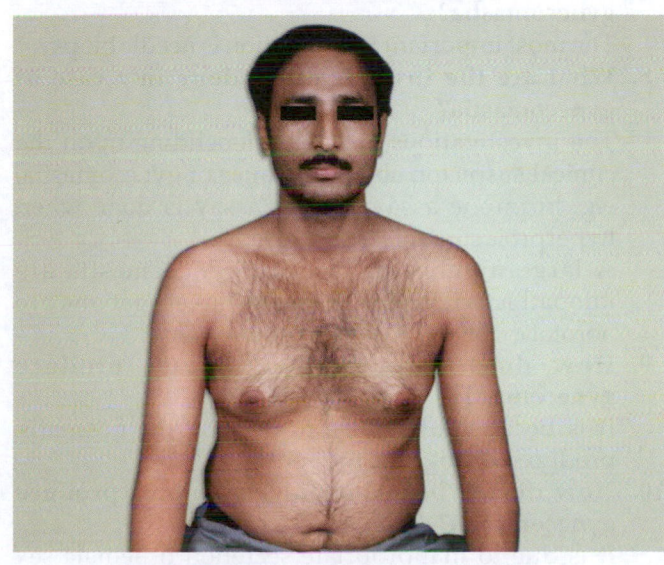

Fig. 1: Bilateral gynecomastia (idiopathic)

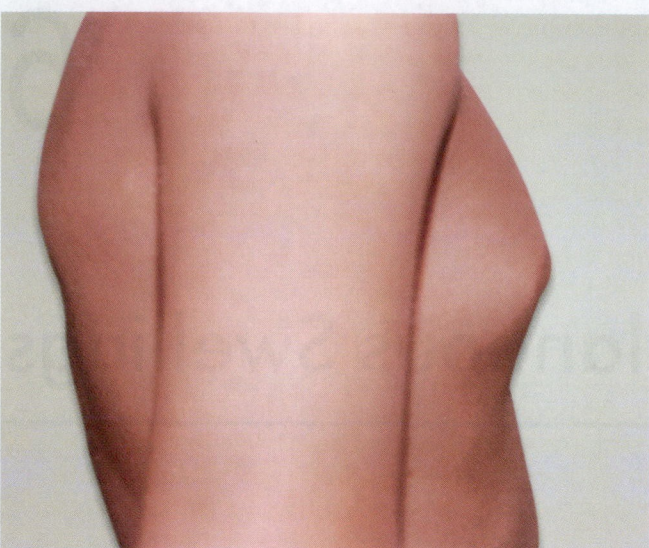

Fig. 2: Gynecomastia as seen by the side

anabolic steroids, HAART (highly active antiretroviral therapy).

4. What are the types of gynecomastia?
It is of two types—fatty gynecomastia and glandular gynecomastia.

5. Can a tumor results in enlargement of male breast?
A tumor, e.g. fibroadenoma or carcinoma can cause enlargement of male breast.

6. How this enlargement is different from gynecomastia?
This enlargement of breast is unilateral, asymmetric and firm or hard.

7. How will you rule out a tumor in a patient of gynecomastia?
The most important investigation is needle biopsy.

8. What are the investigations done in a case of gynecomastia?
The investigations are done depending upon the clinical suspicion about the cause of gynecomastia, e.g. hormone assay as PRL assay is done when hyperprolactinemia is suspected.
A large number of cases of gynecomastia are idiopathic where the results of investigations are normal.

9. How does chronic liver disease produce gynecomastia?
It is because of failure to destroy the normally produced estrogen in the body.

10. How does a bronchogenic carcinoma produce gynecomastia?
It is due to inappropriate secretion of female sex hormones by the cancer. Gynecomastia is one of the paraneoplastic syndrome of bronchogenic carcinoma.

11. How do you treat gynecomastia?
- Prepubertal gynecomastia may resolve spontaneously within 1 to 2 years. Reassurance is the treatment
- If cause is known, it must be treated. For example, drug induced gynecomastia usually resolves if the causative drug is withdrawn
- Painful or persistent gynecomastia is treated by a course of SERM, e.g. raloxifene or tamoxifen. It is more effective in glandular gynecomastia
- If there is no response and the patient is very much concerned surgery may be considered.

12. What is the nature of surgery?
The breast is excised preserving the nipple and areola. A small enlargement is excised by a circumareolar incision (Fig. 3). For large breast a submammary incision may be employed.

13. Is there a less invasive method of treatment available?
Fatty gynecomastia can be treated by endoscopically assisted transaxillary liposuction.

14. What are the complications of operation?
The complications are flap necrosis, wound hematoma and seroma.

DISCUSSION

It is the presence of a female-like breast in a male. It is often asymmetric or unilateral.

Etiology

- Idiopathic, where the cause is not known.
- Physiologic:
  1. Puberty.
  2. Old age.

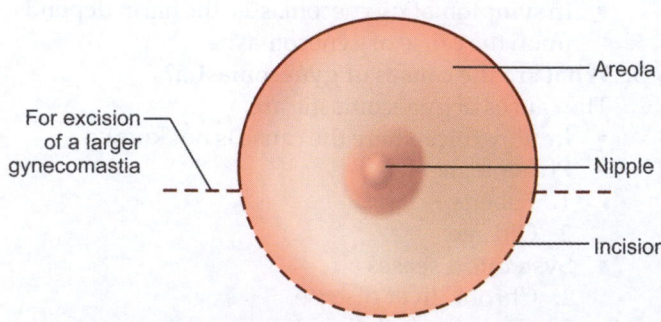

Fig. 3: Circumareolar incision for excision of gynecomastia. In a larger lesion the incision can be converted into an omega incision or it can be excised by a submammary incision

- Systemic diseases:
  1. Chronic liver disease.
  2. Chronic renal disease.
  3. Refeeding after starvation.
- Endocrine disorders:
  1. Androgen resistance syndromes.
  2. Hyperprolactinemia.
  3. Hyperthyroidism.
  4. Klinefelter's syndrome.
  5. Male hypogonadism.
- Tumors: Adrenal tumors, bronchogenic carcinoma, testicular tumors
- Drugs (partial list): Cimetidine, estrogens, spironolactone, chorionic gonadotropins, digitalis, diazepam, isoniazid, methyldopa, calcium channel blockers, phenothiazines, anabolic steroids, HAART (highly active antiretroviral therapy).

Pathology—It is of two types - in fatty gynecomastia, there is excessive deposition of fatty tissue, while in glandular gynecomastia there is proliferation of glandular elements.

Clinical Features

Gynecomastia is common in teenagers who are very tall or overweight. It is common among elderly men, especially when there is associated weight gain.

Fatty gynecomastia is usually diffuse, soft and non-tender while the glandular type may be firm, granular and tender. The pubertal gynecomastia is characterized by a tender discoid swelling 2 to 3 cm in diameter under the areola.

Depending upon the severity, the gynecomastia can be mild (I), moderate (II) and severe (III).

The history of the patient is taken and a careful physical examination is done to find the cause which is not found in a good number of patients.

Investigations

1. Hormone assay:
   - Prolactin is assayed to detect hyperprolactinemia.

- β-hCG: Detectable levels implicate a testicular tumor (germ cell or Sertoli cell), or other malignancy usually lung or liver. Detectable low levels of β-hCG (less than 5 mIU/ml) may be found in men with primary hypogonadism.
- *Plasma testosterone (T) and LH*—A low T and high LH levels are found in primary hypogonadism. High T plus high LH levels are seen in partial androgen resistance.
- *Serum estradiol*—It is usually normal. Increased levels may result from testicular tumors, increased β-hCG, liver disease, obesity and adrenal tumors
- Serum TSH and FT_4 are done to rule out thyroid disease.

2. In Klinefelter's syndrome a karyotype is obtained.
3. Radiography of chest is done for metastatic or bronchogenic carcinoma.
4. In unilateral or asymmetric gynecomastia needle biopsy is done.

These investigations are done depending on clinical suspicion. All the investigations are not done in every case.

Treatment

- Pubertal gynecomastia may resolve by itself within 1 to 2 years.
- Drug-induced disease is treated by withdrawing the causative drug. It usually resolves by doing so. Spironolactone is substituted by eplerenone.
- Painful or persistent gynecomastia is treated by 3 to 9 months course of SERM, e.g. raloxifene or tamoxifen. It is more effective in glandular gynecomastia.
- Surgery—If there is no response and the patient is very much concerned, the operation may be done. The breast is excised preserving the nipple and areola. A small enlargement is excised by a circumareolar (omega) incision (Fig. 3) and a very large lesion is excised by a curved submammary incision.
- Fatty gynecomastia can be managed by endoscopically assisted transaxillary liposuction.

CASE 2: ARTERIAL ANEURYSM

CLINICAL DIAGNOSIS

1. The patient presents with a gradually enlarging swelling along the course of a large artery (Fig. 4).
2. It is pulsatile, the pulsation are expansile and synchronous with the heart beat.
3. It is smooth, tensely cystic and nontender (tender with onset of leak).
4. It can be moved slightly across but not along the long axis of artery.
5. If the artery proximal to the swelling is compressed the size, tension and pulsation of the swelling are reduced. On release of pressure the size, tension and pulsation become as they were before compression.
6. If the artery distal to the swelling is compressed the size and tension may increase.
7. A systolic bruit may be present on auscultation.
8. The pulsation in the artery distal to the swelling may be delayed or diminished.
9. Pressure symptoms such as venous congestion and edema, nerve palsy (e.g. foot drop in popliteal aneurysm), dysphagia (thoracic aortic aneurysm), etc. may be seen.

   (A deep seated aneurysm may be asymptomatic and detected by investigations. Palpation must be done very gently as the aneurysm may rupture).

VIVA VOCE

1. **What is an aneurysm?**

   It is a localized dilatation or a blood filled sac in direct communication with the lumen of an artery (Fig. 4).

2. **What are the causes of an aneurysm?**
   - Congenital
     1. Berry aneurysm of circle of Willis.
     2. Arterial dilatation associated with an arteriovenous fistula.
     3. Marfan's syndrome.
   - Traumatic
     1. Arterial contusion.
     2. Radiation injury.
     3. Penetrating trauma.
   - Infections
     1. Subacute bacterial endocarditis.
     2. Tertiary syphilis.
   - Degenerative arterial diseases
     1. Atherosclerosis.
     2. Cystic medial necrosis.
   - Other causes
     1. Systemic hypertension.
     2. Polyarteritis nodosa.

3. **What are the types of aneurysms?**

   Aneurysms are of two types—true and false (Fig. 5).

4. **What is a true aneurysm?**

   It is a localized dilatation of an artery which is either symmetrical or eccentric. It consists of all the three layers of the arterial wall.

5. **What is a pseudo-aneurysm?**

   The wall of this aneurysm is formed by condensed fibrous tissue. It is a fibrous sac communicating with an artery.

6. **What are the causes of pseudo-aneurysm?**

   The causes of pseudo-aneurysm are:

   1. Penetrating arterial trauma.
   2. Arteriography.
   3. Leakage from suture line following arterial surgery.

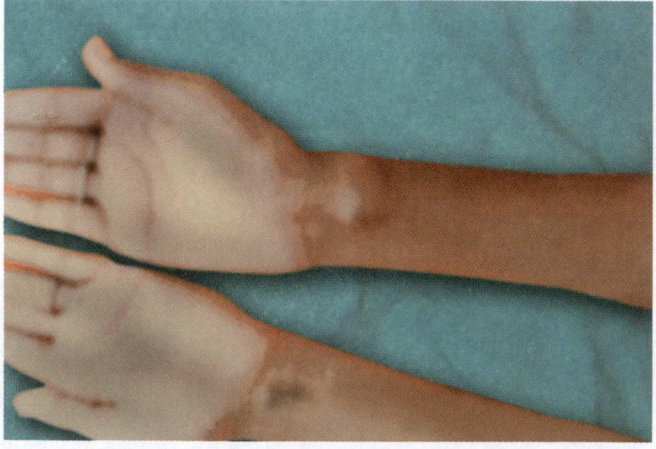

Fig. 4: Aneurysm of right radial artery

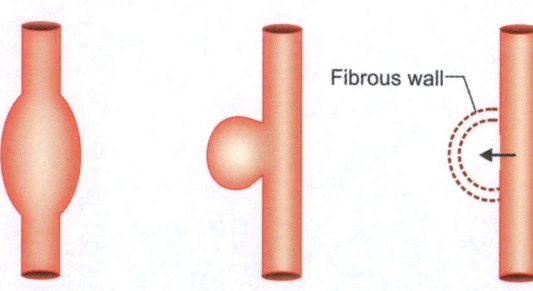

Fusiform aneurysm   Saccular aneurysm   Pseudo-aneurysm

Fig. 5: Types of arterial aneurysm

7. **What is a fusiform aneurysm?**
   It is a type of true arterial aneurysm where there is uniform expansion of the entire circumference of the artery in all the directions along its long axis. It is a spindle-shaped dilalation of the artery.

8. **What is a saccular aneurysm?**
   In this aneurysm there is a spherical expansion of a part of circumference of the arterial wall.

9. **What is a dissecting aneurysm?**
   In this aneurysm the blood stream dissects the wall of the artery in between the medial coat and adventitia. It usually affects aorta.

10. **What are the causes of dissecting aneurysm?**
    The causes of dissecting aneurysm are:
    - Availability of dissecting stress
      1. Systemic hypertension.
      2. Trauma.
      3. Pregnancy.
    - Availability of dissectable wall
      1. Atherosclerosis (atherosclerotic ulcer).
      2. Cystic medial necrosis.
      3. Marfan's syndrome.
      4. Ehlers-Danlos syndrome.
      5. Coarctation of aorta and bicuspid aortic valves.
      6. Aortic stenosis.
      7. Following surgery on aorta.

11. **What are the effects of an aneurysm?**
    The effects of aneurysm are:
    - Due to pressure on organs and structures in the vicinity
      1. Pressure on the vein results in venous congestion and phlebedema in the distal part, for example popliteal arterial aneurysm causing phlebedema of leg.
      2. Pressure on the nerves may cause pain, tingling, numbness and paralysis, for example an aortic aneurysm may cause aphonia by pressing the recurrent laryngeal nerve.
      3. Pressure (pulsation+pressure) on bones such as vertebral body, sternum and ribs may cause erosion or pressure atrophy.
      4. Pressure on other adjacent organs may cause symptoms related to those structures for example an aortic aneurysm may cause dysphagia by compressing the esophagus.
    - Due to distal ischemia
      Ischemia of structures distal to the site of aneurysm is a common manifestation. It is due to many reasons:
      1. Pressure of aneurysm on arterial branches in the vicinity of aneurysm.

2. Thrombosis with occlusion of ostia of emerging arteries.
3. Distal embolism from contained thrombus.
4. Dissection of arterial wall.
   Thus in a case of femoral or popliteal aneurysm the patient may have intermittent claudication, rest pain or gangrene of the toes.

12. **What are the complications of an aneurysm?**
    The complications are:
    1. Rupture and massive hemorrhage.
    2. Ischemia of structures distal to aneurysm.
    3. Pressure an adjacent organs.
    4. Infection.
    5. Thrombosis.
    6. Embolism.

13. **What is the cause of rupture?**
    The causes of rupture are:
    1. Trivial trauma.
    2. Manipulation or pressure.
    3. Spontaneous.

14. **What are the results of rupture?**
    It leads to massive hemorrhage. The patient complains of severe pain and goes quickly into shock and may die soon if nothing active is done.
    Following rupture the blood may go into many directions depending upon the site of aneurysm –
    - It may extravasate into surrounding tissues or tissue spaces, e.g. retroperitoneal hemorrhage, intracerebral hemorrhage.
    - It may rupture into a body cavity, e.g. peritoneal cavity (hemoperitoneum), or pleural cavity (hemothorax).
    - It may leak into a hollow organ, e.g. trachea (hemoptysis) or upper gastro-intestinal tract (hematemesis).

15. **What is the cause of infection in an aneurysm?**
    The source of infection is from the bacteria present in the blood.

16. **What is the result of infection?**
    The aneurysm is thrombosed and may result in an abscess.

17. **What is the danger in an aneurysm-abscess?**
    It may rupture spontaneously or drained surgically resulting in massive hemorrhage.

18. **How do you prevent this disaster?**
    If the patient presents with an abscess near a large artery, the diagnosis must be confirmed with a needle aspiration before drainage is done.

19. **Can an aneurysm have a spontaneous cure?**
    Yes, but rare. It may occur following thrombosis and later on fibrosis.

20. What are the conditions with which an aneurysm may be confused clinically?

The conditions are:

- A swelling over an artery
- A swelling under an artery
- A very vascular or pulsating tumor for example osteosarcoma, metastasis from renal cell carcinoma, aneurysmal bone cyst.

21. What is the example of swelling under the artery confused as an aneurysm?

The usual example is the subclavian artery pushed out by a bony boss of cervical rib.

22. How do you differentiate a swelling over an artery from an aneurysm?

The differences are given in following table:

Differentiating features	Aneurysm	Swelling over an artery
Type of pulsation in knee-elbow position	Expansile No change in pulsation	Transmitted Pulsation is lost or becomes less definite

23. What are the investigations?

The investigations are:

1. Plain X-ray.
2. Ultrasonography, CT scanning.
3. Arteriography.
4. Blood - Hemoglobin counts sugar, urea, creatinine, lipids, serological tests for syphilis.
5. Renal function tests.

24. What do you find in a plain X-ray?

- It may show soft tissue shadow and curvilinear calcification of arterial wall (Fig. 6).

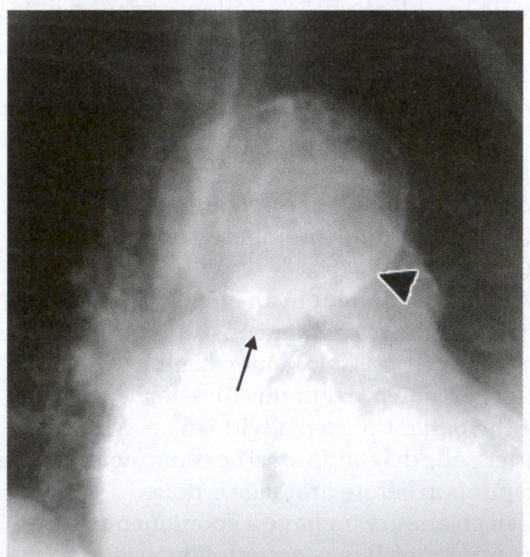

Fig. 6: Radiograph showing the shadow of aneurysm of arch of aorta (*Courtesy:* Dr SS Sarkar, Sarkar Diagnostics)

- There may be erosion or pressure atrophy of the bones in the contact with the aneurysm.

25. What is the role of ultrasound and CT scan?

They are of value to delineate the lesion clearly as the arteriography may not fully visualize, it is due to laminated blood clot.

26. What is the role of arteriography?

It reveals the aneurysm. Further, it shows the collaterals above and below the lesion.

27. What are the disadvantages of arteriography?

The disadvantages are:

1. It may not reveal the full size of aneurysm because of laminated intramural clot.
2. It is an invasive investigation and may result in bleeding and may result in bleeding and pseudo-aneurysm formation.

28. What is the role of MRI?

MRI is substituting the arteriography as it is now used to see the vasculature and detect associated arterial occlusive disease. The angiography shows the size of the lumen as the aneurysm is filled with a circumferential clot.

29. How do you treat an arterial aneurysm?

- An asymptomatic small aneurysm which is not growing rapidly, may be left as such and the patient is kept under ultrasonographic surveillance.
- A symptomatic aneurysm, a large aneurysm and an aneurysm with imminent rupture are operated.
- A ruptured aneurysm needs urgent and quick repair if the life has to be saved.

30. How do you treat a fusiform aneurysm?

It is treated by open surgical repair (EVAR, endovascular aneurysm repair) with a dacron or PTFE graft sutured end-to-end inside the opened aneurysmal sac or by a stent-graft through an arteriotomy (endoluminal procedure) (Fig. 7).

31. How do you treat a sacular aneurysm?

A saccular aneurysm with a narrow neck is excised with repair of vascular defect.

32. What are the indications of excision of an aneurysm?

A small peripheral aneurysm with good collateral circulation may be excised.

33. If collateral circulation is not good what will you do?

The arterial defect is repaired by a vein graft after excision of the aneurysm.

34. How do you treat distal arterial embolism?

It is treated by urgent intra-arterial thrombolysis.

35. How do you treat a popliteal artery aneurysm?

If the aneurysm is more than 25 mm in diameter, it is treated by bypass with ligation of the aneurysm or an inlay graft.

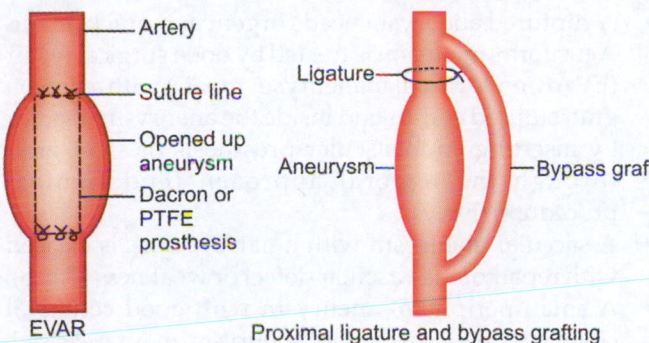

EVAR | Proximal ligature and bypass grafting

Fig. 7: Treatment of arterial aneurysm

36. **How do you treat an infected aneurysm?**
    Bypass clear of the infected area followed by excision of aneurysm may be the treatment of choice.
37. **How do you treat an iliac aneurysm?**
    It is treated by bypass and exclusion of the aneurysm by ligation above and below the dilatation.

DISCUSSION

An arterial aneurysm is a localized dilatation of an artery when it becomes 1.5 times of its normal diameter.

Etiology

The causes of aneurysm formation are:
- Atherosclerosis is the commonest cause (atherosclerotic aneurysm)
- Infections, e.g., bacterial aortitis can produce a mycotic aneurysm while syphilitic aortitis of late syphilis produces a thoracic aortic aneurysm
- Congenital, e.g. congenital or berry aneurysm.

Atherosclerosis—An imbalance of tissue metalloproteinases and metalloproteinase inhibitors is responsible for elastin and collagen degeneration. Genetic predisposition, inflammation and hemodynamic factors may also play a role.

Infection—The arterial wall is usually very resistant to infection but salmonella and treponema pallidum are capable of infecting the aortic wall (aortitis) to make it weak leading to formation of a mycotic aneurysm.

Marfan's syndrome is a systemic connective tissue disease having an autosomal dominant pattern of inheritance and diffuse medial abnormalities.

Pathology

An aneurysm can occur in any large or medium-sized artery but the abdominal aorta, and iliac and femoral arteries are most commonly affected. It has all the layers of arterial wall but they are thin.

Once the aneurysm develops it increases in size in tune with Laplace's law (T=RP, where T is tension on arterial wall, R is radius of artery and P is blood pressure). Increasing size and increasing pressure leads to its rupture, which is its most dreaded complication.

Morphologically, a true aneurysm is of two types—localized (saccular) and diffuse (fusiform). The first one occurs in the thoracic aorta and cerebral arteries, and the second one usually affects abdominal aorta and popliteal artery (Fig. 5).

Clinical Features

Age—Most of the aneurysms are seen in middle-aged or elderly persons.
Sex—They are somewhat more common in females.
Symptoms—It may be asymptomatic and may be detected as an incidental finding. It may present as a swelling or pain or may present when it has ruptured.
Signs—The swelling is smooth, tensely cystic and pulsatile.

Complications

1. Rupture—It results in massive bleeding which may kill the victim.
2. Thrombosis and distal embolism.
3. Compression or stretching of neighboring structures.

Investigations

- Plain radiography may show a soft tissue shadow with curvilinear calcification in its wall by which the size of the aneurysm can be measured.
- Ultrasound is the simplest way of detecting and accurately measuring the size of aneurysms.
- CT scan reveals the details of the aneurysm. It can be done using intravascular contrast. With CT, it is possible to generate three dimensional reconstruction of the vasculature. It is the main investigation to see intracranial and intrathoracic aneurysms.
- Arteriography shows the aneurysm with details of branching and the collaterals, especially when the operation is being planned. It shows the size of the lumen, as the aneurysm is filled with a circumferential clot.
- MR angiography using gadolinium is now used to see the vasculature and to detect the associated arterial occlusive disease.

Treatment

- An asymptomatic, small aneurysm, which is not growing rapidly, may be left as such but the patient is kept under ultrasonographic surveillance.

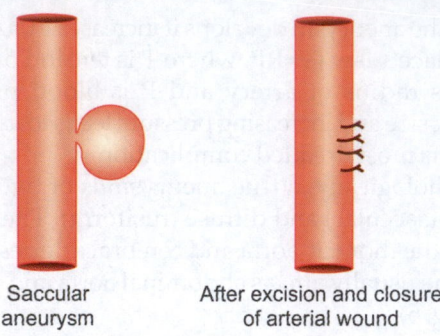

Saccular aneurysm   After excision and closure of arterial wound

Fig. 8: Treatment of a saccular aneurysm

- A symptomatic aneurysm, a large aneurysm and an aneurysm with imminent rupture are operated.

- A ruptured aneurysm needs urgent and quick repair. A fusiform aneurysm is treated by open surgical repair (EVAR, endovascular aneurysm repair) with a dacron graft sutured end-to-end inside the aneurysmal sac, or by inserting endovascular prosthesis or stent graft through the femoral approach (endoluminal procedure) (Fig. 7).
- A saccular aneurysm with a narrow neck is excised with repair of the vascular defect or weakness (Fig. 8).
- A small peripheral aneurysm with good collateral circulation, e.g. radial artery aneurysm, may be excised. If there are no collaterals, the artery is repaired by a vein graft after excision of the aneurysm.

The complications of the operation are bleeding, distal ischemia, endoleaks, prosthetic migration, thrombosis or rupture.

CASE 3: VARICOCELE

CLINICAL DIAGNOSIS

1. The patient is usually an adolescent or young adult who presents with a scrotal swelling with or without dragging pain in the scrotum.
2. The patient is usually tall and thin with a pendulous scrotum.
3. The hemiscrotum on the side of disease is elongated and hanging low.
4. In standing position an ill-defined swelling is felt behind and above the testis like a compressible bag of worms (Figs 9 and 10).
5. Cough impulse may be present.
6. When the patient lies down and the scrotum is elevated, the swelling disappears (not so when it is due to a left renal tumor).
7. On standing the swelling reappears and fills up from the bottom of scrotum.

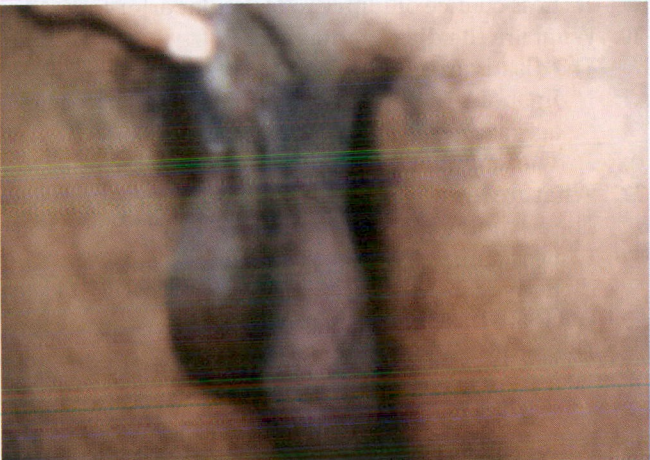

Fig. 9: Varicocele on left side—The left testis is hanging lower than right testis and prominent longitudinally running veins are visible

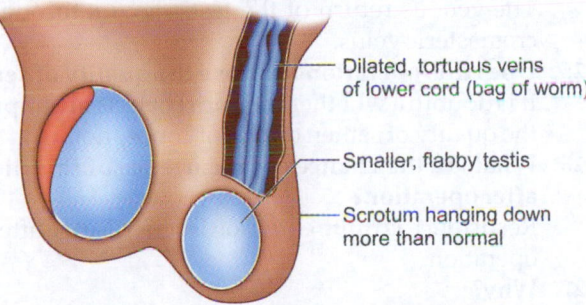

— Dilated, tortuous veins of lower cord (bag of worm)

— Smaller, flabby testis

— Scrotum hanging down more than normal

Fig. 10: Signs of left varicocele

8. If the swelling is held between the finger and thumb and the patient is asked to bow down, the tension within the swelling is reduced markedly (bow sign).
9. The testis may be smaller and softer than normal.

VIVA VOCE

1. **What is varicocele?**
   It is a varicose dilatation of the veins draining the testis (Fig. 10).
2. **What is the etiology of this condition?**
   Etiologically it is of two types:
   1. Primary or idiopathic where the cause is not known. It may be related to absence of valves near the termination of testicular veins.
   2. Secondary, e.g. obstruction of left testicular vein by a renal cell carcinoma.
3. **Why is this disease more common on the left side?**
   This disease is more common (95 percent) on the left side because of many reasons, i.e.
   1. The left testicular vein joins the left renal vein almost at right angle while the right vein joins the inferior vena cava at an acute angle.
   2. The left testicular vein is longer than right, hence it has to bear a long column of blood.
   3. The left-sided vein passes behind the left colon, and a loaded colon may compress the left testicular vein.
   4. The left renal vein is more likely to be obstructed than the right due to:
      - It may be sandwitched between abdominal aorta and trunk of superior mesenteric artery
      - The left testicular artery may be arching over the left renal vein (in 16 percent of persons).
      The left renal vein obstruction eventually hinders the venous return of left testicular vein.
4. **How do you clinically differentiate the primary from secondary varicocele?**
   They can be differentiated by:
   1. The primary varicocity disappears on elevating the scrotum of the patient lying down. This does not occur in a secondary varicocele.
   2. In primary varicocele there are no signs to explain for the cause while in secondary varicocele a cause may be clinically detectable, e.g. a renal lump on the left side.
5. **What is the mechanism of dragging pain?**
   Normally, the weight of testis is borne by scrotum and dartos. In varicocele, it is borne by cord which gives rise to dragging pain.

6. **How do you explain a positive bow sign?**
When the patient bows down, the tension in the varicocele becomes less as the bowing cuts off the continuity of blood inside the varicocele mass with that of testicular vein.

7. **What constitutes the pampiniform plexus of veins?**
The pampiniform plexus of veins consists of three groups of veins:
1. Veins from testis and epididymis.
2. Veins accompanying the vas deferens.
3. Cremasteric veins.

8. **How is carcinoma of left kidney related to varicocele?**
In carcinoma of left kidney, there may be obstruction of left testicular vein due to intraluminal extension of tumor into the left renal vein or thrombosis, as the left testicular vein drains into left renal vein.

9. **How can a varicocele harm its victim?**
A varicocele may disturb the temperature regulating function of scrotum thus reducing both the sperm count and motility. In long-standing cases, the testis is reduced in size and feels soft and flabby.

10. **What are the investigations?**
    - The varicocele can be visualized by Doppler probe
    - For detecting the cause, abdominal ultrasound, intravenous urography or CT scan may be done.

11. **How do you treat a varicocele?**
    - Asymptomatic varicocele does not need any treatment except reassurance and a scrotal suspensory bandage. A high Y front underpants may relieve the dragging pain
    - Symptomatic varicocele is usually treated by ligation of testicular vein.

12. **What are the indications for operation?**
The indications for operation are:
1. Unrelieved unbearable pain.
2. Subfertility.
3. When it is a bar to entry in some services.

13. **What are the approaches for operation?**
The approaches for operation are:
1. Inguinal approach.
2. Scrotal approach.
3. Abdominal extraperitoneal approach (Palomo operation).
4. Laparoscopic ligation.

14. **What do you do in inguinal approach?**
By an inguinal incision the spermatic cord is exposed, and the vas deferens, testicular artery and one or two veins are separated from the main mass of dilated veins. A two inch segment of dilated veins is excised and the cut ends are tied together to bring the testis to a higher level.

15. **What are the merits and demerits of this approach?**
The advantages are:
1. It is effective, convenient and a simple method of treatment.
2. The spermatic cord can be shortened to normal.
The disadvantage includes the chance of damage to testicular artery.

16. **What do you do in scrotal approach?**
Through a scrotal incision, the varicose veins are dissected down to the testis and excised subtotally.

17. **What are the disadvantages of scrotal approach?**
The disadvantages include:
1. Difficulty in dissection of veins.
2. Hemorrhage, scrotal hematoma.
3. Injury to testicular artery.

18. **What do you do in Palomo operation?**
The testicular vein is ligated above the inguinal ligament extraperitoneally where there is only one or two testicular veins.

19. **What are the advantages of Palomo operation?**
The advantages are:
1. The procedure is simple and easy.
2. Less chance of injury to testicular artery.

20. **What are the disadvantages?**
The disadvantages are:
1. In about 10 percent of patients, the varicocele is aggravated.
2. The length of spermatic cord cannot be reduced.

21. **What are the advantages of laparoscopic approach?**
The advantages are:
1. Less cutting of tissues, so pain is less.
2. Early recovery.

22. **What are the disadvantages?**
The disadvantages are:
1. It takes more time to do the procedure.
2. More facilities are required.

23. **If the testicular artery is damaged, how is the arterial supply to the testis maintained?**
In most of the cases the testis continues to get adequate blood supply through the artery to vas.

24. **What is the route of venous drainage of testis after ligation of testicular vein?**
The venous return of the testis occurs through the cremasteric veins.

25. **Does this operation improve the quality of semen?**
It is doubtful whether the varicocelectomy improves the quality of semen or rate of conception.

26. **What are the chances of recurrence of this disease after operation?**
Recurrence is quite common in this disease after any operation.

27. **Why?**
Because there are many collateral veins in this region.

DISCUSSION

Varicocele is a varicose dilatation of the veins draining the testis.

Etiology

The exact cause of this condition is not known. It may be something to do with the valves which are present near the termination of testicular veins. They are often absent.

The left testicular vein may be obstructed by a renal cell carcinoma of left kidney or after nephrectomy resulting in a varicocele in middle life or after.

Pathology

The veins of pampiniform plexus are dilated and tortuous. However, in many cases the dilated vessels are cremasteric veins and not part of the pampiniform plexus.
Oligospermia—Some patients of oligospermia have a varicocele and it is a common practice to blame this for infertility. The varicocele may disturb the temperature regulation function of scrotum which keeps the testis at some 2.5° C below rectal temperature. It is doubtful whether the varicocelectomy improves the quality of semen or rate of conception.

Clinical Features

Age—Most of the patients are abolescents and young adults.
Side—The left side is affected in 95 percent of cases.
Body build—Tall, thin men with pendulous scrotum are frequently affected, whereas short, fat individuals are rarely affected.

It may not cause any symptoms or there may be vague and annoying dragging pain which is relieved, if testis is supported by underwear. The symptoms are more troublesome in hot climates.

The scrotum on the affected side hangs lower than normal. It is enlarged and feels like a bag of worms. A cough impulse may be present.

When the patient lies down, the varicocele disappears. But when it is secondary to a renal tumor, it does not decompress in supine position.

The testis is normal in early stage but in long-standing cases, the affected testis is smaller and softer than the normal.

Varicocele is incriminated as a cause of infertility but statistical evidence is lacking.

Varicocele of Recent Onset

Varicocele of recent onset on the left side may be due to left renal cell carcinoma. Hence, the patient must be examined accordingly.

Varicocele of recent onset on the right side should raise the suspicion of retroperitoneal malignancy.

Intracaval spread and caval obstruction caused by a renal cell carcinoma may lead to bilateral varicocele of recent onset.

The renal veins and inferior vena cava can be seen by MRI.

Investigations

Doppler ultrasound—By this investigation, the varicocele can be visualized.
Ultrasound of abdomen—It should be done to rule out any space occupying lesion in the abdomen which might be compressing the testicular vein. It detects the tumors of the left kidney.
Intravenous urography—By this investigation, the tumors of the left kidney are diagnosed.

Treatment

Asymptomatic varicocele does not need any treatment except scrotal support and reassurance.

Operation is indicated when there are symptoms. The simplest operation is ligation of the testicular vein above the inguinal ligament behind the peritoneum where there is only one or two testicular veins. This operation can be done laparoscopically.

If facilities are available, embolization of testicular vein under radiographic guidance is the modern method of treatment. It is a minimally invasive method of treatment.

Results

Recurrence is common after any operation as there are many collateral veins in this region.

CASE 4: PHARYNGEAL POUCH (ZENKER'S DIVERTICULUM)

CLINICAL DIAGNOSIS

1. The patient is usually an elderly male who presents with gurgling noises in the neck during swallowing, regurgitation of undigested food during next meal or when the patient turns sides, dysphagia and may be swelling in the neck, of insidious onset.
2. The patient may be awakened from sleep by a feeling of suffocation followed by a violent fit of coughing.
3. There is a swelling usually to the left of midline in the neck. It is smooth, cystic, nontender, ill-defined and nonpulsatile (Fig. 11).
4. It is situated below the level of thyroid cartilage behind the sternomastoid.
5. It enlarges when the patient swallows some food.
6. It can be emptied by pressure with a palpable and audible gurgle.
7. Succussion splash may be present.

VIVA VOCE

1. **What is a pharyngeal pouch?**
   It is a protrusion or herniation of pharyngeal mucosa through Killian's dehiscence.
2. **What is Killian's dehiscence?**
   It is potentially a weak area in the posterior wall of pharynx at its lower end between two components of inferior constrictor of pharynx.
3. **What are the components of inferior constrictor of pharynx?**
   Inferior constrictor has two groups of muscle fibres -
   1. The upper fibres run obliquely upwards and backwards (thyropharyngeus).
   2. The lower fibres run horizontally backwards (cricopharyngeus).
4. **What is pharyngeal dimple?**
   It is a depression on the mucosal surface at the site of Killian's dehiscence.

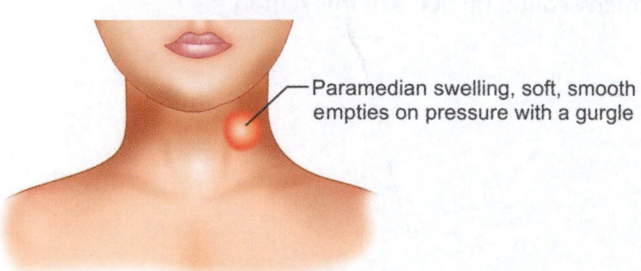

Fig. 11: Signs of a pharyngeal pouch

5. **How does a pharyngeal pouch develop?**
   The thyropharyngeus is propulsive while the cricopharyngeus is sphincteric and remains closed (contracted). The latter opens up when the former is propelling the food bolus down.
   Due to some neuromuscular imbalance, the lower component does not open up (achalasia) when the thyropharyngeus is propelling the food. Thus, the local intrapharyngeal pressure rises pushing the pharyngeal mucosa outside through the Killian's dehiscence (Fig. 12).
6. **What is the course of this pouch?**
   The pouch initially bulges in posterior midline but because of the presence of vertebral column it is deviated to one side, mostly to the left.
7. **What are the stages of this lesion?**
   As it grows a pharyngeal pouch is described to have 3 stages (Fig. 13):
   * *Stage 1 (stage of initial bulging):* The pouch is small, projects horizontally and has a vertical mouth. It is usually symptomless. Sometimes, the patient has a foreign body sensation in the throat
   * *Stage 2 (stage of well formed diverticulum)*—The pouch is large and globular. It projects obliquely downwards but the mouth is still vertical. It is symptomatic

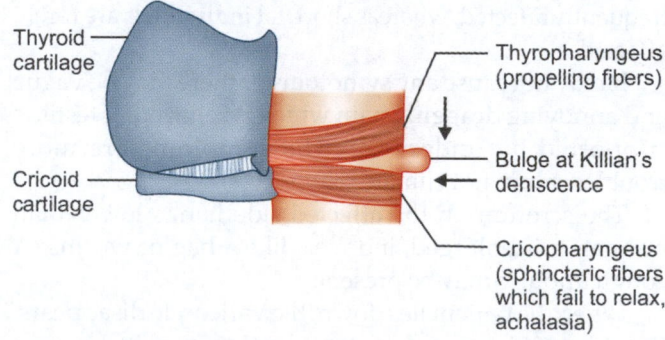

Fig. 12: Pathogenesis of pharyngeal pouch

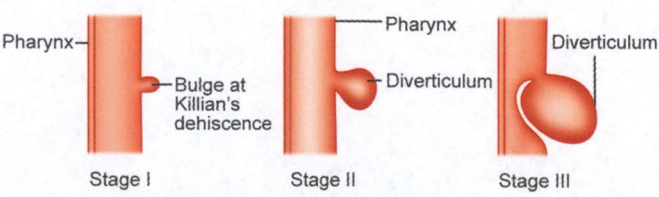

Fig. 13: Pharyngeal pouch

- *Stage 3 (stage of big diverticulum)*—The pouch becomes larger and its mouth becomes horizontal. The fundus of the pouch is big and dependent, hence may cause pressure symptoms.

8. **What type of diverticulum is the pharyngeal pouch?**
   It is a pulsion diverticulum.

9. **What are the differences between a pulsion and traction diverticulum?**
   The differences are given below:

Features	Pulsion diverticulum	Traction diverticulum
Size	May be large	Usually small
Neck	Narrow	Broad
Fundus	Wide	Narrow
Distal obstruction	Present	Absent
Adhesion	Not present	Present at the fundus
Site	Upper or lower third of esophagus	middle third of esophagus
Emptying	Stasis present	Empties well
Complications	Common	Rare
Type	True diverticulum	May be a pseudo-diverticulum

10. **What are the complications of this disease?**
    The complications are:
    - Due to stasis in the pouch:
      1. Diverticulitis.
      2. Peridiverticulitis.
      3. Cellulitis of neck.
      4. Mediastinitis.
      5. Abscess.
      6. Rupture.
      7. Pharyngeal fistula.
    - Due to aspiration of contents of pouch:
      1. Aspiration pneumonitis.
      2. Lung abscess.

11. **What are the investigations in this problem?**
    The investigations are:
    1. Barium swallow to see the pouch radiographically (Fig. 14).
    2. Video-fluoroscopic study.
    3. Chest X-ray.
    4. Routine investigations.

12. **What type of barium is used in barium swallow?**
    Thin type of barium should be given for swallowing.

13. **Why?**
    Because it is difficult for the thick barium to clear from the pouch.

14. **What are the views in which the radiography is done?**
    The radiography is done in anteroposterior and semilateral positions.

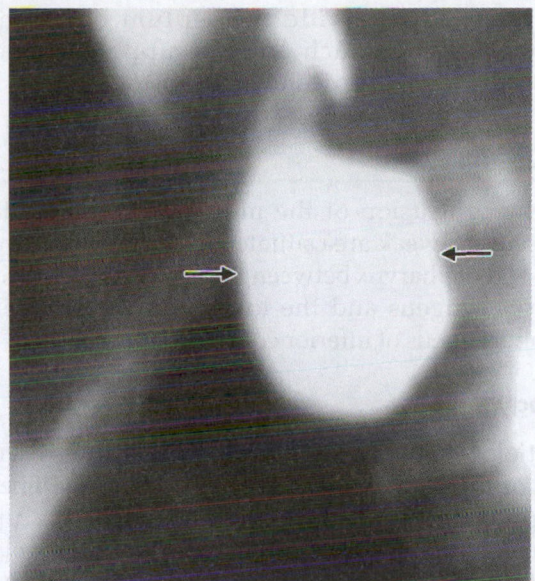

Fig. 14: Barium swallow, lateral view showing a pharyngeal pouch full with barium

15. **What are the radiographic signs?**
    The radiographic signs are:
    1. The pouch is seen filling up with the barium.
    2. It compresses the posterolateral wall of esophagus.
    3. The barium spills into esophagus from the top of the pouch and not from the floor when it fills up with barium.
    4. If the swelling is compresed, the barium is seen spilling into the esophagus.

16. **What is the role of endoscopy?**
    It is not required for detecting this lesion. Further, it may be dangerous as it may perforate the diverticulum.

17. **How do you treat this condition?**
    The essentials of the treatment are:
    - Stage 1 – No treatment is required
    - Stage 2 – Diverticulectomy
    - Stage 3 – Diverticulectomy which may be preceded by feeding gastrostomy.

18. **What are the complications of operation?**
    The complications are:
    - Wound infection
    - Mediastinitis
    - Pulmonary complications
    - Seroma, hematoma
    - Pharyngeal fistula.

19. **What is the endoscopic method of treatment?**
    Now, this disease in being treated by endoscopic linear cutting stapling gun which is passed per orally

and fired to divide the septum between the pharyngeal pouch and the upper esophagus producing a diverticuloesophagostomy.

DISCUSSION

It is the protrusion of the mucosa through Killian's dehiscence, a weak area situated in the posterior wall of lower end of pharynx between the upper oblique fibers of thyropharyngeus and the lower transverse fibers of cricopharyngeus of inferior constrictor of pharynx.

Etiology

The etiology is not clear. During swallowing when the fibers of thyropharyngeus are contracting the fibers of cricopharyngeus and circular fibers of the upper esophagus (upper esophageal sphincter, UES), relax to open the pharyngeal outlet. The pharyngeal pouch may form due to incomplete pharyngeal relaxation, early cricopharyngeal contraction and the abnormalities of pharyngeal contraction wave (cricopharyngeal achalasia).

Pathology

As the diverticulum (pulsion diverticum) comes out and grows in size, the vertebral column situated posteriorly causes it to turn laterally, usually to the left. As the disease progresses it passes through 3 stages:
- Stage 1—The pouch is small and is directed towards the vertebral column.
- Stage 2—The pouch is large and more globular. It's mouth lies in vertical plane.
- Stage 3—The pouch grows further and because of weight the mouth looks horizontally upwards.

Clinical Features

This disease is usually seen in patients more than 60 years of age. It is twice more common in males than females. Initially, it is asymptomatic and may be detected during the course of investigations for any other problem.

The symptomatic disease is characterized by a feeling of something in the throat (globus) and some regurgitation of food and drinks after swallowing (stage 1).

As the pouch increases in size, there is regurgitation of undigested food sometimes after a meal, especially when the patient bends down or turns over in the bed at night. The patient may get up from sleep with a feeling of tightness in the throat and a bout of coughing (stage 2).

As the diverticulum enlarges further in size, there may be gurgling noises in the neck during meals with appearance of a mass in the neck by the side of midline, usually on the left side. The lump may increase in size when the patient takes some food or drink. The patient may present with dysphagia due to extrinsic pressure of pouch on the food passage. The pouch may grow to a large size and may extend into the posterior mediastinum.

The swelling is intermittent appearing at the time of meal with a gurgle. It is smooth, soft and can be emptied by pressure, again with a gurgle.

Complications

- Aspiration pneumonitis, lung abscess
- Diverticulitis, peridiverticulitis, abscess
- Mediastinitis
- Pharyngeal fistula.

Investigations

Plain X-ray of the neck may show a gas shadow and fluid level in the neck.

Barium swallow—The patient is asked to swallow very thin emulsion of barium and radiographs are taken in anteroposterior and semilateral views. The fundus of the sac may be seen invading the mediastinum (Fig. 14).

In the anteroposterior picture the barium filled pouch looks as if a partial septum is obstructing the commencement of esophagus. In semilateral picture the barium is seen overflowing into the esophagus from the top of the pouch (not from the bottom).

The video-fluoroscopic study shows the pharyngeal contraction waves and the intergrity of upper esophageal sphincter.

Esophagoscopy in not required rather it may be dangerous as it may perforate the diverticulum resulting in cellulitis of neck and mediastinum.

Treatment

- Asymptomatic small pouch—No treatment is required
- Symptomatic pouch—Diverticulectomy is done.

The neck is opened with a crease incision at the level of cricoid and the sac is identified which is separated medially from the laryngopharynx and overlying thyroid. The middle thyroid vein is ligated and divided if present. The pouch is dissected up to its neck and excised, and the pharyngeal opening is closed in 2 layers. It is followed by cricopharyngeal myotomy to deal with achalasia. The complications of the operation are wound infection, hematoma, mediastinitis and pharyngeal fistula.

Now, this disease is being treated by endoscopic linear cutting stapling gun which is inserted through the mouth and fired to divide the septum between the diverticulum and the upper esophagus producing a diverticulo-esophagostomy.

Malignant Ulcers

CASE 1: BASAL CELL CARCINOMA (BCC)

CLINICAL DIAGNOSIS

1. The patient is usually a middle-aged or elderly person, commonly a male who presents with a nodule or a chronic ulcer of insidious onset (Fig. 1).
2. It is usually seen on the midportion of face above the line drawn from the angle of mouth to the ear lobule, the commonest site being around the medial canthus of eye ('tear drop' cancer) (Fig. 2).

3. When it is a nodule (nodular or button type):
   - There is a small, painless, slow growing nodule or button-like swelling which is somewhat indurated.
   - The edge is slightly elevated.
   - There may be a network of flery-red vessels on its surface.
   - It may have a pearly or gray-blue translucent color as if it is containing water (cystic type).
   - It may be a pigmented nodule.

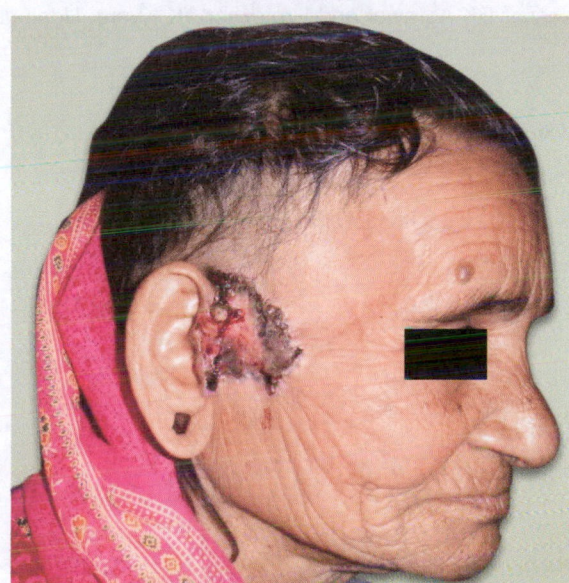

Fig. 1: Basal cell carcinoma of right parotid region (*Courtesy:* Professor Sandeep Kumar)

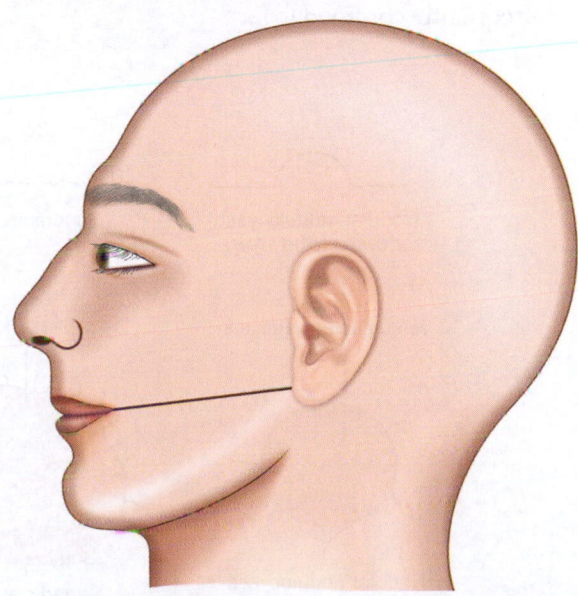

Fig. 2: Basal cell carcinoma commonly occurs above the line joining the angle of mouth with the lobule of the ear

4. When it is a chronic ulcer:
   I. a. The patient may present with a nonhealing ulcer of variable size which tends to burrow deeply (rodent ulcer) (Fig. 3).
      b. It tends to destroy the structures coming its way, i.e. nose, eyelids, pinna, skull, etc.
      c. It has an irregular shape and raised edge.
      d. It discharges serosanguineous fluid.
   II. a. The patient may present with a chronic lesion that is large, flat, superficial and serpiginous in shape.
      b. The edge is raised and beaded like a motor car tyre and actively spreading into the neighboring areas (field fire).
      c. The central area appears inactive and healed but never heals, and keeps scabbing over and breaking down.
      d. It discharges serosanguineous fluid.
5. It may be single or multiple.
6. The regional lymph nodes are not enlarged.

VIVA VOCE

1. **What is basal cell carcinoma?**
   It is a malignant tumor arising from basal cell layer of epidermis.
2. **Can it arise from any other cell?**
   Yes, it can also arise from basal cells of hair follicles and sweat glands.
3. **What is the cause of this cancer?**
   The exact cause is not known. The risk factors are:
   • Chronic sun exposure that is why the lesion is frequently confined to face

• Inorganic arsenic exposure (arsenical dermatitis)
• Light complexion as it is more common in fair skin persons and red heads. It is seldom seen in dark skin people.

4. **What are the macroscopic types?**
   There are many macroscopic types of basal cell carcinoma (Fig. 4):
   1. *Localized type:* Nodular, nodulocystic, cystic, pigmented and nevoid.

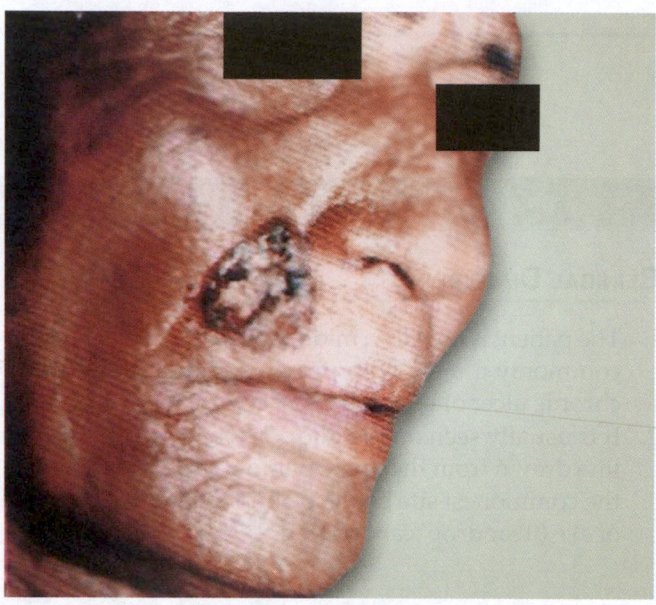

Fig. 3: Basal cell carcinoma (rodent ulcer) (*Courtesy:* Professor RK Agrawal and Professor AK Khare, Udaipur)

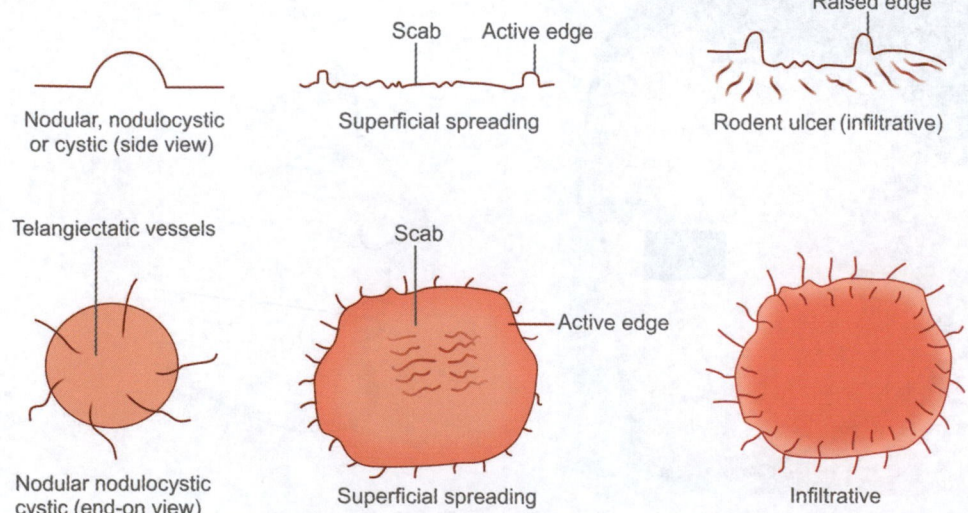

Fig. 4: Types of basal cell carcinoma

2. *Generalized type:*
  • Superficial—Multifocal and superficial spreading ('field-fire' type)
  • Infiltrative—Morpheic, ice pick and cicatrizing.

5. **Why one of its types is called as rodent ulcer?**
The common ulcerative form of this cancer *gnaws* the neighboring tissues like a rodent (a type of rat) and destroys deeper tissues like muscle, cartilage and bone producing severe disfigurement.

6. **What is 'field-fire' type lesion?**
It is called as 'field-fire' type cancer because it is active and spreading at the edge and healing in the center, i.e. spreading centrifugally like 'field-fire'.

7. **What are the constituents of the 'scab' of a 'field-fire lesion'?**
It consists of dry serum and epithelial cells.

8. **What is the character of fluid in the cystic type lesion?**
The cystic type appears as if it contains water but it is a solid lesion.

9. **What is a 'tear-drop' cancer?**
This cancer commonly occurs in the region of the face where the tears roll down, i.e. near the medial canthus and nasolabial fold.

10. **What are the microscopic features of this cancer?**
  • It is composed of closely packed islands of uniform basophilic epithelial cells disposed in rounded masses or columns set in a stroma of cellular connective tissue.
  • The peripheral cells are columnar, more deep staining and have a palisade arrangement, and the central cells are polyhedral. Prickle cells and cell nests are absent.

11. **How does this cancer kill its victim?**
The patient dies due to:
1. Meningitis caused by direct intracranial extension
2. Hemorrhage due to erosion of a major blood vessel.

12. **What is sclerosing or morphea carcinoma?**
It is an uncommon type of basal cell carcinoma consisting of elongated strands of basal cells that infiltrate the dermis, with the intervening corium being unusually compact. The lesion is usually flat, whitish or waxy and firm, and looks like localized scleroderma.

13. **How does this tumor spread?**
It is locally malignant and erodes into the neighboring tissues. It does not spread by lymphatics and very rarely by blood stream.

14. **What are the investigations?**
  • Shave or punch biopsy under local anesthesia is the main investigation which confirms the diagnosis.
  • If there is suspicion of involvement of bone, radiography of the part is required.

15. **How do you treat this cancer?**
Surgery is the main method or treatment of choice. The other methods of treatment are radiotherapy, topical 5-fluorouracil, cryosurgery and curettage and electrodesiccation.

16. **What is the surgical treatment of a BCC?**
As this cancer is located commonly in the areas where one must try to maximize conservation of surrounding normal tissue and minimize the chances of recurrence. This aim of treatment is achieved by Mohs' micrographic surgery.

17. **What is Mohs' micrographic surgery?**
It is the excision of the tumor under microscopic control followed by flap reconstruction after confirmation of clear margin.

18. **Can you find the margin of the tumor preoperatively?**
The margin of the tumor can be assessed and marked under loupe magnification. It varies between 2 to 15 mm depending upon the gross appearance of the tumor.

19. **What is the technique of Mohs' surgery?**
Under local anesthesia saucerising excision of the visible tumor is done and the excised tissue and the defect are marked and orientated. A map of excised tissue is made which is then examined histologically for the presence of cancer and more tissue is removed from the corresponding area in the wound. Thus, the wound is completely cleared off the tumor from the lateral and deep margins (more than 99% tumor is removed).

20. **What are the results of Mohs' surgery?**
If the cancer is completely excised it gives 90 percent cure rate, But if the margins are grossly involved the recurrence rate is 67 percent, and 33 percent if there is microscopic involvement.

21. **What are the indications of Mohs' surgery?**
Mohs' surgery is appropriate for tumors of the eyelids, nasolabial folds, canthi, pinna, temple, recurrent cancers and cancers of other areas of cosmetic importance.

22. **What is the role of wide excision?**
  • It can be done if the cancer is situated in the areas where more tissue can be sacrificed, e.g. chest or back of the trunk.
  • Deeper infiltrative and morphea type of lesions, especially when bone is involved, are also treated by wide excision.
  • A radio-recurrent cancer is best treated by wide excision.

23. **What do you mean by wide excision?**
    It is the three dimensional excision which is 3 to 5 mm beyond the edge of the tumor through the healthy tissues.

24. **What are the indications for radiotherapy?**
    It is indicated in patients of over 65 years of age who are not fit for surgery.

25. **What are the results of radiotherapy?**
    It is curative in 90 percent of patients.

26. **What are the disadvantages of radiotherapy?**
    The disadvantages of radiotherapy are:
    1. It a very expensive method of treatment.
    2. It leaves behind a bad scar.
    3. The radiorecurrent tumors are more difficult to treat and may be more aggressive.

27. **How do you treat an early superficial cancer?**
    It can be treated by topical 5-FU, imiquimod, cryosurgery.

28. **What do you do in curettage and electrodesiccation?**
    The lesion with 2 to 3 mm around is curetted under local anesthesia, and the wound is desiccated with an electrosurgical unit to destroy the residual lesion. Usually 3 cycles are required. The wound heals by granulation tissue in 4 to 6 weeks.

29. **What is the role of curettage and electrodesiccation?**
    It is not recommended for head and neck lesions as it leaves a bad scar, but it is a simple, quick and inexpensive method.

DISCUSSION

Basal cell carcinoma (BCC) is a malignant neoplasm of pleuripotent epithelial cells originating from basal epidermis and hair follicles. Therefore, it affects the pilosebaceous skin. 95 percent of BCCs occur at 40 to 80 years of age, and more commonly in males.

Etiology

It is not known exactly. The risk factors are:
1. Chronic sun exposure—The most important risk factor is chronic exposure to ultraviolet rays. Hence, its incidence rises with proximity to equator and the lesion is mostly confined to the face. In 90 percent of patients it occurs above the line joining the angle of mouth to the lobule of the ear, the commonest site being around the inner canthus of the eye.
   This cancer is common in people who work on the sea (seamen's disease) as their face is exposed whole day to dual exposure—direct exposure and the reflected light from sea surface.
2. Exposure to arsenicals, coal tar and aromatic hydrocarbons.
3. Complexion of skin—It is more common in fair skin people and red heads. It is seldom seen in dark skins.

Pathology

Gross appearance—Depending upon the gross appearance this tumor is divided into many types (Fig. 3).

The nodular and nodulocystic types having a central scab or erosion account for 90 percent of patients. There is a waxy, "pearly" appearance with telangiectatic vessels easily visible. It is the pearly or translucent appearance that is most diagnostic, a feature best seen if the local skin is stretched.

Micropathology—There are densely packed islands of darkly stained cells which extend down from the epidermis, though no connection with the epidermis may be seen. The peripheral cells of the islands are more deeply staining and have palisade-like arrangement. It is only this outer layer of cells which divides actively. There is no keratinization, no pickle cells and no mitotic figures.

Spread

This cancer grows slowly attaining a size of 1 to 2 cm or more in diameter, usually only after many years of growth. As it grows, it ulcerates, invades and gnaws the local tissues like a rodent. Hence, it is called rodent ulcer. It is a locally malignant tumor and does not produce metastases.

Investigations

1. Biopsy—A lesion suspected to be a BCC should be biopsied by shave or punch to confirm the diagnosis.
2. X-ray of the affected part if there is clinical suspicion of involvement of the bone.

Treatment

- **Surgery:** Surgical excision is the treatment of choice. As the tumor is situated commonly in the areas where one must try to maximize conservation of the surrounding normal tissue and minimize the chances of recurrence, one must be careful in sacrificing the tissues. The margin of the tumor is assessed and marked under loupe magnification. It varies between 2 to 15 mm depending upon the gross tumor type.
  Mohs' micrographic surgery—It is the excision of the tumor under microscopic control followed by flap reconstruction after confirmation of clear margin under local anesthesia. 'Saucerising excision' of the visible tumor is done and the excised specimen and the wound are marked and orientated. A map of the excised tissue is made and it is studied histologically for the presence of cancer and more tissue is removed from the corresponding area in the wound. Thus, the wound is

completely cleared of the tumor from the lateral and deep margins (more than 99 percent clearance). The wound is closed with a flap.

The results of complete excision are good (90% cure rate), but if the margins are grossly involved there is 67 percent recurrence rate, and 33 percent if there is microscopic involvement.

Mohs' surgery is appropriate for tumors of the eyelids nasolabial fold, canthi, pinna, temple, recurrent cancers and cancers of other areas of cosmetic importance.

- **Radiotherapy:** It can be given in patients over 65 years of age otherwise unfit for surgery. It cures 90 percent of lesions. The disadvantages of radiotherapy are:
  1. The radiorecurrent tumors are more difficult to treat and may be more aggressive.
  2. It is the most expensive method of treatment.
  3. It leaves behind a bad scar.
- **Other methods of treatment:**
  1. Superficial cancers can be treated by topical 5-fluouracil, imiquimod or cryotherapy.
  2. Three cycles of curettage and electrodesiccation. It is not recommended for head and neck lesions.

Results

The results of Mohs' surgery are good. It is nearly curative but it is a time consuming procedure.

About 50 percent of patients are likely to develop a second lesion. Hence, the patients are followed-up to detect a new or recurrent tumor for early management.

CASE 2: CUTANEOUS SQUAMOUS CELL CARCINOMA (CSCC)

CLINICAL DIAGNOSIS

1. The patient is usually a middle-aged or elderly person who presents with a nodule, a non-healing ulcer or an ulcerated swelling of insidious onset.

2. It can occur anywhere in the skin, especially dorsum of hand, face and extremities, or junctional areas, e.g. lip, penis, vulva, and anus.

3. When it presents as a nonhealing ulcer:
   • It is irregular in shape, size and surface.
   • The edge is everted (Figs 5 and 6).
   • The base is indurated.

4. When it presents as an ulcerated swelling:
   • It is sessile.
   • The surface is irregular with bosselation and fungation giving a cauliflower like appearance (Fig. 6).

5. It may rarely present as a hard and irregular nodule or mass, or an indurated fissure.

6. It may be friable and bleed on touch.

7. The regional lymph nodes:
   • Not enlarged in early disease.
   • Enlarged mild to moderate in size, hard, mobile and nontender
   • Enlarged moderate to massive in size, hard, fixed to underlying structures or overlying skin and tender or nontender (late disease).

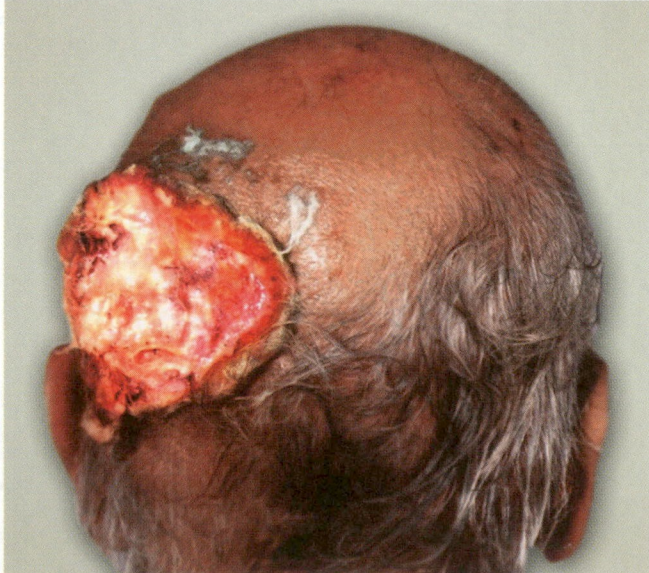

Fig. 5: Squamous cell carcinoma of scalp. The eversion of the edge can be seen (*Courtesy:* Professor Rajiv Agarwal)

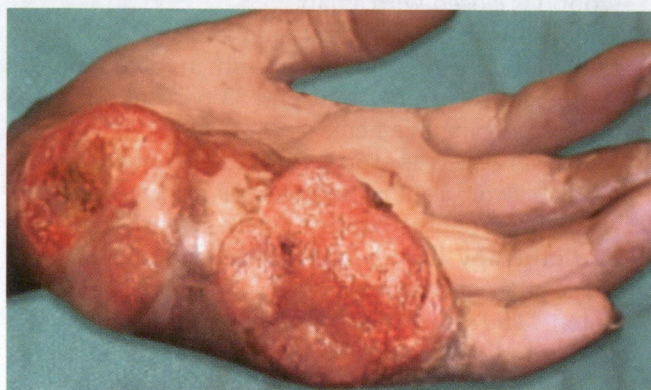

Fig. 6: Squamous cell carcinoma of palm (*Courtesy:* Professor Sandeep Kumar)

VIVA VOCE

1. **What is cutaneous squamous cell carcinoma (CSCC)?**
   It is a malignant neoplasm of keratinizing cells of the epidermis or its appendages, and also of the stratum basale of the epidermis of complex etiology, and characterized by a nonhealing ulcer or an ulcerated mass.

2. **What is the incidence of this cancer?**
   • It is the second most common skin cancer after basal cell carcinoma. It is four times less common than the basal cell cancer.
   • It is usually seen in elderly persons.

3. **What is the cause of this cancer?**
   1. Cumulative sun exposure—This cancer is strongly related to chronic actinic skin damage. It is twice as common in men and in whites living near the equator.
   2. SCC can occur in chronic sinus tracts, e.g. chronic osteomyelitis, fistula tracts, e.g. anorectal fistula, and ulcers, e.g. venous ulcer.
   3. Pre-existing scars—Here the SCC is known as a Marjolin's ulcer.
   4. Vaccination points.
   5. Immunosuppression—It is common in organ-transplant recipients.
   6. Radiation exposure—The time of onset of the cancer is related to the wave length of radiation.
   7. Chemical carcinogens, e.g. arsenicals, tar.
   8. Viral infection with HPV 5 and HPV 16.
   9. Tobacco use—It doubles the risk.
   10. Others examples are senile keratosis, actinic keratosis, lupus vulgaris, xeroderma pigmentosum, and chronic exposure to heat, e.g. kangri cancer of abdominal wall of Kashmiris,

Kang cancer of buttocks, heels and elbows in Tibetans.

4. What is Bowen's disease?

It is a type of endo-epidermal carcinoma in which dyskeratosis and intracellular vacuolation occurs. It is characterized by single or multiple brownish or reddish plaques on the skin, often on covered surfaces.

5. What is erythroplasia of Queyrat?

It is almost identical to Bowen's disease clinically and histologically, but is confined to glans penis and vulva, where the lesion appears as red, velvety, irregular and slightly raised plaque.

6. What is senile keratosis?

It is a lesion of the skin or mucocutaneous junction occurring in elderly people in which the epidermis is usually atrophic and shows hyperkeratosis and parakeratosis. It is more frequently a form of actinic keratosis than it is due merely to old age.

7. What is actinic keratosis?

A premalignant lesion caused by much exposure to sunlight or actinic rays.

8. What is lupus vulgaris?

It is a granulomatous type of cutaneous tuberculosis characterized by 'apple jelly' granules.

9. What is xeroderma pigmentosum?

A disease of skin which commences in infancy or very early childhood, involves chiefly the exposed parts, and is characterized at first by erythema and vesiculation after exposure to sunlight, followed by freckle-like pigmentation and telangiectasis, later by superficial ulceration, warty growths and formation of small areas of atrophy and finally by squamous cell carcinoma and death.

10. What are the gross types of SCC?

Grossly it is of three types (Fig. 7):

1. Smooth nodular lesion.
2. Verrucous, papillomatous or proliferative lesion.
3. Ulcerative lesion.

   All these types ulcerate as they grow with the passage of time.

11. What are the microscopic features?

This cancer consists of solid columns of epithelial cells which grow down into the dermis separated from one another by connective tissue. They expand into bulb-like masses which on section may appear detached. Later, the cells in the center being the oldest

degenerate and change into a structureless hyaline mass of keratin (keratinization), which looks red with eosin stain. It is surrounded by normal looking squamous cells presenting the characteristic 'prickle cell appearance arranged in concentric manner like onion skin. This whole structure is called cell nest or 'epithelial pearl' which is a characteristic feature of a squamous cell carcinoma.

12. What are ' cell nests' ?

'Cells-nests' are spherical structures with some hyaline structureless mass of keratin in the center surrounded by epithelial cells in a concentric manner giving onion peel like appearance.

13. How does a 'cell-nest' develop?

The epithelial cells of epidermis proliferate into the dermis in columns separated from one another by the connective tissue. Later, the central cells degenerate into keratin.

14. What do the 'cell-nests' indicate?

The presence of 'cell-nests' indicates that:

1. The tumor is relatively slowly growing.
2. There is a high degree of cell differentiation.
3. It is poorly radiosensitive.

15. Do you know of some tumors other than squamous carcinoma where cell-nests are present?

The tumors are:

1. Pleomorphic adenoma of parotid.
2. Teratoma of testis.

16. What is the special staining characteristic of this cancer?

This cancer stains positive for cytokeratins 1 and 10.

17. What are the special points which are to be included in the histopathological report?

The histopathological report of this cancer should include the following:

- Pathological pattern, e.g. adenoid
- Cellular morphology, e.g. spindle
- Broders grade
- Depth of invasion, including perineural or vascular invasion
- Deep and peripheral margin clearance.

18. What is Broders grading?

Depending upon the degree of anaplasia and the number of mitotic figures SCC is of four grades:

- Grade I—Upto 25 percent cells are undifferentiated
- Grade II—25 to 50 percent cells are undifferentiated
- Grade III—50 to 75 percent cells are undifferentiated
- Grade IV—More than 75 percent cells are undifferentiated.

For practical purposes the SCC is of three grades.

- G1—Low grade
- G2—Moderately differentiated
- G3—High grade or anaplastic.

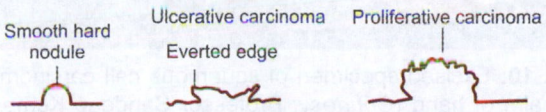

Fig. 7: Three gross types of SCC

19. **What is the difference in the histological picture depending upon the grade of malignancy?**

In low grade cancers, the individual cells may be quite well differentiated resembling uniform mature squamous cells having intercellular bridges. Keratinization may be present and the layers of keratinizing squamous cells may produce 'cell-nests', 'horny-pearls' or 'epithelial pearls'.

In tumors of high grade malignancy, the epithelial cells may be extremely atypical, abnormal mitotic figures are common, intercellular bridges are not present and keratinization does not occur.

20. **What are the modes of origin?**

The modes of origin are:

1. Arising de novo from normal skin.
2. Secondary to some pre-existing lesion of skin like actinic keratosis, scar of burn.

21. **How does this tumor spread?**

This cancer spreads by:

1. Local infiltration by continuity and contiguity into the local tissues or structures.
2. Lymphatic spread by both embolism and permeation into the local or regional nodes.
3. Hematogenous spread is rare and late.

22. **What are the investigations?**

Apart from routine investigations the most important investigation is biopsy.

If the regional lymph nodes are enlarged FNAC or biopsy may be done.

23. **What is the TNM staging of SCC?**

T	—	Tumor
T1	—	Less than 2 cm in size
T2	—	2 to 5 cm
T3	—	More than 5 cm
T4	—	Muscle or bone invasion
N	—	Nodes
N0	—	No nodal metastases
N1	—	Nodal metastases present
M	—	Distant metastasis
M0	—	No metastasis
M1	—	Distant metastasis present.

24. **How do you treat this cancer?**

This cancer is treated by surgical excision which is the main method of treatment, or radiotherapy.

25. **What is the nature of surgical excision?**

Usually two types of surgical excisions are employed:

1. Three dimensional wide excision—The tumor is excised beyond the visible and palpable margin of the lesion in all the three dimensions. The margins of primary depend on the surface size. This is further assessed by surgical loupe magnification. If the tumor measures less than

2 cm across a 4 mm clearance margin is achieved. If it measures more than 2 cm, a 1 cm clearance margin is achieved (Figs 6, 8, 9 and 10).

2. Amputation—The tumors of the limbs involving bone, tendons, muscle or neurovascular bundle, or of the penis are usually treated by amputation of the affected part.

26. **What instruction will you give to the pathologist who will examine the excised specimen?**

Apart from doing the accurate histology the margins of excision are to be seen for any evidence of disease.

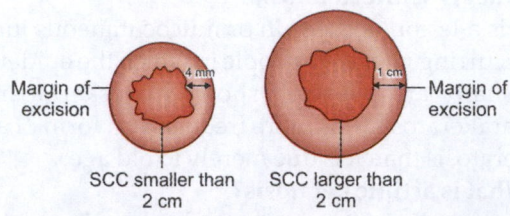

Fig. 8: Surgical treatment of cutaneous SCC

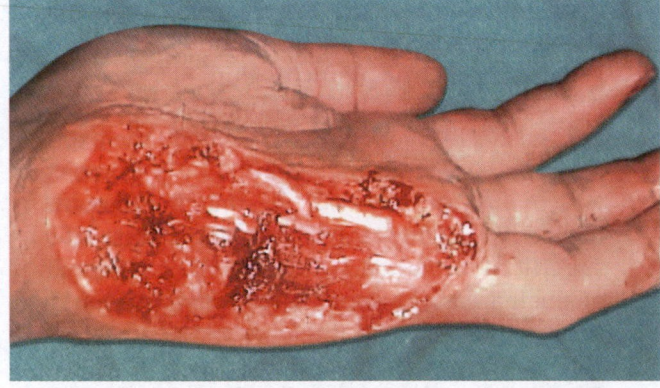

Fig. 9: Hand after wide excision of a squamous cell carcinoma (*Courtesy:* Professor Sandeep Kumar)

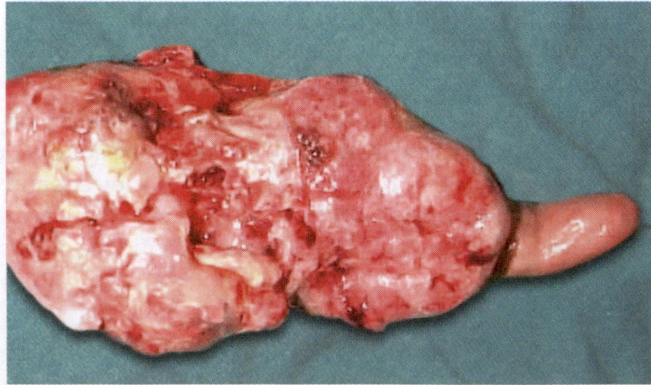

Fig. 10: Excised specimen of squamous cell carcinoma of palm of hand (*Courtesy:* Professor Sandeep Kumar)

27. **What are the indications of radiotherapy?**
The indications are:
1. Early lesions—It is curative in more than 80 percent of cases without mutilation.
2. Late lesions—When surgery is not possible, for palliation.

28. **What are the methods of radiotherapy?**
The methods are:
1. Superficial radiotherapy.
2. Deep X-ray therapy.
3. Electron beam.
4. Iridium implants or moulds.

29. **What are the contraindications of radiotherapy?**
They are:
1. Tumors of pinna or nose for fear of radionecrosis of cartilage.
2. When bone is involved for fear of osteonecrosis.
3. Lesions are very near the eye for fear of damage to the eye.
4. Carcinoma of scalp for fear of permanent alopecia.

30. **How do you treat local/regional lymph nodes?**
The essentials of treatment are:
1. If the nodes are not palpable, the patient is kept in regular follow up or the involvement is detected by sentinel node biopsy.
2. If the nodes are palpable or subsequently become palpable a biopsy is done. If it shows metastasis, a block dissection is carried out.
3. If the nodes are enlarged and fixed to the surrounding structures palliative radiotherapy is given.

31. **What are the factors that determine the prognosis?**
The prognosis depends upon invasion (local, perineural and vascular), Broders grade, site, etiology and the immunological status of the patient.

32. **How does the prognosis depend on invasion?**
Invasion is the most important factor on which prognosis depends:
- Depth of the lesion—If the depth is less than 2 mm the metastasis is highly unlikely. If it is more than 6 mm, 15 percent of cancers will have metastasized.
- Surface area—If the lesion is larger than 2 cm, the prognosis is worse than in a smaller one.
- A tumor with a perineural invasion has a worse prognosis as compared to noninvolving tumor.

33. **How does the site modify the prognosis?**
- Cancers of the lips and pinna have a higher local recurrence rate than tumors of other places.
- Cancers of the limbs are worse than those of the trunk.

34. **How is the prognosis related to the etiology?**
The carcinomas that occur in oteomyelitic skin sinuses, chronic ulcers and irradiated skin areas have a higher metastatic potential.

35. **How is the prognosis related to immunosuppression?**
In patients with immunosuppression, the tumor is more invasive.

36. **What is the prognosis?**
- Small early low-grade cancers have a very good prognosis.
- The metastases usually occur to the regional nodes. The overall rate of metastasis in 2 percent.
- 95 percent of local recurrence and regional metastases occur within 5 years.

37. **What is the duration of follow-up?**
The follow-up is not required beyond 5 years.

DISCUSSION

Squamous cells carcinoma (SCC) is a malignant neoplasm of the keratinizing cells of the epidermis or its appendages, of complex etiology and characterized by a nonhealing ulcer or a proliferative mass. It can also arise from the stratum basale of the epidermis.

Etiology: The etiology is not exactly known, but the risk factors are:
1. *Exposure to sunlight*—It is strongly related to cumulative sun exposure and cutaneous damage (actinic keratosis). Hence, it is twice as common in men and in white skinned persons living near the equator than others.
2. *Chronic inflammations*—This cancer can occur in a chronic sinus tract of osteomyelitis, fistula tract of an ano-rectal fistula, pre-existing scars, burns, vaccination points, lupus vulgaris and venous ulcer.
3. *Immunosuppression*—It can occur in organ-transplant recepients.
4. *Radiation exposure*—It is one of the complications of chronic radiation damage and the time taken to develop the lesion is proportional to the wave length of radiation.
5. Chemical carcinogens, e.g. arsenicals, tar.
6. Infection with HPV5 and HPV16.
7. *Tobacco*—The chronic tobacco-use (current and previous) doubles the relative risk of cutaneous squamous cell cancer.
8. Chronic thermal injury, e.g. Kangri cancer of abdominal wall of Kashmiris and Kang cancer of buttocks, heels and elbows of Tibetans.

Pathology

Sites of occurrence—This cancer can occur at any place where there is squamous epithelium. However, the common sites are:

1. Dorsum of hand, face, extremities.
2. Junction of skin and mucous membrane, e.g. lip, nostril, eyelid, penis, vulva.

Gross appearance—This tumor may vary from a smooth hard nodule to a proliferative or ulcerative lesion. However, all gross types eventually ulcerate as they grow with passage of time (Fig. 7).

Origin—Depending upon the method of origin this cancer is of two types:

1. De novo from the skin.
2. Secondary to some pre-existing lesion of skin like leukoplakia, scar of burn.

This cancer arises from the prickle cell layer of epidermis.

Microscopic appearance—This tumor contains solid columns of epithelial cells which grow down into the dermis separated from one another by connective tissue. They expand into bulb like masses which on section may appear detached. Later, the cells in the center being the oldest degenerate and change into a structureless hyaline mass of keratin (keratinization), which looks red with eosin stain. It is surrounded by normal looking squamous cells presenting the characteristic 'prickle cell' appearance and are arranged in a concentric manner like onion skin. This whole structure is called 'cell nest' or 'epithelial pearl', which is a characteristic feature of epidermoid carcinoma, but may be absent in a rapidly, growing carcinoma.

This carcinoma almost always shows infiltration of dermis by chronic inflammatory cells especially plasma cells which may be an immune defensive phenomenon.

This cancer stains positive for cytokeratins 1 and 10.

Spread of Disease

1. Infiltration by continuity and contiguity into the local tissues.
2. Lymphatic spread occurs by both embolism and permeation into the local or regional lymph nodes. The lymph node involvement depends upon the site of primary. It is late in cancers of hand, and early in cancers of foot, face and neck.
3. Hematogenous spread is uncommon and occurs late.

Clinical Features

1. The patient is usually a middle-aged or elderly person who presents with a smooth hard nodule, non-healing ulcer or an ulcerated swelling of insidious onset. It is four times less common than a basal cell carcinoma.
2. It can occur anywhere in the skin especially dorsum of hand, face and extremities.
3. When it presents as a nonhealing ulcer:
   - It is irregular in shape, size and surface
   - The edge is everted
   - The base is indurated.
4. When it presents as an ulcerated swelling:
   - It is sessile
   - The surface is irregular with bosselation and fungation giving a cauliflower like appearance.
5. It may rarely present as a hard and irregular nodule or mass, or an indurated fissure.
6. It may be friable and may bleed on touch.
7. The regional lymph nodes are:
   - Not enlarged in early disease
   - Enlarged, mild to moderate in size, hard, mobile and non-tender, or
   - Enlarged, moderate to massive in size, hard, fixed to underlying structures or overlying skin and tender or nontender.

The lymph node enlargement may be due to secondary infection or metastasis. In about 33 percent of cases, the enlargement is due to secondary infection and usually subsides after treatment of primary cancer. But palpable nodes should be taken as malignant until proved otherwise.

Investigations

1. Biopsy from the edge of the lesion, may be done under local anesthetic. The biopsy report should include information on the pathological pattern, e.g. adenoid, shape of the cells, e.g. spindle shaped, the Broders grade and the depth of invasion and evidence of perineural or vascular invasion.
2. FNAC of enlarged nodes to confirm for metastasis. The nodes may also be biopsied.
3. Chest X-ray, if there is suspicion of hematogenous spread.
4. CT scan—To find out the extent of disease, especially the nodal involvement or if there is local infiltration into muscles and or bone.

Treatment

- **Primary cancer**
  i. *Surgery*—It is the treatment of choice for most of the cancers, and wide excision should be performed, with some normal tissue in three dimensions

surrounding the tumor. The margins of excision are marked depending on the surface size. Ideally it should be confirmed by surgical loupe magnification.

If the tumor measures less than 2 cm across, a 4 mm clearance margin should by achieved.

If it measures more than 2 cm, a 1 cm clear margin should be the aim (Figs 6, 8, 9 and 10)

The surgical specimen is sent for detailed histopathology especially to see the margin of clearance. If the cancer is involving a finger or toe, or penis amputation of affected part is the right choice. Surgial treatment is especially indicated in the following situations:

1. When the lesion is quite large.
2. When it has invaded muscle, cartilage or bone.
3. Radiorecurrent cancers.

ii. *Radiation treatment*—Radiotherapy is a very effective method of treatment as it cures about 80 percent of early cancers. The indications of this treatment are:

1. When the tumor is small and not invading muscle, cartilage or bone.
2. In patients not fit for surgery or when surgery is refused.

Different types of radiotherapy may be applied according to the site, size and type of lesion, and the methods are – superficial radiotherapy, deep X-ray therapy, radon seeds, iridium wire, etc.

- **Secondary nodes:**
  1. If the nodes are not palpable, the patient is kept on regular follow-up. If the nodes do not enlarge, no treatment is advised. If they get enlarged, a biopsy is done. If metastases are present, a block dissection is done. In this phase, now the treatment of the nodes is decided by sentinel node biopsy.
  2. If the nodes are palpable, a biopsy should be done. If it shows metastases, a block dissection is done.
  3. If the nodes are enlarged and fixed to the surrounding structures palliative radiotherapy is given.

Prognosis

The prognosis depends upon the size of SCC, Broders grade, site of the lesion, depth of the lesion, and etiology.

Early low-grade lesions without invasion have excellent prognosis following excision.

Late disease, anaplastic cancers with invasion have a poor prognosis with early local recurrence or metastases.

CASE 3: MARJOLIN'S ULCER

CLINICAL DIAGNOSIS

1. The patient is usually a middle-aged or elderly person who presents with a nonhealing ulcer developing on a scar, especially of a burn (Figs 11 and 12).
2. It is growing very slowly.
3. The size and shape are variable.
4. It is usually very shallow.
5. The edge is everted.
6. It is nontender with an indurated base.

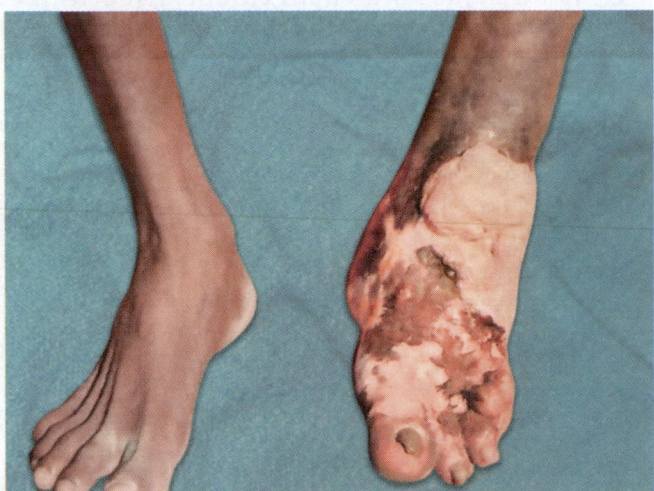

Fig. 11: Marjolin's ulcer (carcinoma on a scar of old burn)

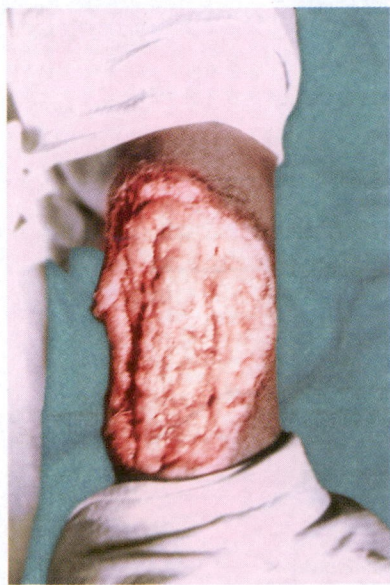

Fig. 12: Squamous cell carcinoma of leg occurring on a scar of burn (Marjolin's ulcer)

7. The regional lymph nodes are not enlarged so long as ulcer is limited to the scar.

VIVA VOCE

1. **What is Marjolin's ulcer?**
   It is a low-grade squamous cell carcinoma arising from the epithelium covering the scar tissue or keloid, the scar of the burn being the commonest.
2. **What are the sites of occurrence?**
   This cancer can occur in:
   1. Burn scars, other scars.
   2. Keloid.
   3. Long-standing venous ulcer.
   4. Chronic osteomyelitic sinus.
3. **Why does this tumor progress very slowly?**
   It grows very slowly because of relative avascularity of the scar tissue.
4. **Why is this lesion often painless?**
   Because the scar tissue has very poor nerve supply.
5. **Why does this tumor not spread to lymph nodes readily?**
   Because the scar tissue does not have lymphatics.
6. **Does this cancer ever spread to lymph nodes?**
   When this cancer grows into healthy skin around the scar, it spreads to the lymph nodes like an ordinary squamous cell carcinoma.
7. **What are the investigations?**
   Apart from routine investigations, biopsy is the main investigation.
8. **How do you treat this condition?**
   - It is usually treated by wide three dimensional excision followed by skin grafting.
   - The margin of the tumor is assessed by surgical loupe magnification. If the lesion is less than 2 cm in size, a 4 mm clearance margin is achieved and if it measures more than 2 cm, a 1 cm clearance margin is required. The orientated excised specimen is examined histologically for complete clearance.
   - If the lesion is affecting a limb and is very extensive amputation may be indicated.
9. **Can you treat this cancer by radiotherapy?**
   No, as this tumor is radioresistant.
10. **Why?**
   Because of relative avascularity.

DISCUSSION

Marjolin's ulcer is a squamous cell carcinoma arising in a chronic benign ulcer or scar (Figs 11 and 12).

Etiology

The cause is not known. The commonest benign ulcer to change into carcinoma is a long-standing venous ulcer. The scar of burn is the commonest scar to change into malignancy.

Pathology

The special pathological features of this lesion are:

1. It is a slow growing cancer. It may be because of less vascularity of the region of the ulcer.
2. It is less malignant than a usual squamous cell carcinoma.
3. It does not cause lymphatic metastasis as the local lymphatics are destroyed in scarring. The lymphatic spread occurs later on when surrounding normal skin is invaded.

Clinical Features

The special clinical features of this lesion are:

1. The edge of the ulcer is not always raised or everted.
2. It is usually a painless disease, hence the treatment is frequently delayed.

The diagnosis can be confirmed by biopsy.

Treatment

Before excision the margin of the tumor is assessed by using surgical loupe magnification.

It is treated as a squamous cell carcinoma arising de novo by wide excision with a margin of at least one centimeter in all the three dimensions. The raw area is skin grafted.

The orientated excised specimen is examined histologically for complete removal of cancer before the raw area is skin grafted.

If the tumor is quite big and involving the distal part of an extremity, amputation is recommended.

If the tumor is quite big and lies in the proximal part of an extremity, excision of tumor with surrounding tissue leaving the part of the ulcer which is still benign may be tried. The raw area is covered by skin grafts. If the disease recurs, amputation is the only solution.

This tumor is radioresistant, hence radiotherapy has no place in the treatment.

CASE 4: CARCINOMA OF LIP

CLINICAL DIAGNOSIS

1. The patient is usually an elderly person more commonly a male who presents with a nonhealing ulcer of the lip.
2. In 95 percent of patients, it is the lower lip that is affected (Fig. 13).
3. It is commonly situated at the vermilion border.
4. The ulcer is irregular with an everted edge and indurated base.
5. The submental and submandibular lymph nodes may be enlarged, hard. nontender and may be mobile of fixed.

VIVA VOCE

1. **What is carcinoma of lip?**
   It is an epithelial malignant tumor of the lip.
2. **What is the cause?**
   The most important risk factor is actinic exposure (actinic cheilitis).
3. **What is the gross pathology?**
   Grossly, it is of two types:
   - Ulcerative carcinoma—It is the commonest form of this cancer. There is an irregular hard ulcer.
   - Proliferative carcinoma—It is an irregular ulcerated mass.
4. **What is the micropathology?**
   It is a squamous cell carcinoma.

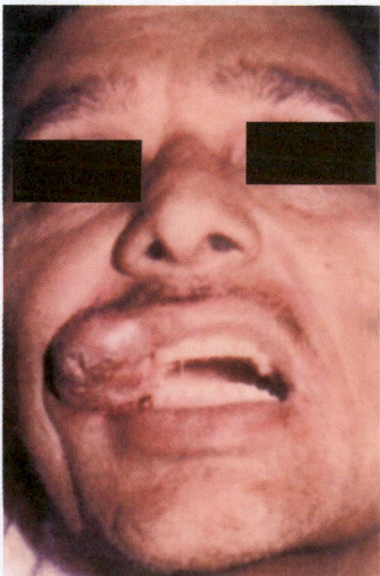

Fig. 13: Carcinoma of upper lip (*Courtesy:* Professor RK Agrawal and Professor AK Khare, Udaipur)

5. **How does this cancer spread?**
   It spreads by local invasion, and by lymphatic route to the regional lymph nodes (submental and submandibular).
6. **How will you confirm the diagnosis?**
   By doing biopsy of the primary and FNAC of enlarged cervical nodes.
7. **How do you stage the primary tumor?**
   The staging of the primary tumor is given below:
   T1—Less than 2 cm in greatest dimension
   T2—More than 2 but less than 4 cm
   T3—More than 4 but less than 6 cm
   T4—Invasion of adjacent structures, e.g. mandible.
8. **How do you treat lip carcinoma?**
   - The carcinoma of lip is treated both by surgical resection and radiotherapy.
   - The extent of resection depends upon the size of the lesion.
9. **How do you treat a small tumor (T1)?**
   It is managed with either a V- or W-shaped excision with a clear margin of resection. It can be done under local or general anesthesia.
10. **How do you repair the defect?**
    The defect is repaired in 3 layers—mucosa, muscle and skin. The aligment of the vermilion border should be restored.
11. **What is the criteria for suture closure?**
    The defect should not be more than one third of the total lip size.
12. **How do you treat T2-T3 tumors?**
    These tumors are excised with a clear margin of resection and the defect is repaired with local flaps.
13. **Can you do V- or W- excision of these tumors?**
    Excision is this manner results in a microstoma.
14. **How do you reconstruct a big central defect?**
    It is reconstructed by using Johansen step technique which permits repair of the defect by symmetrical advancement of soft-tissue flaps, utilizing the excess skin in the labiomental grooves.
    Bernard rotational flap is another method.
15. **How do you treat T4 lesions?**
    Depending upon the extent of disease, it is treated by total excision of lower lip and chin with unilateral or bilateral selective lymph node dissection (as there is a great possibility of nodal involvement).
16. **How do you repair the defect?**
    It is reconstructed employing a forearm flap.
17. **What is selective lymph node dissection?**
    It involves only certain cervical lymph node levels, e.g. level I, II and III.

18. **What is the role of radiotherapy?**
    - Early lesions can be cured with radiotherapy.
    - Advanced large volume lesions usually require a combination of surgery and radiotherapy.

19. **What are the complications of radiotherapy?**
    The complications are mucositis, xerostomia and radionecrosis of mandible.

20. **What are the results of treatment?**
    The cure rate are 90 percent for T1 lesions and for 65 to 75 percent T2 cancers.

21. **How do you treat premalignant change in the lower lip?**
    It is treated by lower lip shave and closure of vermilion defect by advancement of lower labial mucosa.

22. **What is keratoacanthoma?**
    It is a rapidly growing hyperkeratotic papule occurring on sun-exposed skin of face, head and neck and dorsum of hands in persons more than 40 years of age.

23. **What are its clinical features?**
    It appears as a rapidly growing reddish papule which reaches its full size in 1 to 3 months. It is 1 to 2 cm in size, firm with a raised rolled edge and a central keratin plug.

24. **How will you confirm the diagnosis?**
    It is done by biopsy for which a wedge resection of the lesion from one side to the other, deep into the subcutaneous tissue is done.

25. **How do you treat it?**
    - It may undergo spontaneous regression.
    - It may regress following biopsy.
    - If the lesion persists it may be excised – shave excision down to the deep dermis.

DISCUSSION

Carcinoma of the lip is a common type of oropharyngeal cancer. As this cancer is visible, it presents early for treatment. Ninety five percent of cancers occur on the lower lip, and usually arise as an ulcer on the vermilion border.

Exposure to sunlight is most important risk factor, tobacco and alcohol may also be contributing. Chronic hyperplastic candidiasis is another high-risk factor.

Grossly, it is of two types—Ulcerative and proliferative. The former is the common type. Microscopically, it is a squamous cell carcinoma.

It tends to spread laterally over the mucosal surface, and invade the adjacent tissues. Lymphatic spread occurs late, and occurs to submental and submandibular nodes. The metastases may go to level I, II and III lymph nodes.

The diagnosis can be confirmed by biopsy. In large tumors or when the lymph nodes are palpable FNAC is done to confirm nodal involvement.

Treatment

Premalignant changes are treated by lower lip shave as the changes are usually extensive. The vermilion defect is repaired by advancement of the lower labial mucosa.

T1 lesions are treated by V or W-excision under local or general anesthesia, and the defect is closed in 3 layers—mucosa, muscle and skin. As the defect is smaller than one-third of total lip size it can be sutured without causing microstoma.

T2 and T3 tumors are excised with clear margin of resection and the repair is done by local flaps. As the defect is larger than one third width of the lip, it cannot be closed by suturing for fear of producing a microstoma.

Big defects are repaired by Johansen step technique which allow repair of the defect by symmetrical advancement of soft tissue flaps, utilizing the excess skin in the labiomental groves. Another method is the use of Bernard rotational flap.

T4 lesion is treated with total excision of lower lip and chin with unilateral or bilateral selective (level I,II, III) lymph node dissection as there is high incidence of nodal metastases. The lower facial defect is repaired with a forearm flap.

Radiotherapy—T1 cancers can be treated by radiotherapy with the same cure rates as given by surgery. In late disease or bulky tumors, the radiotherapy is combined with surgery.

The complications of radiotherapy are mucositis, xerostomia and radionecrosis of the mandible.

Prognosis

T1 cancers have 90 percent cure rates following surgery or radiotherapy. As the ulcer is visible, most of the patients come early for treatment.

Five-year cure rates for T2 cancers is 65 to 75, for T3 cancer is 40 to 50 percent and for T4 cancer is 30 percent.

CASE 5: CARCINOMA OF TONGUE

CLINICAL DIAGNOSIS

1. The patient is usually a middle-aged or elderly person who presents with a nonhealing ulcer or a warty swelling in the tongue.
2. There may be pain referred to the ear, excessive salivation and difficulty in speech, mastication and protrusion of tongue (ankyloglossia).
3. When the lesion is an ulcer:
   - It is usually single, situated on the lateral border or dorsum of tongue, and variable in size (Fig. 14).
   - It is irregular in shape and has an everted edge and yellowish-gray slough
   - It is hard, friable and bleeds on touch.
4. When the lesion is a papilliferous or warty swelling:
   - It may look like a cauliflower.
   - It has a wide and indurated base.
5. There may be clinical signs of chronic superficial glossitis.
6. The regional lymph nodes:
   - May not be palpable, or
   - May be hard, nontender and mobile, or
   - May be markedly enlarged and fixed.

VIVA VOCE

1. **What is carcinoma of tongue?**
   It is an epithelial malignant tumor of tongue, usually a squamous cell carcinoma.
2. **What is the commonest site of occurrence?**
   Near the edge of anterior two thirds of tongue where it occurs in nearly 50 percent of patients.

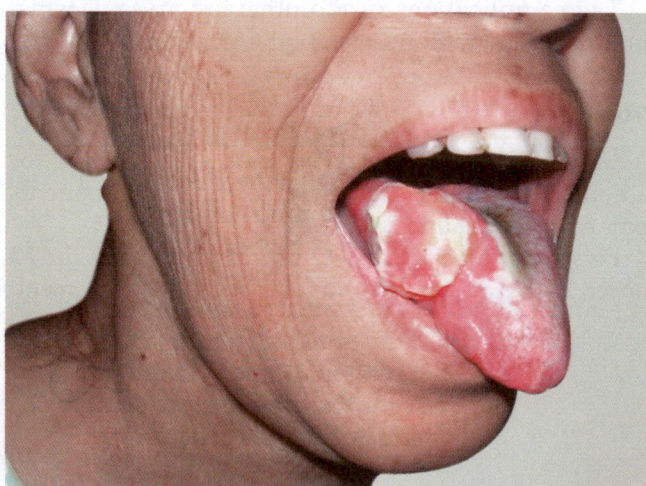

Fig. 14: Carcinoma of tongue (*Courtesy:* Professor Sandeep Kumar)

3. **What is the relative frequency of sites of occurrence?**
   It occurs as follows:
   1. Near the edge of anterior two thirds   50%
   2. Posterior one third   20%
   3. Tip   10%
   4. Dorsum   10%
   5. Undersurface   10%.
4. **What are the clinical appearances of this cancer?**
   It has four clinical appearances:
   - A nonhealing ulcer
   - A raised papilliferous plaque or warty mass
   - A deep fissure
   - A lobulated hard mass
5. **What is the cause of this cancer?**
   - The main etiological agents are tobacco (both smoking and chewing) and alcohol. Synergism between these agents is well established.
   - Other risk factors are betel nut, pan masala, human papillomavirus, Epstein-Barr virus and Plummer-Vinson syndrome.
   - The whole of the oral cavity is exposed to the damaging effect of prolonged exposure resulting in cancerization. But the disease usually manifests at one point (relatively most exposed area).
6. **What are the precancerous lesions?**
   The precancerous lesions are:
   - Chronic superficial glossitis
   - Leukoplakia
   - Dental ulcer
   - Sessile papilloma
   - Syphilis.
7. **Why is the pain referred to the ear?**
   It is because the tumor invades the lingual nerve.
8. **What are the symptoms of carcinoma of posterior one third?**
   The symptoms are:
   1. Pain during swallowing
   2. Pain in the back of tongue
   3. It may be entirely asymptomatic or the patient may present with cervical lymphadenopathy.
9. **What is the cause of excessive salivation?**
   It is a reflex phenomenon.
10. **What is ankyloglossia?**
    It is the inability to protrude the tongue out.
11. **Is it an inability?**
    It is not a true inability as the patient can protrude the tongue out.
12. **What is the problem with protrusion, then?**
    If the lesion is limited to one side, that side of tongue will not come out. Hence, on protrusion the tip points to the side of the lesion.

If the tongue is totally infiltrated it cannot be protruded out.

13. What is cause of this symptom?

This symptom is due to infiltration of musculature of tongue.

14. How does this tumor spread?

This tumor spreads by the following methods:

1. Local.
2. Lymphatic.
3. Blood-born.

15. How does it spread locally?

Locally it spreads by anatomical continuity and contiguity of tissues, and perineural invasion.

16. What are the parts affected by local spread?

A carcinoma of lateral border reaches the floor of mouth before it extends across the midline. A tumor of junction of anterior two-thirds with posterior one-third may invade the mandible. A lesion of posterior one-third spreads laterally into the tonsil, side of pharynx and cervical spine and up into soft palate; posteriorly into the epiglotitis; and downwards into the larynx; and across to the other side of tongue.

17. What is the lymphatic drainage of tongue?

It is as described below:

1. From the tip, the lymphatics pass through the floor of mouth to submental lymph nodes of both sides. One set of lymphatics also go to jugulo-omohyoid gland.
2. From the anterior two-thirds the lymphatics drain into submandibular nodes which may be embedded in the submandibular salivary glands.
3. The lymphatics of posterior third of tongue drain into jugulo-digastric nodes of both sides. A few lymphatics pass to jugulo-omohyoid group.
4. The central lymphatics from either side of median raphe of tongue pass vertically downwards in the midline of tongue between the two genioglossi which often decussate and then pass some to the left and some to right to jugulo-digastric nodes. The jugulo-digastric group of upper deep cervical nodes ultimately receive the efferent lymphatics from the submadibular and submental groups.

18. What is the significance of jugulo-digastric group?

In later stages of disease, the jugulo-digastrics group is involved regardless of the original site of tumor.

19. Which is the commonest lymph node to be involved in the metastatic process?

The submandibular lymph node.

20. What does the involvement of submandibular lymph node mean?

It means that the cancer is present very close to periosteum of the mandible and the resection of relevant segment of the lower jaw may be required to ensure surgical clearance.

21. Are distant metastases common in this cancer?

The patient usually dies as a result of uncontrollable primary tumor or lymphatic metastases before the distant metastases are able to manifest.

22. Cancer of which part of tongue is more likely to metastasize by blood stream?

Cancer of posterior third.

23. What are the investigations?

The investigations are:

- Biopsy from the tumor
- FNAC or biopsy of enlarged nodes, may be done under ultrasound guidance
- Radiography of jaw (orthopantomogram) if the lesion is near the jaw
- MRI to see the soft tissue infiltration by the tumor.

24. How do you stage the primary tumor according to TNM staging?

It is done as given below:

T1—Tumor less than 2 cm in size

T2—Tumor 2 to 4cm

T3—Tumor 4 to 6 cm

T4—Tumor invading mandible, skin.

25. How do you treat this cancer?

It can be treated by surgery or radiotherapy, but surgery is the treatment of choice. Up to 30 percent of cases of T1 cancer have occult nodal metastases. Hence, they are also treated at the same time.

26. What are the essential steps of surgical resection?

The primary tumor is excised 2 cm away from the lesion in the three dimensions with either a cutting diathermy or laser. The clear margin of resection must have a histological confirmation.

The excision of cancer may result in partial or hemiglossectomy.

27. How do you treat a T3 lesion?

It requires a wide resection of tongue, floor of the mouth and mandible. The cervical nodes are resected at the same time. This step resects the lingual lymph nodes which are present between the primary tumor and submandibular (level I) nodes.

28. How do you treat a T4 tumor?

It requires total glossectomy.

29. How do you approach the tongue for excision?

- Small anterior tumors—Transoral excision
- Large tumors—Splitting the lip with paramedian or median mandibulotomy, or Visor approach.

30. How do you reconstruct the tongue?

- Small lateral defects—Suture closure or left to granulate

- Large defects—Radial forearm flap utilizing microvascular anastomosis
- Total glossectomy—Rectus abdominis flap

31. What will you do to the hypoglossal nerves during total glossectomy?

If possible one or both hypoglossal nerves are preserved.

32. What is the role of radiotherapy?

- A small tumor may be treated by primary radiotherapy.
- Advanced disease is better treated by a combination of surgery and radiotherapy.
- Advanced carcinoma with fixed nodes is treated by palliative radiotherapy.

33. What is chemoradiotherapy?

It is a combination of chemotherapy with radiotherapy. It is a very powerful method of treatment, but the patient must be fit to tolerate this combination.

34. What do you do if there is bilateral lymph node involvement?

The following measures are employed:

1. Bilateral node dissection with preservation of internal jugular vein of least involved side. The side in which the vein is to be retained is operated first.
2. Alternatively low dose preoperative radiotherapy is given to worst side followed by block dissection and therapeutic radiation to other side. The metastatic nodes respond to megavoltage radiation.
3. Or, a full block dissection on involved side and a suprahyoid block dissection on the opposite side.

35. Why don't you remove both the internal jugulars in bilateral disease?

Both cannot be excised as it will result in postoperative cerebral venous engorgement, and edema of head and face. The patient may die due to these problems.

DISCUSSION

Carcinoma of the tongue is an epithelial malignant tumor of the tongue of complex etiology and characterized by a nonhealing ulcer or a mass in the tongue (Fig. 15).

It is an uncommon cancer in the western world but in India it is one of the types of oropharyngeal cancer which accounts for 40 percent of all cancers.

Etiology

The main etiological agents are tobacco (both smoking and chewing) and alcohol; synergism between these agents is

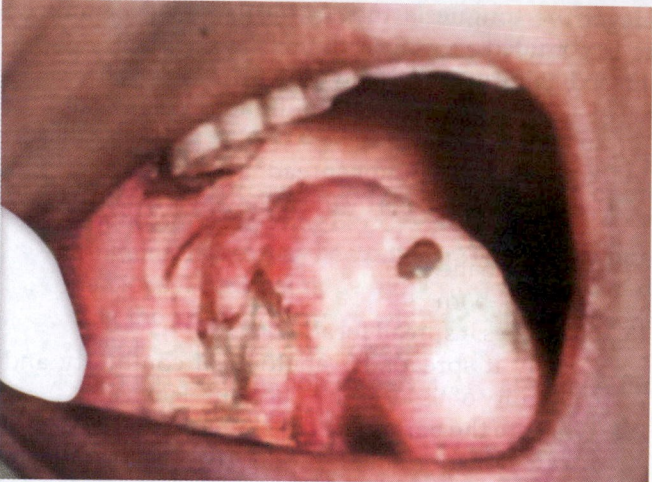

Fig. 15: Carcinoma of tongue involving the adjacent area (*Courtesy:* Professor RK Agrawal and Professor AK Khare, Udaipur)

well established. Other risk factors are – betel nut, pan masala, human papillomavirus, Epstein–Barr virus, Plummer-Vinson syndrome and poor nutrition.

Repeated trauma by a sharp tooth may produce a dental ulcer which may become cancerous. Leukoplakia of the tongue is another premalignant lesion of tongue.

Other risk factors are erythroplakia, chronic hyperplastic candidiasis, oral submucous fibrosis and syphilitic glossitis.

Pathology

- **Site**—The commonest site is near the edge of anterior two thirds which is seen in 50 percent of patients. The other sites are posterior third (20%), tip (10%) dorsum (10%) and undersurface (10%).
- **Macroscopic types**—It has four gross types:
  1. *Ulcerative type*—It is the commonest type, and almost always seen near the edge. The ulcer is irregular in shape and size. The edge is raised and everted. The floor is covered by yellowish gray slough. The base is indurated and even in a shallow ulcer it extends more deeply as the cancer is invasive.
  2. *Proliferative or warty type*—It usually occurs on leukoplakia and has a broad and indurated base. There is an ulcerated mass which may look like a cauliflower.
  3. Indurated plaque or mass.
  4. *Fissure*—There is a crack or fissure having the lesion in the depth of the fissure.

Micropathology—In the anterior, two-thirds of the tongue, it is a squamous cell carcinoma with cell nest formation. It is a less differentiated lesion as compared to carcinoma of the lip.

In the posterior third it may be a basal cell or transitional cell carcinoma or a lymphoepithelioma. It is because there is no cornification, abundant racemose glands and numerous lymphocytes near the basal layer of cells.

Spread

- *Local*—Though the fascial planes including the periosteum serve as barriers to local spread of this cancer, the perineural invasion acts as a conduit for the direct spread. The cancer of the lateral border invades the floor of mouth, and the cancer of posterior third tends to invade the corresponding tonsil, epiglottis and soft palate.
- *Lymphatic*—It spreads to the cervical lymph nodes usually by embolism. Hence, the intervening tissues are not involved. Initially it involves the submental and submandibular nodes. Later on jugulodigastric nodes are involved regardless of the site of tumor.

  The cancer of posterior third may present with lymph node metastases as the primary may remain occult for quite some time.
- *Hematogenous*—Angio-invasion is a rare and late phenomenon. It may be seen in the posterior lesions.

Clinical Features

- *Age and sex*—It usually occurs after 50 years of age with peak incidence in 6th decade. It is a little more common in males.
- *Early disease*—The patient presents with a nonhealing ulcer in the tongue usually along its lateral border.
- *Late disease*—It is a common presentation in our country. The common clinical features are excessive salivation, fetor oris (halitosis), ankyloglossia, pain which may be referred to the ear of same side and cervical lymph node enlargement.

  The commonest presentation is an irregular ulcer along the lateral border with raised or everted edge, yellowish gray slough and indurated base. It may bleed on touch. The cervical lymph nodes may not be palpable, or palpable, mobile, hard and nontender. Later on they may get fixed.

Investigations

- Biopsy—It can be taken under local anesthesia from the edge of the lesion.
- FNAC of enlarged nodes
- Radiography of the jaw may be required if the growth is very near the jaw. Orthopantomogram gives better information.

- In grossly infected lesions culture of the swab may be done.
- MRI provides excellent visualization of soft tissue infiltration by the tumor.

TNM Staging

T1	—	Tumor less than 2 cm in size
T2	—	Tumor 2 to 4 cm in size
T3	—	Tumor 4 to 6 cm in size
T4	—	Tumor invading adjacent structures, e.g. mandible, skin
N1	—	Metastasis in a single ipsilateral lymph node less than 3 cm in size
N2a	—	Metastasis is a single ipsilateral lymph node more than 3 cm but not more than 6 cm
N2b	—	Metastases in multiple ipsilateral lymph nodes, none more than 6 cm in size
N2c	—	Metastases in bilateral or contralateral nodes none greater than 6 cm in size
N3	—	Metastases to any node more than 6 cm
Mo	—	No distant metastasis
M1	—	Distant metastases present

Stage Groups

I	—	T1 NO MO
II	—	T2 NO MO
III	—	T3 NO MO, T1 T2 T3 N1 MO
IV	—	T4 NO MO, Any T N2 MO Any T N3 MO, Any T any N M1

Treatment

Surgery

The treatment of choice is surgical resection. Up to 30 percent of cases of T1 cancer have occult nodal metastases. Hence, they should also be treated at the same time.

The primary tumor is excised 2 cm away from the lesion in all the planes. The excision can be done with either a cutting diathermy or laser. The clear margin of resection must have a histological confirmation.

The resection of the lesion may result in partial or hemiglossectomy.

T3 cancer—It might have involved the floor of the mouth and may be mandible. It requires a major resection of the tongue, floor of mouth and mandible.

T4 tumor often crosses the midline, hence total glossectomy has to be done.

A lesion of posterior third may be treated by total glossectomy.

If the lymph nodes are being treated at the same time, they are excised in continuity with the primary. This step removes the lingual lymph nodes, which are present between the primary tumor and level I (submandibular) nodes.

Appraoch—Small anterior tumors can be excised transorally. For larger tumors splitting the lip with paramedian or median mandibulotomy or Visor approach is followed.

Reconstruction—Small lateral defects may be suture closed or are left to granulate.

Large defects are reconstructed by a radial forearm flap utilizing microvascular anastomosis.

Following total glossectomy the tongue may be reconstructed by rectus abdominis free flap. If possible one or both hypoglossal nerves are preserved.

Radiotherapy

1. A small tumor may be treated by primary radiotherapy.
2. Advanced disease is better treated by a combination of surgery and radiotherapy.
3. Carcinoma of posterior third can be treated by radiotherapy.
4. Chemoradiotherapy is the combination of chemotherapy and radiotherapy which is a powerful method of treatment but the patient must be fit to tolerate its toxicity.
5. In advanced disease with fixed nodes palliative radiotherapy is given.

CASE 6: CARCINOMA OF PENIS

Clinical Diagnosis

1. The patient is usually a middle-aged or elderly person who has not been circumcised and comes from lower sections of society.
2. There is a foul-smelling serosanguinous discharge from the prepucial orifice
3. There is an ulcer or ulcerated swelling in the prepucial sac (Fig. 16).
4. The ulcer is irregular is shape with everted edge and indurated base, or
5. The swelling is cauliflower-like (Fig. 17) irregular, and hard or variable in consistency.

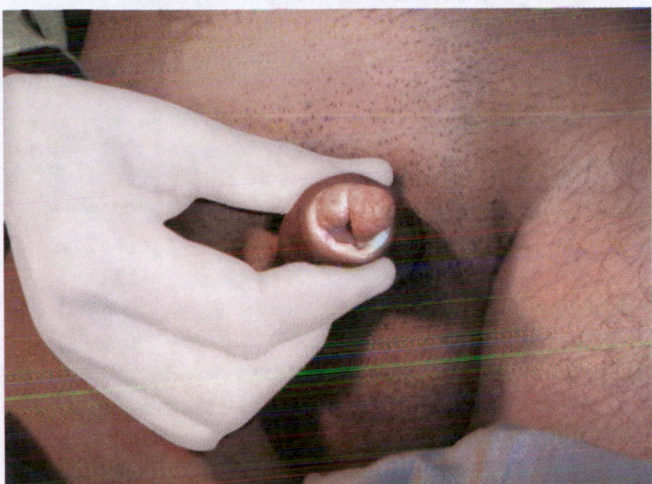

Fig. 16: Prepucial carcinoma. This patient was having phimosis. The lesion was extirpated by circumcision with clear margin of excision.

6. The inguinal nodes may not be enlarged, or enlarged and mobile or fixed. They are nontender and firm or hard in consistency.

Viva Voce

1. **What is carcinoma of penis?**
   It is a squamous cell carcinoma usually occurring in the prepucial sac.
2. **What are the common sites of occurrence?**
   The common sites are glans, inner layer of prepuce, coronal area and postcoronal sulcus.
3. **What is the appearance of external meatus?**
   It is normal if the lesion is away from meatus. If it is involving the meatal area it is difficult to see it. It can be seen only if the patient is asked to pass urine.
4. **What is the clinical status of inguinal nodes?**
   The nodes may not or may be palpable.
5. **What is the cause of impalpable nodes?**
   The lymph nodes are not palpable because of the following reasons:
   1. There are not involved by the disease process.
   2. They are involved in the disease process but too small to be palpable.
   3. Obesity.
6. **What is the cause of palpable nodes?**
   The palpable nodes may be due to following reasons:
   1. Secondary infection
   2. Metastatic involvement (Fig. 18).

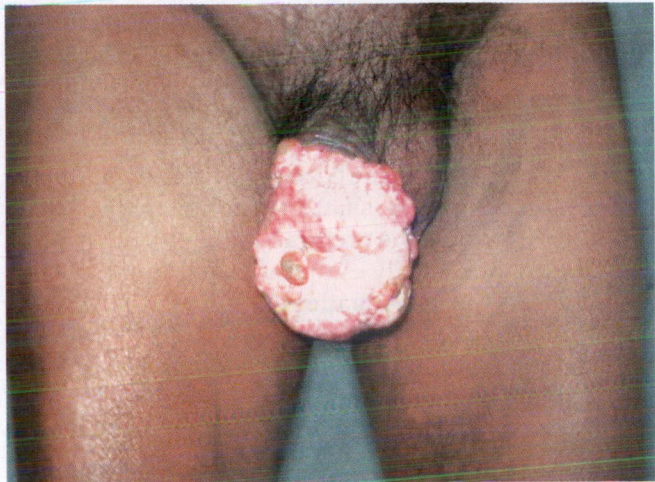

Fig. 17: Cauliflower-like carcinoma of penis (*Courtesy:* Professor Sandeep Kumar)

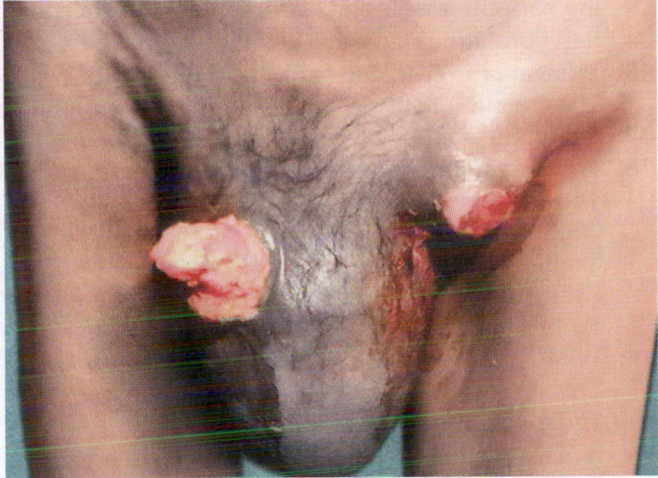

Fig. 18: Carcinoma of penis which has nearly destroyed the shaft of penis with ulcerating left inguinal nodal metastases. (*Courtesy:* Professor RK Agrawal and Professor A K Khare, Udaipur)

7. What is autoamputation?
Sometimes the penis is totally destroyed by the carcinoma. This phenomenon is known as auto-amputation.

8. What is the relationship of this cancer with circumcision?
- Circumcision performed soon after birth as in Jews confers almost total immunity against this cancer. Circumcision done soon after in early infancy (as in Muslims) does not provide the same degree of protection.
- Thus, carcinoma of penis occurs in those men who are not circumcised (Hindus, Christians).

9. How does circumcision prevent this cancer?
It helps in maintaining penile hygiene, and also prevents the occurrence of chronic balanoposthitis.

10. What are the precancerous states?
The precancerous states are—leukoplakia, long standing genital warts, Paget's disease of penis (erythroplakia of Queyrat).

11. What is Paget's disease of penis?
It is the persistent rawness of glans like a long standing balanitis.

12. What are the gross types of this cancer?
It is of two gross types—flat or infiltrating and papilliferous.

13. What is the difference in these types ?
- The flat type commonly presents with an ulcer and may be associated with leukoplakia.
- The proliferative type presents with a cauliflower-like mass and may commence in a long standing papilloma.

14. Is there any difference in treatment and prognosis of these types?
Treatment-wise there is no difference. Prognostically, the papilliferous lesions are considered better than flat types, though it is not always true.

15. What are the essential features of micropathology?
The essential features are—keratinizatin, epithelial pearls and mitotic figures (Figs 19 and 20).

16. What are the histological grades of this tumor?
The histological grades are:
Grade I—Well differentiated tumor (47.5%)
Grade II—Moderately differentiated tumor (41.7%)
Grade III—Poorly differentiated or undifferentiated tumor (10.8%).

17. What are the modes of spread of this cancer?
This tumor spreads by:
1. Direct infiltration or local spread.
2. Lymphatic spread mostly by embolism.
3. Blood stream (rare).

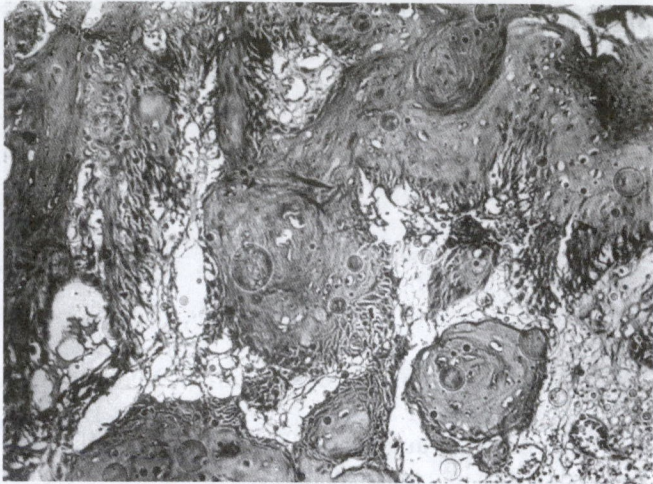
Fig. 19: Carcinoma of penis grade I

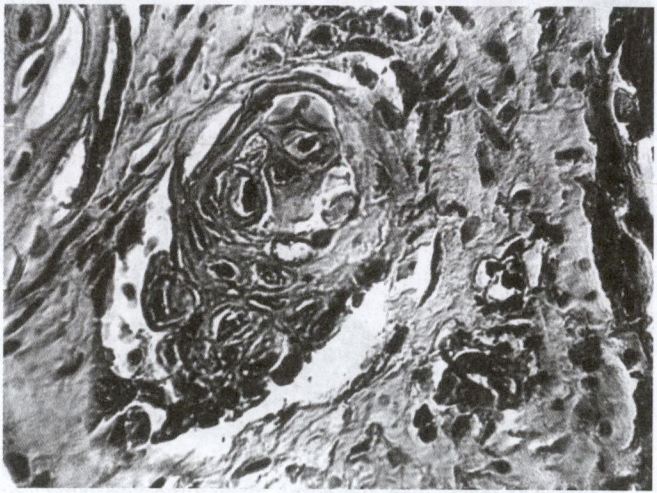
Fig. 20: Carcinoma of penis, inguinal metastases

18. How does it spread directly?
- It spreads directly by continuity and contiguity. The fascial sheath of corpora acts as a barrier for quite sometime against spread.
- When the fascial barrier is broken the tumor spreads into the shaft and grows rapidly.

19. Does it involve the urethra?
The urethra usually escapes.

20. What are the investigations?
The investigations are:
1. Preputiotomy if lesion is covered by phimosis.
2. Biopsy of primary.
3. Lymph node biopsy or FNAC.
4. Ultrasound/CT scan for pelvic and abdominal lymph node involvement.

21. **What is preputiotomy?**
It is slitting open the prepucial sac for clinical examination and taking a biopsy.
22. **What is the role of FNAC?**
It can be employed for finding out lymph node involvement. It is of limited value as it gives only the cytological diagnosis not tissue diagnosis.
23. **What are the indications of lymph node biopsy?**
It is indicated in the following situations:
1. High grade tumor.
2. Highly invasive lesion.
3. Lesion more than 5 cm in size.
4. Lesion involving more than 75 percent of shaft.
5. Lymphadenopathy with lymph node more than 3 cm in size.
6. Persistent lymphadenopathy.
24. **What is sentinel lymph node?**
It is a specific lymph node amongst the inguinal nodes which is said to be always involved if there is lymph node involvement in carcinoma of penis.
25. **What do you know of clinical staging of penile carcinoma?**
There are many methods of staging a penile carcinoma clinically, but in practice two are popular.
1. Jackson staging
2. TNM staging.
26. **What is Jackson staging?**
It is as described below:
Stage I or A—The lesion is limited to glans, prepuce or both.
Stage II or B—The shaft is involved.
Stage III or C—The inguinal nodes are positive but operable.
Stage IV or D—The inguinal nodes are inoperable (fixed).
27. **What is TNM classification?**
It is as given below:
Primary tumor (T)
TIS — Tumor in situ
T1 — Upto 2 cm, superficial, exophytic
T2 — 2 to 5 cm, minimal infiltration
T3 — More than 5 cm, deep infiltration
T4 — Infiltration of surrounding structures
Regional lymph nodes (N)
No — Impalpable nodes
N1 — Palpable, mobile, unilateral nodes
N1a – Clinically uncertain
N1b – Clinically certain
N2 — Palpable, mobile, bilateral (a,b) nodes
N3 — Fixed nodes
Distant metastases (M)
Mo — No distant metastasis
M1 — Distant metastasis at one site

28. **How do you treat this cancer?**
1. Stage I disease is treated by partial amputation or iridium implant.
2. Stage II disease is treated by subtotal or total penectomy.
3. Stage III disease is treated by partial or total (radical) amputation with bilateral ilioinguinal lymph node dissection.
4. Stage IV disease is treated by palliative radiotherapy and or chemotherapy.
29. **What are the indications of partial penectomy?**
Jackson stage I or A cancer
30. **What do you do in partial penectomy?**
The penis is amputated 2 cm above the lesion. At least a 3 cm stump of penis must be available after operation (Fig. 21).
31. **What are the complications of this operation?**
The complications are—Hemorrhage, wound infection, meatal stenosis.
32. **What are the indications of total amputation?**
The indications are:
1. Jackson stage II disease.
2. Failure of radiation treatment, radionecrosis.
33. **What do you do in total penectomy?**
The total penis including its triradiate root is removed. The urethra is divided 5 cm distal to perineal membrane.
34. **What do you mean by radical amputation?**
In this operation, apart from removing the whole penis including its triradiate root, the testis and scrotum are also removed (Fig. 22).
35. **What is the rationale of this procedure?**
Two reasons are given for doing this operation:
1. When penis is not there, no useful purpose is served by retaining the testis.

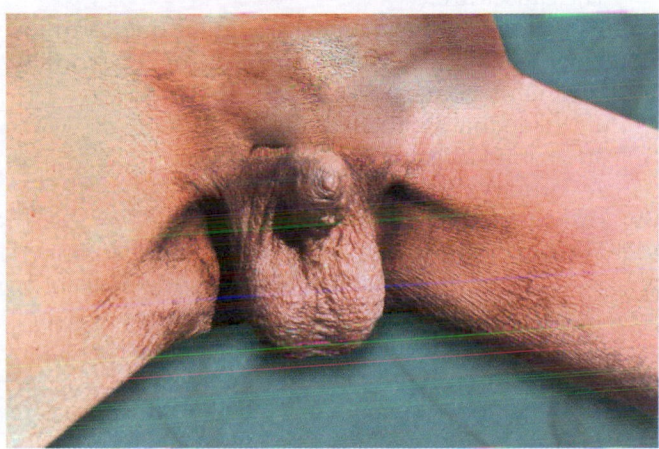

Fig. 21: After partial amputation for penile carcinoma

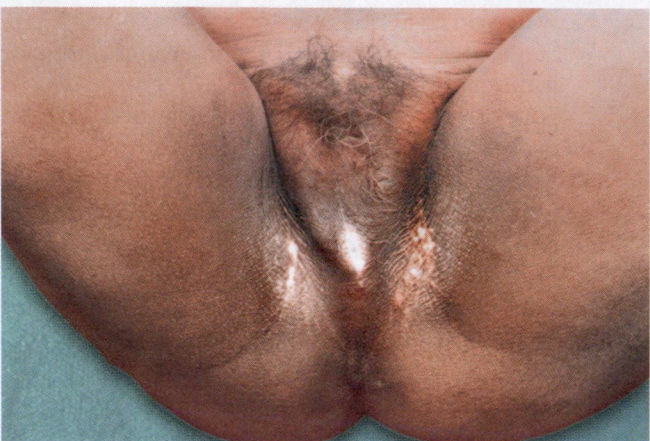

Fig. 22: After emasculation for carcinoma penis

2. The retained scrotum hangs down in front of neourethrostoma and gets wet during each act of micturition.

36. How can you overcome these problems?

These problems can be overcome by:

1. A new penis can be reconstructed, and then the retained testis and scrotum may serve useful function.
2. Prepubic advancement of the scrotum will prevent the second problem.

37. How does this cancer alter the urinary functions of penis?

The alterations in the functions of micturition are –

- Disease-induced alterations
  1. Dysuria.
  2. Retention (rare).
- Treatment–induced alterations
  1. Stenosis of neourethrostoma.
  2. Urethral fistula.
  3. Inability to urinate in standing position.

38. What are the causes of stenosis of neourethra?

The causes are:

1. Continued mechanical irritation due to drain, catheter, and scrotum hanging in front of urethrostoma.
2. Inadequate epithelial cover.
3. Wound infection.
4. Urinary dermatitis.

39. How do you treat inguinal nodes?

The treatment of inguinal nodes is described below:

1. If the nodes are not palpable the patient is kept on regular follow up, or the involvement of lymph nodes is detected by sentinel lymph node biopsy at the time of primary surgery.
2. If the nodes are palpable but clinically uncertain (N1a) the patient is given antibiotics for 3 weeks

following treatment of primary to eliminate infection. If they persist, bilateral ilioinguinal lymphadenectomy is done.

3. If the nodes are palpable and clinically certain (N1b) they are treated by bilateral ilioinguinal lymphadenectomy.
4. If the nodes are fixed (N3) they are treated by radiotherapy.

40. What is the treatment of choice for metastatic nodes?

Surgical block dissection is the treatment of choice as it gives better results than other forms of treatment.

41. Can you treat them by radiotherapy?

Yes, they can be treated by radiotherapy also.

42. How do you treat them by radiotherapy?

The following is the line of treatment:

1. Impalpable nodes—Radiotherapy by 5000 rad in 5 weeks.
2. Palpable mobile nodes—Megavoltage + interstitial treatment of residual by 6000 rad in 6 weeks.
3. Fixed nodes—Megavoltage radiotherapy by 3000 to 4000 rad in 2 to 3 weeks.

43. What are the indications for ilioinguinal lymph node dissection?

The indications are:

1. Persistent lymphadenopathy for more than 4 weeks.
2. Confirmed nodal metastases.
3. Subsequent lymphadenopathy in a treated patient.
4. Extensive disease of base of penis.
5. Involvement of corpora cavernosa.

44. Will you do unilateral or bilateral ilioinguinal lympadenectomy?

It should be a bilateral procedure.

45. Why?

Because half the patients with involved lymph nodes also have tumor in contralateral nodes and 30 percent have iliac node involvement. Hence, bilateral ilioinguinal lymph node dissection is recommended.

46. What is the upper limit of this dissection?

The nodal clearance should be done upto the bifurcation of iliac artery.

47. What are the complications of lymph node dissection?

The complications are:

1. Skin flap necrosis.
2. Wound infection.
3. Lymphorrhea.
4. Lymphedema of lower extremity.
5. Hemorrhage.
6. Inguinal hernia.

48. What do you mean by prophylactic node dissection?

Removal of nonpalpable nodes with the aim of

improving the cure rates is called as prophylactic node dissection.

49. Does it improve the survival rates?
No

50. What is the present status of this procedure?
Majority of surgeons do not do it.

51. What are the indications of radiotherapy?
The indications of radiotherapy are:
1. Jackson stage I or T1 lesion (curative radiotherapy).
2. Advanced or inoperable disease.

52. Are there any contraindications of radiotherapy?
The contraindications of radiotherapy are:
1. Involvement of urethra.
2. Involvement of shaft of penis.

53. What may happen if radiotherapy is given to above patients?
The patient may have the following complications:
1. Urethral fistula.
2. Meatal stricture.
3. Radionecrosis of penis

54. What are the results of radiotherapy?
The results of radiotherapy are:
1. Almost 100 percent in T1 lesions.
2. Large lesions limited to distal end 75 to 80 percent response.
3. Overall cure rate—65 percent.

55. How do you treat T1 lesions by radiotherapy?
They are ideally treated by Ir^{192} implant or mould, with a dose of 5000 to 6000 rad in 5 to 6 days.

56. What are the advantages of radiotherapy?
The main advantage is minimal or no mutilation of penis.

57. What are the disadvantages of radiation treatment?
The disadvantages are:
1. Higher morbidity.
2. The lesion is always infected which reduces its effectivity.
3. Risk of radionecrosis of penis, which is difficult to differentiate from local recurrence.
4. Treatment is time consuming.

58. What is the role of Laser?
Early lesion can be treated effectively by Neodymium YAG laser.

59. What are the results?
The results are as good as those of surgery or radiotherapy. There is no mutilation.

60. What is the role of chemotherapy?
- As such chemotherapy has no role, but in advanced cases it may be tried.
- In early cases if it is combined with surgery or radiotherapy the results may improve.

61. What are the drugs used?
The drugs are:
1. Bleomycin 15-30 mg IV Bi-weekly to a total of 300 mg.
2. A combination of bleomycin, vincristine and cisplatin.

62. What is the toxicity of bleomycin?
Pulmonary fibrosis.

63. Can you reconstruct a new penis after excision?
Yes.

64. How do you reconstruct?
The methods of reconstruction are –
- Partial penile loss
    1. Abdominal flap phalloplasty.
    2. Scrotum recession phalloplasty.
- Total penile loss
    1. Pedicled tissue transfer phalloplasty.
    2. Free tissue transfer phalloplasty.

65. What is the prognosis?
The five year survival rates are:
1. Noninvasive lesions localized to penis—86 percent
2. Inguinal nodal involvement—50 percent
3. Distant metastases—Nil

DISCUSSION

Carcinoma of penis is an epithelial malignant tumor of penis of complex etiology and characterized by a varying degree of subprepucial discharge and ulceration (Fig. 23).

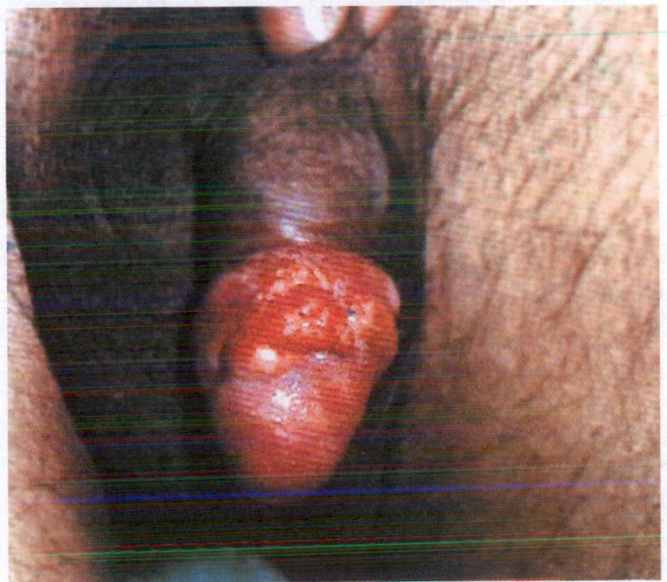

Fig. 23: Carcinoma of penis extending into the shaft (*Courtesy:* Professor RK Agrawal and Professor AK Khare, Udaipur)

It constitutes 2 to 3 percent of all urological cancers of male.

Etiology

This disease is related to local penile hygiene that is why it is commonly seen in people of dirty habits ('stinking disease of stinking men').

Relation with circumcision – If it is done immediately after birth this disease does not occur as in Jews. Circumcision done later in life (e.g. at 4 to 9 years of age as in Muslims) reduces the chances of this disease but does not prevent it completely.

It is etiologically related to phimosis and chronic balanoposthitis, and may be human papilloma virus.

The following are definite precancerous states—leukoplakia of glans, long-standing genital warts and Paget's disease of penis (syn. erythroplasia of Queyrat).

Pathology

It may occur any where in the prepucial chamber, the commonest site being the corona or postcoronal sulcus. The lesion may be flat and infiltrating (ulcerative) or papillary, the former occurring on a leukoplakic patch and the latter on a papilloma.

Microscopically, it is usually a squamous cell carcinoma (Figs 19 and 20).

Spread

1. *Lymphatic*—The earliest lymphatic spread is to the inguinal and then to the iliac nodes. From there it may go to the abdominal nodes.
2. *Local*—It infiltrates the neighboring penile tissue. Initially the facial sheath of corpora cavernosa resists invasion. But when this barrier is broken the lesion spreads rapidly.
3. *Hematogenous*—It is rare and late, hence, the distant metastatic deposits are infrequent.

Clinical Features

This disease commonly occurs in middle aged or elderly people but 40 percent of patients are 40 years of age.

The earliest symptoms are mild discomfort and light subprepucial discharge. They are often neglected, hence the disease progresses slowly. By the time the patient comes the lesion is often large and discharges foul bloody serum. There is hardly any pain or disturbance in micturition. **Inguinal nodes**—Sixty percent of patients have inguinal lymphadenopathy when they present but in 50 percent of patients it is reactive enlargement due to infection.

In most of the patients, the prepuce is nonretractile. If it is not treated in time the whole of the glans penis is replaced by a fungating mass and the penis is gradually destroyed ('auto-amputation'). The lesion in the nodes may fungate through the inguinal skin. It may erode the femoral or external iliac artery with torrential hemorrhage and death.

Investigations

1. Biopsy—The prepuce may require a slit open (preputiotomy) for doing biopsy.
2. The inguinal nodes may be studied by FNAC or lymph node biopsy. Sentinel node biopsy may be required during the primary surgery with injection of patient blue violet and a radio-isotope into the lesion.
3. Ultrasound examination of pelvis and abdomen for finding out nodal metastases.

Treatment

1. **Radiotherapy**—It is ideal for a small lesion in a relatively young patient.
   The patient is circumcised and then the tumor is treated by radioactive iridium-192 wire, external beam radiation or radioactive mould applicator.
   60 to 70 percent of patients survive for 5 years.
2. **Surgical treatment**—It is indicated for a large anaplastic cancer, if the shaft is infiltrated or when radiation treatment has failed.
   - Partial penectomy is done in a distal cancer when adequate clearance is possible without sacrificing the whole penis. The margins of excision must be confirmed histologically (Fig. 21).
   - Total penectomy—If the lesion is infiltrating, advanced or anaplastic total removal of the penis with its triradiate root with a perineal urethrostomy is indicated (Fig. 22).
   - Inguinal lymphadenopathy—They are managed as described below:
     1. If not palpable—The patient is kept on regular follow up.
     2. If the nodes are palpable and mobile—If FNAC is positive for malignant cells they are removed by block dissection. The 5-year survival rate is 35 percent.
        If FNAC is not positive, the patient is given a course of antibiotic therapy, and reassessed after three weeks. If the nodes do not subside further investigations are done.
3. If the nodes are significantly enlarged and fixed they are treated by palliative radiotherapy.

Prognosis

- Localized lesion without metastasis—60 to 90 percent 5-year survivals.
- Inguinal nodes involved—30 to 50 percent 3-year survivals.
- Iliac nodal involvement—20 percent 5-year survivals.

CASE 7: MALIGNANT MELANOMA

CLINICAL DIAGNOSIS

1. The patient is usually between 20 to 30 years and presents with an ulcer or ulcerated mass of insidious onset.
2. It usually occurs in the foot (sole) and hand (palm), subungual region, head and neck and the pigmented layer of the eye (Figs 24 to 26).
3. There is a dark brown or black ulcer or fungating swelling with foul smell.
4. It is soft or firm and nontender.
5. It may have scabbing on the surface. It bleeds if the scab is rubbed off.
6. A halo of brown pigment may be present in the skin around the lesion.
7. There may be small, multiple and hard nodules around the lesion (satellite nodules) especially in the direction of lymphatic drainage. They may also be surrounded by a depigmented halo.
8. The regional lymph nodes may be enlarged (Fig. 24).
9. There may be signs of distant metastases in the liver (hepatomegaly, melaninuria), lung (cough) and bones.

VIVA VOCE

1. **What is a malignant melanoma?**
   It is a malignant tumor arising from melanocytes of unknown etiology and characterized by a pigmented ulcer or fungating mass.

2. **What is the incidence of melanoma?**
   - It accounts for 3 percent of all cancers all over the world. One in 4 patients of melanoma occurs before the age of 40.
   - The incidence of cutaneous melanoma is much higher in whites than in blacks, equal in men and women, extremely low in children, and increases with age in adults.

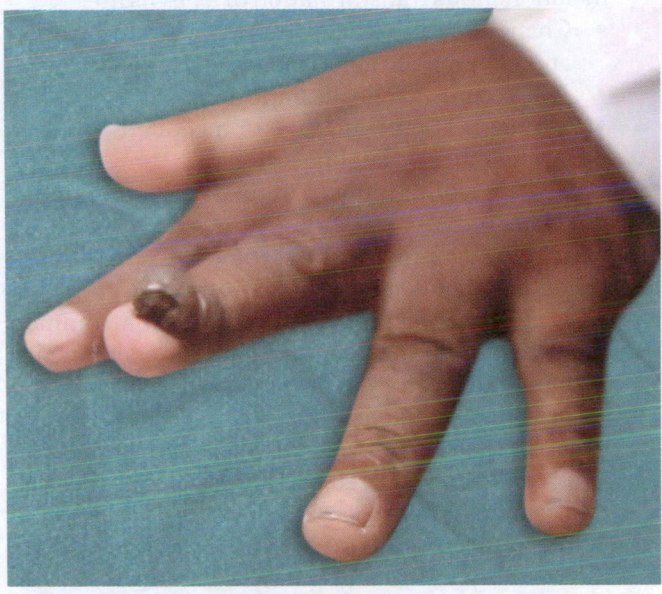

Fig. 25: Subungual melanoma of middle finger lifting up the nail

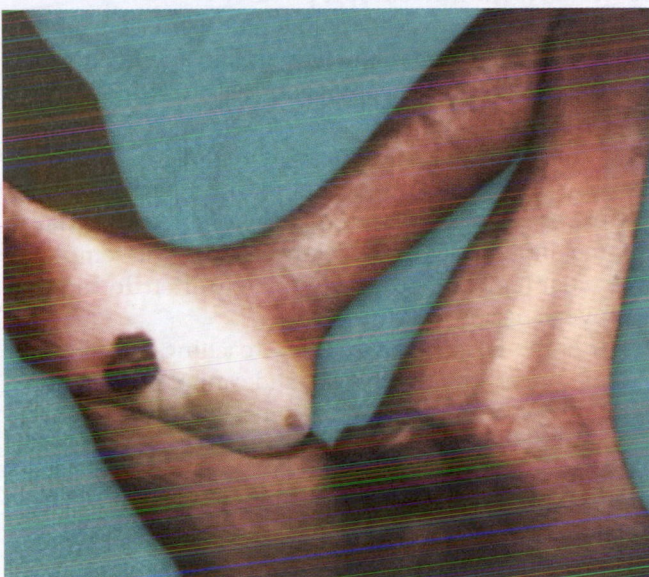

Fig. 24: Malignant melanoma of sole of foot with inguinal nodal metastases (*Courtesy:* Professor R K Agrawal and Professor A K Khare, Udaipur)

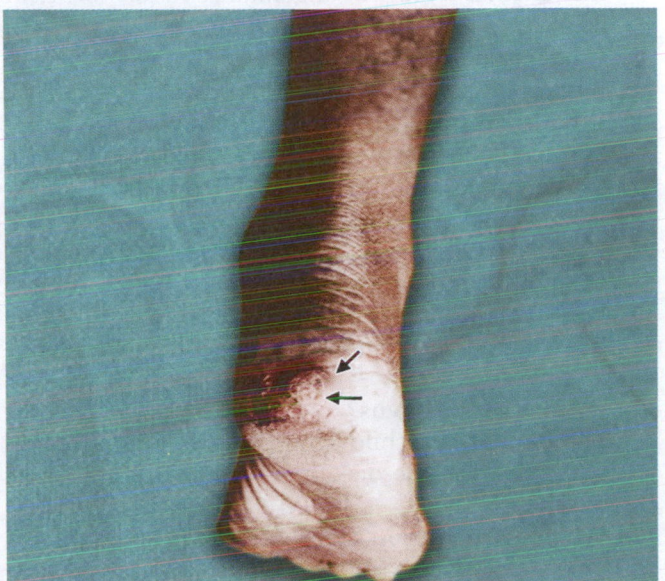

Fig. 26: Malignant melanoma of right heel (Late Professor SC Misra's case)

3. **What is the etiology of this tumor?**
   It is not known, but the risk factors are:
   1. Exposure to ultraviolet radiation.
   2. Xeroderma pigmentosum, past medical or family history of malignant melanoma, large number of nevi, dysplastic nevi, red hair, tendency to freckle and immunosuppression secondary to drugs or HIV infection.

4. **What are the features in a pigmented lesion to arouse a suspicion of malignant change?**
   The features suggestive of a melanoma or melanomatous transformation of a nevus are:
   - Change in size—A nevus more than 6 mm is suspect and more than 10 mm is more likely to be malignant.
   - Any recent change in shape or color
   - Surface becoming nodular or ulcerated
   - Appearance of satellite lesions
   - Presence of tingling, itching or serosanguinous discharge
   - Having 'Doppler-positive' blood supply.

5. **What do you mean by dysplastic nevus?**
   - It is slightly larger (5-12 mm) than a common nevus. It has macular and papular components, variegated color (tan brown) on a pink base, and indistinct irregular edge.
   - Contrary to common nevi, dysplastic nevi are most prevalent on covered body areas though they can occur anywhere.

6. **What is a congenital nevus and what is its relationship with a malignant melanoma?**
   It occurs in about 1 percent of neonates. It is a small lesion and a precursor of melanoma. The risk of malignant change in a congenital nevus of more than 20 mm is 5 to 20 percent.

7. **What is a mole?**
   It is a benign pigmented lesion of skin.

8. **What are the types of moles?**
   A mole is of four types—hairy mole, nonhairy or smooth mole, blue nevus and Hutchinson's lentigo.

9. **What is a hairy mole?**
   It is a flat or very slightly raised patch which is smooth or slightly warty with a tuft of hair.

10. **What is a nonhairy or smooth mole?**
    It is a pigmented spot which is smooth, not elevated and hairless.

11. **What is a blue nevus?**
    The patient is a child who presents with a bluish patch deep in the dermis with smooth and shiny overlying skin.

12. **What is Hutchinson's lentigo?**
    There is a large area of dark pigmentation on the face and neck with a smooth or rough nodular surface. The patient is in late adult life.

13. **What are the high-risk locations of a melanoma?**
    The high-risk locations are:
    1. Upper back.
    2. Posterolateral arm.
    3. Posterior and lateral neck.
    4. Posterior scalp (BANS region).

14. **What are the types of melanoma?**
    The types of melanoma are:
    1. Superficial spreading (70%).
    2. Nodular (15-20%).
    3. Lentigo maligna (5-10%).
    4. Acral lentiginous (rare).

15. **What are the clinical features of a superficial spreading melanoma?**
    It is the commonest type, slightly elevated and brown with small discrete nodules of black, gray, blue or pinkish hue, and seen most frequently on the back of both sexes and lower limbs in women. Nearly half of these cancers arise from a preexisting mole.

16. **What is the microscopic picture?**
    Microscopically, the malignant melanocytes are fairly uniform with a prominent intraepidermal component and a variable degree of dermal invasion.

17. **What is a nodular melanoma?**
    - It is a dense black or reddish blue black elevated and firm nodule occurring anywhere. If it occurs at a site the patient cannot see, it may become quite large and may ulcerate before it is noticed.
    - It may occur in a pre-existing nevus, and is the most dangerous type of melanoma.
    - A distinct convex nodular development indicates deep dermal invasion.

18. **What is the microscopic picture?**
    Microscopically, the malignant cells arise from the epidermal-dermal junction and invade deeply into the dermis and subcutaneous tissue with relatively little lateral intradermal invasion.

19. **What is lentigo maligna melanoma?**
    This lesion usually occurs in older patients on an exposed surface of the body. It is often seen as a large melanotic freckle (Hutchinson's) on the temple or malar region. It grows very slowly often developing over a period of years.
    It is the largest in size often reaching 5 to 6 cm in diameter. Initially it is flat and cannot be felt and as the disease progresses it becomes slightly raised with a palpable thickening. The edge is irregular. There may be discrete brown nodules in the lesion.

20. **What is micropathology?**
    The malignant change is scattered irregularly throughout the lesion, corresponding with elevated areas and color changes. Malignant melanocytes appear to concentrate in the darker areas.

21. What is acral lentiginous melanoma?

It occurs in the hairless skin of the sole and palm, or subungual region (Figs 24 and 25). It is the commonest melanoma of pigmented races.

22. What is the microscopic picture?

Microscopically, the intraepidermal component is that of a lentiginous proliferation of typical or malignant cells at the margin of tumor. In contrast to lentigo maligna the epidermis is hyperplastic.

23. What are Breslow levels?

The Breslow levels are (Fig. 27):

Level I — 0.75 mm or less

Level II — 0.76 to 1.5 mm

Level III — 1.51 to 3 mm

Level IV — Greater than 3 mm

24. What are the investigations?

- The main investigation is limited excisional biopsy to make a tissue diagnosis. Full thickness incisional or punch biopsy may be used in large lesions.
- If the lymph nodes are enlarged they may be studied by FNAC or biopsy. The extent of spread in the lymph nodes may be assessed by lymphoscintigraphy.
- If there is suspicion of spread to the liver, ultrasonography is indicated. Similarly chest X-ray is done to detect pulmonary metastases.

25. Have you heard of spontaneous regression of a melanoma?

Yes, a cutaneous melanoma and even visceral metastases may rarely undergo spontaneous regression.

26. What is the mechanism of regression?

It is not known. Probably, it is due to activation of immune mechanisms.

27. How do you treat this tumor?

The primary lesion is treated by wide surgical excision.

28. What do you mean by wide excision?

- Lentigo maligna—Excision with a clinical 5 mm margin
- Lesion less than 1 mm deep—Excision with a 1 cm margin
- Deeper lesions—Excision with 2 cm margin

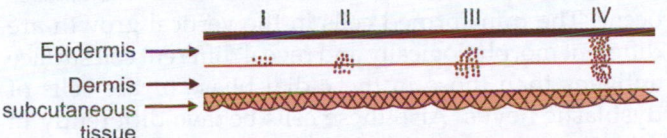

Fig. 27: Breslow levels of malignant melanoma

29. What is the extent of excision in the depth?

The depth of excision has been traditionally upto deep fascia more because it is an easily identifiable landmark rather than for any therapeutic value.

30. How do you make up for tissue defect?

The defect is closed by skin grafting or flap.

31. How do you treat the melanomas of digits?

They are treated by ray amputation without attempts at local excision.

32. How do you deal with nodal metastases?

- All clinically positive nodes are excised by regional nodal dissection for cure or palliation.
- If the nodes are not clinically involved a sentinel node biopsy (SNB) is done at the time of primary surgery as it is predictive of nodal status in 99 percent of patients.

33. What is the extent of lymph node dissection in lower limb melanomas?

In groin the deep (iliac) nodes are also excised alongwith the superficial (inguinal) nodes.

34. What is extent of dissection in axilla?

In axilla, the nodes medial to pectoralis minor must be removed.

35. What is the additional step in the operation of cervical lymph node dissection for melanoma of face?

When the cervical node dissection is being done for melanoma of face a superficial parotidectomy is also done as the preparotid lymph node may contain cancer before the cervical nodes.

36. What is prophylactic node dissection?

If the lymph nodes are removed before they are palpable in early disease, it is called prophylactic node dissection.

37. What is the role of prophylactic node dissection?

As the disadvantages are more than the advantages, the prophylactic node dissection is not recommended.

38. How do you treat distant metastases?

Resection of surgically accessible metastatic lesions or solitary pulmonary metastasis may provide significant palliation or even may cure in rare cases. Disseminated melanoma is treated by chemotherapy or immunotherapy.

39. What are the factors on which depends the prognosis?

The prognosis depends on:

- Breslow thickness of the primary tumor
- Mitotic index—The higher the mitotic index the poorer the prognosis.
- Nodal metastasis is the most important prognostic factor as 78 to 85 percent of patients with clinical nodal metastases have occult distal metastases.

40. Have you heard of a secondary melanoma without a primary lesion?

It accounts for 4 percent of metastatic melanomas. Primary melanoma may be in the gastrointestinal tract.

41. What is amelanotic melanoma?

It is a melanoma with no visible pigmentation. It carries a poor prognosis either from a delay in diagnosis or aggressive behavior or both.

DISCUSSION

Malignant melanoma is a malignant tumor of melanocytes of unknown cause characterized by an ulcerative or nodular lesion of insidious onset (Fig. 28).

Melanoma affects around 62,000 persons per year in USA, resulting in 7910 deaths. It is the fifth most common cancer in men (5% of cancers) and the 6th most common in women (4% of carcers). The lifetime risk is 1:53 in males and 1:78 in females.

Other types—Amelanotic melanoma is not pigmented, it usually occurs in gastrointestinal tract and presents with obstruction or as a metastasis from an unknown primary.

Desmoplastic tumor usually occurs in head and neck and has a propensity for perineural infiltration hence more likely to recur locally.

Etiology

This cancer is etiologically related to exposure to ultraviolet light which reflects occupational and recreational exposure to sunlight especially in white skinned people. Thus

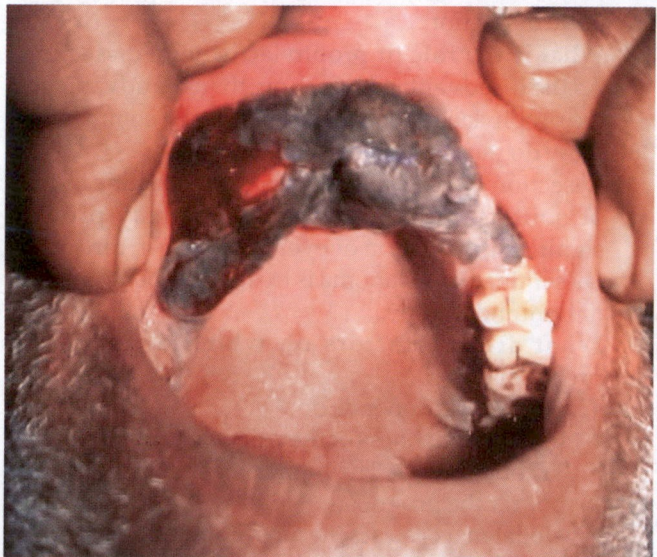

Fig. 28: Malignant melanoma of upper alveolus (*Courtesy: Professor Sandeep Kumar*)

cumulative exposure results in the occurrence of lentigo maligna, while the 'flash fry' exposure (holiday tanning of skin) favors the development of other types.

The risk factors are xeroderma pigmentosum, past medical or family history of malignant melanoma, large number of nevi, dysplastic nevi, red hair, tendency to freckle, immune suppression secondary to drugs or HIV infection.

Nevi and malignant melanoma—About 10 to 20 percent of melanomas develop in pre-existing nevi. The rest (majority) develop de novo in normally pigmented skin. The junctional and compound types of nevi are most likely to develop a malignant melanoma. The features that arouse a suspicion of malignant change are:

- Change in size—A nevus more than 6 mm is suspected and more than 10 mm is more likely to be malignant
- Any recent change in shape or color
- Surface becoming nodular or ulcerated
- Appearance of satellite lesions
- Presence of tingling, itching or serosanguineous discharge
- Having 'Doppler-positive' blood supply.

Pathogenesis

This lesion arises from transformed melanocytes; thus apart from skin it can occur anywhere where melanocytes migrated during embryogenesis, i.e. eye (retina) central nervous system (leptomeninges), gastro-intestinal tract and even gall bladder. More than 90 percent melanomas occur in skin. 7 percent of melanomas occur as metastases without the primary being identified which is probably completely regressed (immune phenomenon) as tumor regression is known to occur in this cancer.

In the skin of many people, nevi are found which are benign melanocytic neoplasms. There are dysplastic nevi also which contain a focus of atypical melanocytes. This nevus probably represents an intermediate between a benign nevus and a malignant melanoma. The risk of developing a malignant melanoma is proportionate to the number of dysplastic nevi as the number of colonic polyps is related to occurrence of colonic carcinoma.

Growth and metastases: A melanoma grows radially in the plane of epidermis. In this phase microinvasion of dermis is seen but metastases do not occur. When the melanoma cells form nests in the dermis then metastases occur. The transformed cells in the vertical growth are different morphologically and reveal different cell surface antigens than those in the radial phase or the cells of dysplastic nevus. Also these cells behave differently in cell culture and can grow in a less enriched medium and have a longer life span.

Types: The four common types of melanoma in the order of decreasing frequency are—superficial spreading, nodular, lentigo maligna and acral lentiginous.

1. **Superficial spreading** is the most common type (70%), most likely to arise in a pre-existing nevus and can occur anywhere on the skin except hands and feet. It is flat, 1 to 2 cm in diameter and commonly contains areas of regression. It has a long radial growth phase before vertical growth begins.
2. **Nodular type** (15-20%) is darker and raised. It arises in normal skin, commonly seen in middle-aged men and usually on the trunk, head or neck (Fig. 29). Histologically there is lack of radial growth peripheral to the area of vertical growth. Hence all types of lesions are in the vertical growth phase at the time of diagnosis. Though it is aggressive, prognostically it is like the first type.
3. **Lentigo maligna** (5-10%) commonly occurs on the back of hands, neck and face of elderly individuals. It presents as a slow-growing, variegated brown macule (a lentigo). These tumors are always surrounded by dermis with heavy solar degeneration. They tend to become quite large before a clinical diagnosis is made but have best prognosis because invasion is a late occurrence.
4. **Acral lentiginous** (rare) occurs on the palm, sole and subungual regions. Melanoma in dark skinned people is relatively uncommon, this lesion is more common in them. The subungual tumor appears as blue black

discolouration of the posterior nailfold and is most commonly seen on the great toe or thumb.

Other types—Amelanotic melanoma is not pigmented. It usually occurs in gastrointestinal tract and presents with obstruction or as metastasis from an unknown primary.

Desmoplastic tumor usually occurs in head and neck, has a propensity for perineural infiltration, hence more likely to recur locally.

Micropathology

The malignant change occurs initially in the melanocytes of the basal epidermis, and the abnormal melanocytes are limited to dermo-epidermal junction without any dermal involvement (in situ lesion)

- *Horizontal growth phase*—The abnormal cells spread along the dermo-epidermal junction. Though they may breach the dermis, the spread is mainly horizontal (radial).
- *Vertical growth phase*—The cells spread in the depth invading the dermis increasing the thickness of the lesion. The more is the depth of invasion the more is the metastatic potential of the tumor.

Breslow Levels

Breslow modified the Clark's method by the use of ocular micrometer. The lesions are measured from the granular layer of the epidermis or the base of the ulcer to the greatest depth of tumor:

Level I	—	0.75 mm or less
Level II	—	0.76 mm to 1.5 mm
Level III	—	1.51 mm to 3 mm
Level IV	—	More than 3 mm

Investigations

- Clinical photograph of the lesion should be taken when one chooses to observe the lesion.
- Dermoscopy—It is the use of a special magnifying device which is used to see the lesion. It helps to select the lesions that require biopsy. It has a 85% specificity and 95% sensitivity.
- Biopsy—An excision biopsy is done with a 2 mm margin of skin and a cuff of subdermal fat. In large lesions an incisional biopsy may be done. The thickness of the lesion is measured to nearest 0.1 mm from the granular layer to the base of the tumor. It is the first step when the biopsy specimen is being examined.
- Sentinel node biopsy (SNB) is recommended for the patients of stage II disease with the help of local intradermal injection of technetium-99 m sulfur colloid and sulfan blue dye.

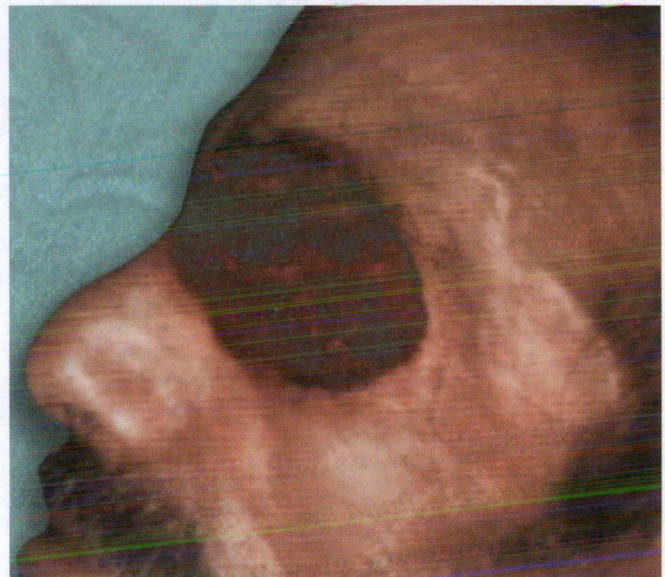

Fig. 29: Malignant melanoma of the eye (*Courtesy:* Professor RK Agrawal and Professor AK Khare, Udaipur)

- Other investigations are dependent on clinical presentation to detect metastases (CT scan, LDH).

Staging

IA   :   Lesion less than 1 mm without ulceration (T1a).

IB   :   Lesion less than 1 mm with ulceration (T1b).
Lesion more than 1 mm, less than 2 mm without ulceration (T2a).

IIA   :   Lesion more than 1 mm, less than 2 mm with ulceration (T2b).
Lesion more than 2 mm, less than 4 mm without ulceration (T3a).

IIB   :   Lesion more than 2 mm, less than 4 mm with ulceration (T3b).
Lesion more than 4 mm without ulceration (T4a).

IIC   :   Lesion more than 4 mm with ulceration (T4b).

IIIA   :   Any Breslow, no ulceration, micrometastases in nodes.

IIIB   :   Any Breslow, with ulceration, micrometastases in nodes
Any Breslow, without ulceration, ≤ 3 palpable nodes.
Any Breslow, with or without ulceration, in transit metastases/satellites.

IIIC   :   Any Breslow, with ulceration, ≤ 3 palpable nodes. Any Breslow, with or without ulceration, ≤ 4 palpable or matted nodes or nodes with in transit metastases.

IV   :   Any of the above plus distant metastasis (M1-skin, subcutaneous or distant: M2 - lungs: M3 - all other sites or any site with elevated LDH).

Treatment—It is primarily surgical excision of the tumor:

- The lentigo maligna (melanoma in situ) is excised with a clinical 5 mm margin all round it to prevent the risk of it entering into the vertical growth phase which will make it lentigo maligna melanoma.
- A melanoma less than 1 mm deep, wide local excision with a 1 cm margin is recommended.
- For deeper melanomas, a 2 cm margin of excision is required including the depth.
- *Nodal disease*—The likelihood of nodal metastasis is proportional to the Breslow thickness of the lesion.
  If the melanoma has clinically spread to the nodes, the lymph node dissection has to be done.
  In those cases where there is no clinical evidence of nodal involvement, sentinel node biopsy (SNB) should be done as it is predictive of nodal status in 99 percent of patients. It is not done if the primary lesion is thinner than 1 mm. With a Breslow thickness of less than 1.25 mm, only 4 percent of the sentinel nodes are positive for metastases 70 to 80 percent of patients with positive sentinel nodes usually do not have involvement of other regional nodes. But if nodal dissection is done all the lymph nodes are removed in the regional basin.
- *Adjuvant therapy*—None of them is useful. Work is going on vaccine and interferon treatments.

Prognosis—It depends upon:

- Breslow thickness of the primary lesion (Fig. 27).
- Mitotic index—The higher the mitotic index the poorer the prognosis.
- Nodal metastasis—It is the most important prognostic factor. 78 to 85 percent of patients with clinical nodal metastases have occult distant metastases.

CASE 8: PAGET'S DISEASE OF BREAST

CLINICAL DIAGNOSIS

1. The patient is usually a middle-aged or elderly female who presents with burning or itching, erosion or ulceration of nipple and areola of insidious onset.
2. It is a unilateral disease.
3. The nipple may be destroyed completely (Fig. 30).
4. An ill-defined lump may be palpable behind the nipple in a late case.
5. The axilla is usually clear, but may have enlarged lymph nodes in late stages of disease.

VIVA VOCE

1. **What is Paget's disease of breast?**
   It is a rare disease of the breast characterized by unilateral eczematoid lesion of the nipple that may result in erosion, ulceration and later on disappearance of nipple (Fig. 30).
2. **What is the cause of this disease?**
   The cause of this condition is not known. It is a manifestation of a well-differentiated infiltrating duct carcinoma or duct carcinoma in-situ.
3. **What is the incidence?**
   It constitutes 1% of all cancers of breast.
4. **How will you confirm the diagnosis?**
   By biopsy.
5. **What is the biopsy report?**
   The biopsy shows superficial ulceration of the epidermis that has proliferated deeply with an increase in the size of inter-papillary processes in which large hydropic Paget's cells are seen (Fig. 31).

6. **What are Paget's cells?**
   The Paget's cells are large ovoid cells with abundant clear, pale-staining cytoplasm in the Malpigian layer of epidermis (Fig. 31).
7. **Does it metastasize?**
   The axillary metastases are seen in less than 5 percent of cases, but when a lump appears, it produces local and distal metastases like a frank cancer.
8. **What is the danger in this disease?**
   It may not be recognized as cancerous and a clinician may treat it like eczema without any benefit, but with silent advancement of disease.
9. **How do you treat this disease?**
   - It is treated like T1 carcinoma of breast with local control of disease by simple mastectomy. No adjuvant treatment is required
   - If a lump is present it is treated on the lines of a frank carcinoma of the breast depending upon the stage of disease.
10. **Will you like to do sentinel lymph node biopsy?**
    It may be done as axillary nodal metastasis are present in less than 5 percent of patients.
11. **What is the prognosis?**
    - The prognosis is excellent before the appearance of the lump
    - If the lump is present, the prognosis depends upon the stage of the disease. Overall it is bad.

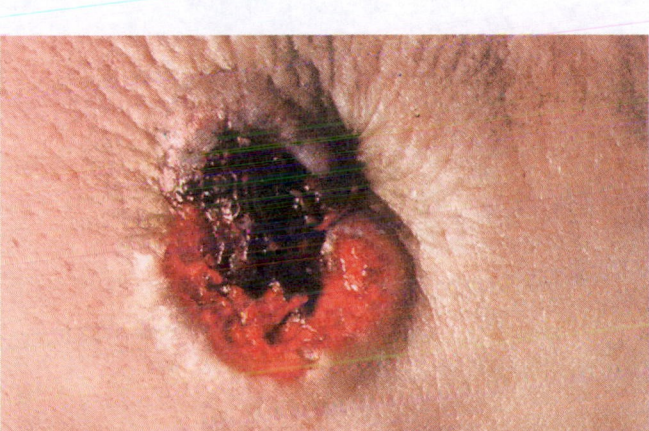

Fig. 30: Advanced Paget's disease of nipple with nipple destruction

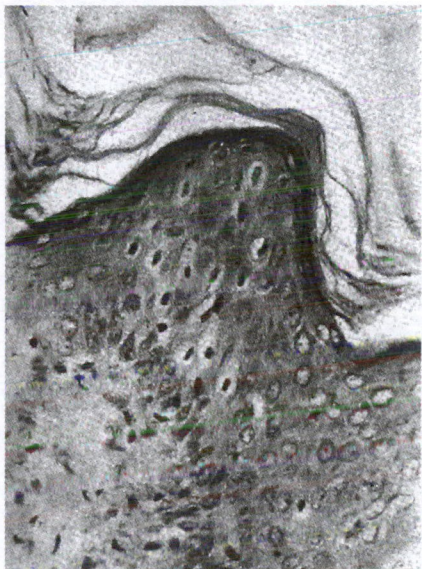

Fig. 31: Paget's disease of nipple with Paget's cell infiltrating epidermis

DISCUSSION

Paget's disease of the breast is a unilateral eczematoid lesion of the nipple that is a manifestation of a well-differentiated infiltrating duct carcinoma or duct carcinoma in situ (DCIS) that grows towards the skin to produce erosion and ulceration. It constitutes 1% of breast cancers.

The ducts of the nipple are infiltrated. The epidermis is ulcerated superficially and proliferated deeply with an increase in the size of interpapillary processes that contain Paget's cells. They are large cells with abundant pale staining clear cytoplasm and dark nuclei.

The patient is usually a middle-aged woman who presents with itching or burning of the nipple with red nipple and areola covered with scales. Gradually the scales are lost and the nipple is destroyed. Finally the nipple is completely destroyed leaving a flat bright red weeping surface. The condition looks like eczema or bacterial dermatitis and may be treated accordingly with delay in detecting the underlying carcinoma. The differences between eczema and Paget's disease are given below:

Features	Eczema	Paget's disease
Laterality	Often bilateral	Unilateral
Time of occurrence	In a lactating breast	Menopausal breast
Itching	Prominent symptom	May be absent; burning is more common
Vesicles	Usually present	Absent
Nipple	Remains intact	Gradually destroyed
Lump	No lump	Lump may be present deep to nipple

The axilla is clear in most of the cases. Axillary nodal metastases are present in less than 5 percent of patients. When a lump is present, the incidence of metastases rises. The diagnosis is established by biopsy. It is treated like a T1 cancer of breast with local control by simple mastectomy. Sentinel lymph node biopsy may be done. When it presents as a lump, it is treated on the lines of a frank carcinoma of the breast depending upon the stage of the disease.

Benign Ulcers

CASE 1: TUBERCULOUS ULCER

CLINICAL DIAGNOSIS

1. The patient is usually a young person (a little more common in females) who presents with a chronic non-healing ulcer of insidious onset.
2. It can occur anywhere but commonly in the neck, axilla or groin.
3. It is usually painless, except when it occurs on the tongue.
4. It may be single or multiple (Fig. 1).
5. It is oval or circular in shape, variable in size and has a undermined edge (Fig. 2).
6. The floor is covered with pale slough or watery granulation tissue.
7. It discharges thin syrup-like pus or watery fluid.
8. The regional lymph nodes may be enlarged, firm and matted.

VIVA VOCE

1. **What is an ulcer?**
   An ulcer is a raw area in the lining skin or epithelium of the body caused by molecular death of tissue. It is always infected and lined by granulation tissue.
2. **How do you differentiate it from a sinus?**
   The structure of the ulcer is such—wide mouth and lesser depth—that the floor of the ulcer is visible. The sinus, on the other hand, has a narrow mouth and considerable depth, hence it is a blind track, i.e. the floor or limit cannot be seen.
3. **What is the mechanism of ulceration?**
   Initially there is a focus of tuberculous infection in the skin or underneath which necroses and ruptures out on the skin producing an ulcer.
4. **Why is the edge undermined?**
   Because more tissue is destroyed by tuberculous infection in the depth than the surface.

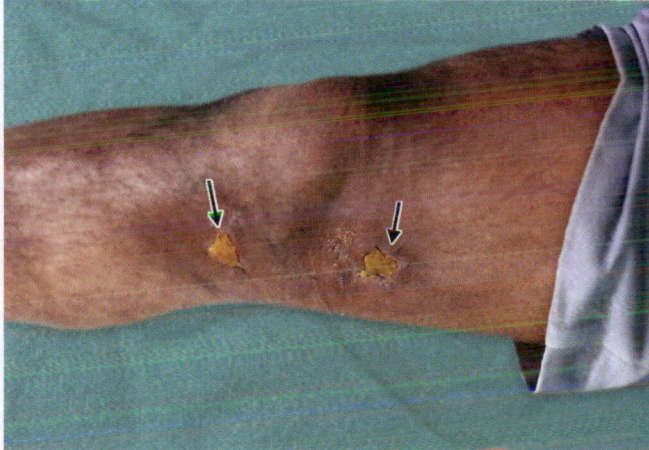

Fig. 1: Chronic encrusting ulcers (two) in knee region—biopsy revealed it to be tuberculous. They healed following antituberculous treatment

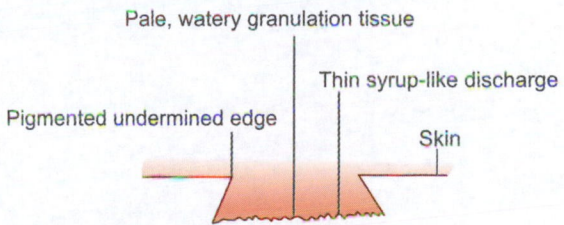

Fig. 2: Signs of a tuberculous ulcer

5. **What is the nature of discharge of a tuberculous lesion?**
It is thin pus or thin syrup-like discharge with curdy flakes.

6. **What is the nature of curdy flakes?**
They are small pieces of caseous necrotic tissue.

7. **What is the mechanism of tuberculous sinus formation?**
When a cold abscess of deep-seated tuberculous lesion ruptures on the skin it may result in a sinus formation.

8. **What are the signs of a tuberculous sinus?**
The patient has a single or multiple openings of insidious onset discharging thin pus. The edge of the sinus is pigmented and undermined.

9. **What are the investigations?**
The investigations are:
- Blood—Blood counts, ESR
- X-ray chest
- Tuberculin skin test
- Culture of discharge, especially for mycobacteria
- Biopsy, a part of biopsy piece may be sent for culture of mycobacteria
- Nucleic acid (DNA and RNA) amplification for M tuberculosis in the discharge or biopsy specimen gives results within hours.

10. **How do you treat this ulcer?**
The essentials of the treatment are:
- Antituberculous drugs—Majority of ulcers heal with a full course of antituberculous drugs
- Dressing of ulcer
- Surgery—If the ulcer fails to heal (rare) or there is residual lesion, it may be excised and skin grafted.

DISCUSSION

Tuberculous ulcer is a chronic ulcer that is caused by tuberculous infection and commonly seen in young patients (Fig. 1).

Etiology

It is due to rupture of a tuberculous necrotic lesion of the skin (e.g. tuberculoma) or structures just under the skin (lymph node, bone or joint).

Pathology

This ulcer can occur anywhere in the body but commonly seen in the neck, axilla or groin. Multiple ulcers may be present. It is usually ovoid or circular. The edge is pigmented and undermined. It contains tuberculous granulation tissue in the floor.

Clinical Features

Majority of patients are young, more commonly females, and present with a chronic nonhealing ulcer that has an undermined edge with pigmented surroundings. It discharges pus or thin syrup-like discharge may be with curdy flakes.

The regional lymph nodes may be enlarged, firm and matted. When the ulcer heals it may leave a thin tissue paper-like scar.

Investigations

- Culture and sensitivity of discharge: It may be done for mycobacteria
- Biopsy—It shows tuberculous granulation tissue. The tissue may also be cultured for tubercle bacilli
- Tuberculin skin test
- X-ray of chest for any evidence of pulmonary tuberculosis
- Nucleic acid amplification for M tuberculosis in the discharge of ulcer.

Treatment

Majority of ulcers heal with antituberculous chemotherapy, a full course of which should be given. Locally, it requires daily dressing. The general health of the patient should be improved. If the ulcer fails to heal or there is residual lesion, it may be excised and skin grafted.

Prognosis

The results of treatment are good. A majority of ulcers heal with chemotherapy alone.

CASE 2: ANAL FISSURE

CLINICAL DIAGNOSIS

1. The patient presents with sharp agonizing anal pain occurring during defecation and lasting an hour or so after the act.
2. The stool may be streaked with blood corresponding to the site of fissure. It may be narrow and short with nipped off appearance.
3. There is a canoe-shaped ulcer in the posterior (more common) or anterior midline (Figs 3 and 4).
4. The ulcer may not be visible because of tight closure of anus (anal spasm). It happens in acute fissure.
5. There is a tag of skin at the lower end of ulcer ('sentinel pile').
6. The ulcer may have tender and indurated edge that may feel like a button-hole.
7. At the upper end of the ulcer an enlarged papilla may be present.
8. An abscess or cutaneous fistula may be present near the lower end of ulcer (Fig. 4) (5 to 8 are the signs of a chronic fissure).

VIVA VOCE

1. **What is an anal fissure?**
   It is a longitudinal split in the anoderm of the lower anal canal extending from anal verge proximally towards the dentate line, and not above it (< 5 mm).
2. **What are the sites of fissure in the anal canal?**
   * The commonest site is posterior midline as seen in > 90 percent of patients
   * The next common site is anterior midline that is seen in women who have given birth to children via vaginal delivery
   * Rarely a fissure can occur at the atypical sites.

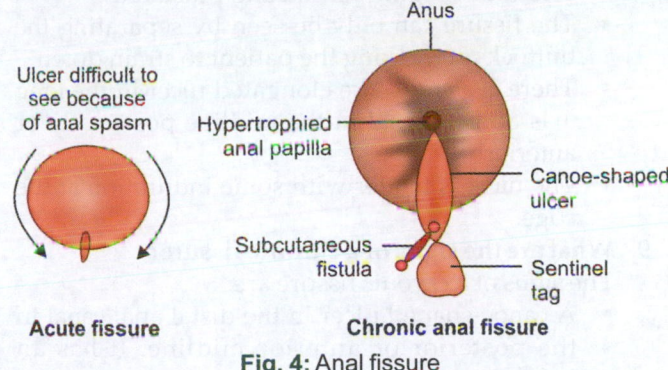

Acute fissure   Chronic anal fissure

Fig. 4: Anal fissure

3. **What is the etiology?**
   * Most fissures are believed to occur from trauma to anal canal during defecation caused by straining, constipation, and frequent stools of diarrhea or high internal sphincter tone
   * The anterior fissure occurs during vaginal delivery due to overstretching of anterior wall
   * Atypical (and multiple) fissures can occur in Crohn's disease, HIV/AIDS, tuberculosis, syphilis, ano-receptive intercourse, chlamydia, lymphogranuloma venereum, chancroid, HSV, cytomegalovirus and anal carcinoma.
4. **Why is the fissure so painful?**
   An anal fissure is very painful (tearing pain) because of its location below the dentate line, as it is stretched and traumatized with every act of defecation.
5. **How is it related to constipation?**
   It may be caused by constipation, and it may cause constipation as the patient may postpone defecation for fear of pain during defecation.
6. **What is the mechanism of chronicity?**
   Due to chronic subepithelial infection the torn edges of anoderm are undermined and the ulcer deepens exposing the fibers of internal sphincter. A vicious cycle ensues in which the subepithelial inflammation causes spasm of the internal sphincter preventing free drainage and permitting continued inflammation.
7. **Why does it occur commonly in the posterior midline?**
   The stretching of anoderm of the posterior anal verge during defecation as this area is less supported by muscle and the anterior curvature of posterior wall of rectum to join the anal canal is the most likely reason for the fissure to occur in the posterior midline.

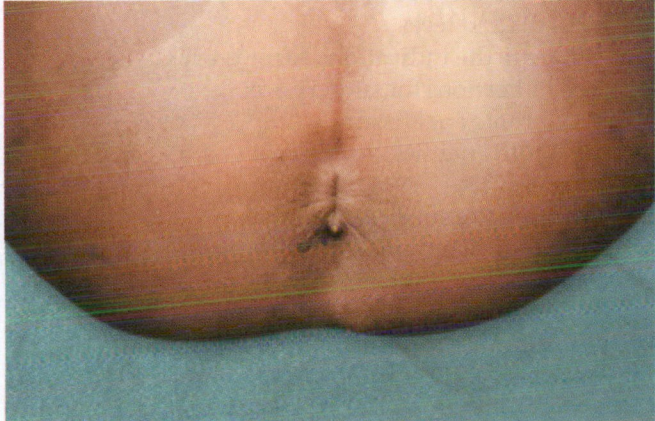

Fig. 3: Posterior midline anal fissure

8. **What are the signs of an acute fissure?**
   The signs are:
   - The anus is tightly closed and puckered
   - The fissure can only be seen by separating the buttocks and asking the patient to strain down
   - There is a crack-like elongated ulcer in the long axis of anal canal in the midline posteriorly or anteriorly
   - The ulcer is tender with some induration at the edge.

9. **What are the signs of a chronic fissure?**
   The signs of a chronic fissure are:
   - A canoe-shaped ulcer in the distal anal canal in the posterior or anterior midline. It has an indurated undermined edge
   - Lower edge of internal sphincter may be visible in the floor
   - Sentinel pile is present at the lower end
   - Hypertrophied anal papilla may be present at the upper end
   - A subcutaneous fistula may be present connected to the lower end (Fig. 4).

10. **What is the cause of hypertrophy of anal papilla?**
    It is because of chronic or recurrent edema of anal papilla that occurs due to inflammation of anal crypt adjacent to papilla.

11. **What is sentinel pile?**
    It is a fibrotic nubbin of skin situated at the anal verge just below the lower end of fissure.

12. **Why is it called sentinel pile?**
    It is so called because it stands as a sentinel just below the fissure.

13. **How is it produced?**
    It forms because of chronic inflammation and interference with lymphatic drainage of the skin at the lower angle of ulcer.

14. **Do you need any investigation for confirming the diagnosis?**
    The diagnosis is made by good clinical examination and investigations are not needed.

15. **What are the indications for sigmoidoscopy?**
    Sigmoidoscopy is indicated to exclude any specific cause of anal fissure such as inflammatory bowel disease.

16. **How do you treat an anal fissure?**
    - An acute anal fissure is usually treated by conservative measures
    - A chronic fissure usually requires surgical help.

17. **What is the conservative treatment?**
    It includes:
    - Alteration of stool consistency by giving celvac 10 ml twice daily
    - Warm sitz bath and local anesthetic cream
    - Dietary bran
    - Glyceryl trinitrate (GTN) 0.2 percent locally four times daily or diltiazem 2 percent twice daily may reduce spasm
    - Injection of botulinum toxin 20 units into the anal sphincter.

18. **What are the results of conservative treatment?**
    - Healing occurs within 2 months in up to 45 percent of patients
    - Recurrence occurs in 40 percent of relieved patients.

19. **What is the role of anal dilatation?**
    It helps by relieving the spasm of anal sphincter.

20. **What are the types of anal dilatation?**
    It is of 2 types:
    - Simple dilatation with the use of anal dilator
    - Maximal anal dilatation (Lord's procedure) under anesthesia.

21. **How is the dilatation done by anal dilator?**
    It is done by the patient himself. The patient is instructed to smear local anesthetic ointment on to the dilator, to lie on the left side and to insert the dilator up to its hilt, whilst retaining hold of the dilator. The dilator should be kept in this position for 30 to 60 seconds, removed and washed.

22. **How do you do maximal anal dilatation?**
    It can be performed under local or general anesthesia. The index and middle fingers of each hand are inserted simultaneously into the anus and are pulled gently apart to give maximal dilatation.

23. **What are the results of maximal dilatation?**
    It gives immediate relief in anal pain and spasm in 75 to 95 percent of patients. The recurrence rate is around 10 percent.

24. **What are its complications?**
    They include bleeding and prolapse of hemorrhoids, and there may be a temporary impairment of control of flatus and feces.

25. **What are the indications for surgery?**
    The indications for surgery are:
    - Chronic anal fissure
    - Acute anal fissure not relieved by conservative measures.

26. **What are the surgical options?**
    The surgical options are:
    - Lateral anal sphincterotomy
    - Fissurectomy and median sphincterotomy.

27. **What is lateral sphincterotomy?**
    In this operation the internal sphincter is divided away from the fissure in any lateral positions. The sentinel pile is excised.

28. How do you do sphincterotomy?

The procedure can be done by an open or a closed method. The internal sphincter is identified in the lateral position in the intersphincteric groove and its lower portion is transected.

29. What are the advantages of this procedure?

The advantages are:
- The fissure heals promptly within 21 days
- Hardly any complication
- It can be performed on an outpatient basis.

30. What is done in fissurectomy and median sphincterotomy?

The fissure along with the sentinel pile and hypertrophied papilla is excised and the internal sphincter is divided in the floor of the wound.

31. What are the disadvantages of this procedure?

The disadvantages include:
- More chances of stress incontinence
- More chances of recurrence.

32. How do you treat a fissure complicating Crohn's disease?

The treatment is conservative with the treatment of causative disease. Sphincterotomy risks sepsis and should be avoided.

33. What are the results?

The majority (70%) heal spontaneously with or without resection of affected intestine.

DISCUSSION

An anal fissure is a longitudinal split or ulcer in the lower anal canal extending from the anal verge proximally towards, but not beyond the dentate line (Fig. 5).

Etiology

- The etiology of this disease is not clearly understood.
- An acute anal fissure occurs from the injury caused by strained evacuation of a hard stool. Less commonly, the crack arises from repeated passage of stool in diarrhea.

  In a female, the anterior anoderm of distal anal canal may tear during vaginal delivery.

  Anoderm of stenotic anus following hemorrhoidectomy may crack during defecation. Anoreceptive intercourse may also result in an anal fissure.
- Chronicity of anal fissure may be due to repeated trauma, anal hypertonicity and vascular insufficiency due to raised sphincter tone, or due to normal less perfusion of posterior commissure
- Site of fissure—Most of the fissures occur in the posterior midline. Anterior anal fissures account for 10 percent of those encountered in females but only 1 percent in men.

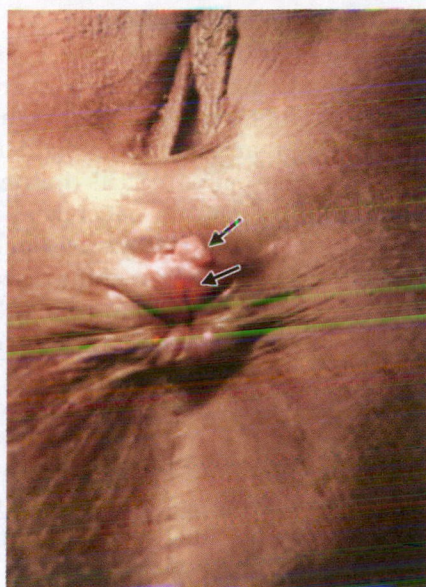

Fig. 5: Anterior midline anal fissure in a female. The upper arrow points to the sentinel tag

The stretching of overlying epithelium of posterior anal verge during defecation as this area is relatively unsupported by muscle, and the anterior curvature of posterior wall of rectum in the hollow of sacrum to join the anal canal is the most likely explanation of occurrence of posterior fissure.

The anterior anal fissure develops during vaginal delivery due to overstretching of anterior wall. Rarely fissures may occur at other sites, may be multiple, or may have atypical features. The causes of these fissures are Crohn's disease, tuberculosis, AIDS, syphilis, Chlamydia, chancroid, lymphogranuloma venereum, HSV, cytomegalovirus, Kaposi's sarcoma, B-cell lymphoma and squamous cell carcinoma.

Pathology

- *Acute fissure*—It is a deep ulcer with inflammatory edema and induration of the edge. The anal sphincter is in spasm. Hence the ulcer can be seen under anesthesia with relaxation.
- *Chronic fissure*—It is a canoe-shaped ulcer with a skin tag (sentinel pile) at the lower angle, scar tissue or lower border of internal sphincter in the base of ulcer, and may be a hypertrophied anal papilla at the upper angle. In the lower angle or pocket a small abscess may form that may rupture on the skin in the vicinity giving rise to a subcutaneous fistula (Fig. 4).

Clinical Features

- *Age and sex*—Most of the patients are young adults, but it can occur at any age. It occurs equally among men and women.

- Pain is the main symptom. Anal fissure is the most important cause of anal pain. It occurs during defecation. It is sharp, agonizing and often overwhelming in intensity. It lasts for an hour or so following defecation and then stops suddenly. Then the patient may be pain-free till the next act of defecation. Because of pain, the patient may postpone the urge to defecate and may become constipated. There may be remissions in the course of the disease when the patient may be pain-free for days or weeks.
- Bleeding is usually slight and is in the form of streaks on the stool.
- Pruritus: In a chronic fissure there may be itching due to presence of sentinel tag and discharge from ulcer or fistula.
- The ulcer is situated in the posterior midline in most of the patients. It may be situated in anterior midline, especially in women.

Investigations

- Usually no investigations are required
- Atypical fissure needs biopsy and culture depending upon the clinical suspicion of the cause.

Treatment

- **Acute fissure:**
  1. Normalization of bowel habit by adding fiber to the diet, using stool softeners and adequate water intake.
  2. Warm baths and topical local anesthetic agents may relieve pain.
  3. Glyceryl trinitrate (GTN) 0.2 percent locally four times daily, or diltiazem 2 percent twice daily: They help by reducing spasm, relieving pain and increasing vascular perfusion. GTN may cause headaches in up to 40 percent of patients.
  4. Injection of botulinum toxin 20 units (Botox) into the anal sphincter may be helpful.

  Almost all fissures heal following this treatment. A few do not respond and some recur after sometime.
- **Chronic fissure:** In the first go the treatment described above is given. A large number of fissures heal following

conservative approach. If it does not respond or recurs operative intervention is indicated. There are many methods of treatment:

1. *Lord's procedure:* This is the simplest procedure. Under general anesthesia the index and middle finger of each hand are introduced into the anal canal and gently pulled apart to dilate the anus to four to six finger-breadth. Overstretching must be avoided as it may cause disruption of sphincter at multiple sites. It is good in young men with very high sphincter tone. Postoperatively there may be some temporary fecal incontinence.

2. *Lateral anal sphincterotomy (Notaras):* Under local, regional or general anesthesia and in lithotomy or prone jack-knife position, the distal sphincter is palpated with a bivalve speculum at the intersphincteric groove.
   - In the closed method a number 11 blade is advanced parallel to the sphincter in the groove and then rotated with sharp edge towards the internal sphincter which is divided along its distal third. Pressure is applied to stop bleeding.
   - In the open method the anoderm of distal internal sphincter is cut to expose the internal sphincter that is divided. The wound is closed by absorbable sutures after hemostasis. The papilla and skin tag are excised and if there is a fistula it is opened.

   The complications are hemorrhage, perianal abscess, fistula and incontinence in 30 percent of patients, especially in women who have a shorter and weaker sphincter compromised by child birth.

3. *Dorsal fissurectomy with sphincterotomy:* The exposed fibers of the sphincter are divided so that a smooth wound is left. It is indicated when it is associated with a fistula. The complications are delayed healing and leakage from keyhole gutter deformity.

4. *Anal advancement flap:* After excision of the fissure the raw area is covered by an inverted house-shaped flap of perianal skin and sutured with interrupted absorbable sutures.

CASE 3: PRESSURE SORES (BED SORES, DECUBITUS ULCERS)

CLINICAL DIAGNOSIS

1. The patient presents with a nonhealing ulcer or ulcers at the greater trochanter, ischium or sacral area (Figs 6 and 7).
2. The patient is confined to the bed for quite some time or immobilized due to some disease, trauma or operation.
3. He/she is unable to change or does not want to change the sides.
4. The ulcer or ulcers vary in size and depth and have nonspecific features.

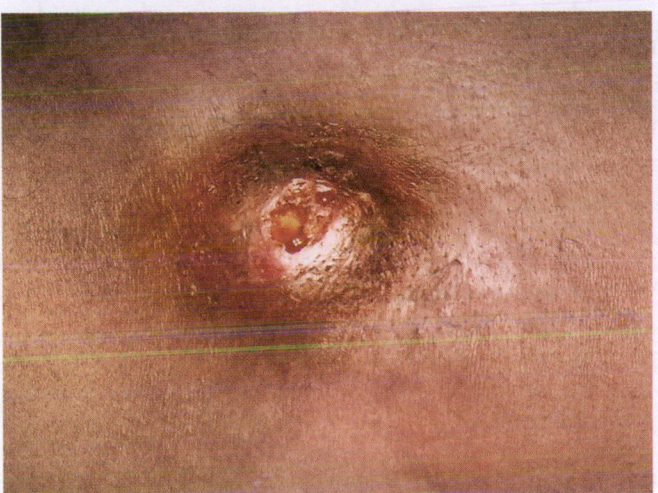

Fig. 6: Pressure sore of sacral region (Grade II)

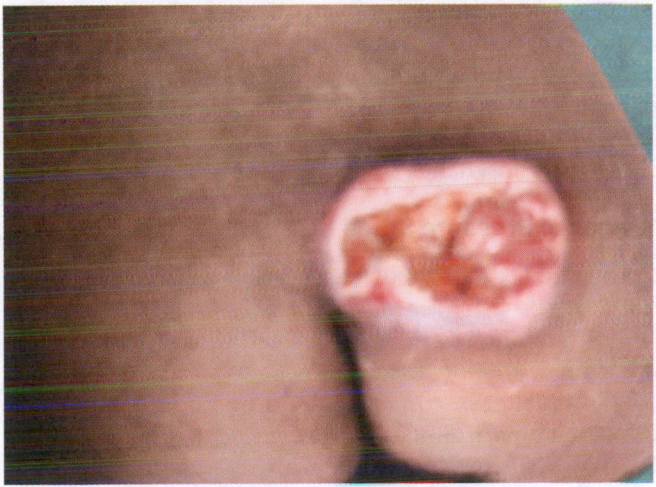

Fig. 7: Sacral pressure sore (Grade III)

VIVA VOCE

1. **What is a pressure sore?**
   It is an ulcer that occurs due to prolonged pressure on a bony point in patients who are confined to bed for quite some time.
2. **What is the incidence?**
   Bed sores occur in 5 percent of all hospitalized patients, with a higher incidence in paraplegics, elderly and seriously ill patients who are confined to bed.
3. **What is the etiology?**
   They occur due to persistent or prolonged pressure at a point which robs the local tissue of its blood supply resulting in its ischemic necrosis and ulceration.
4. **What are the predisposing factors?**
   Prolonged contact with moisture, urine and feces contribute to ulceration. Other predisposing factors are poor nourishment, paraplegia, immobile elderly patient after a major operation and drug addicts who lie immobile for hours under the effect of drugs. Denervation of tissues is another factor.
5. **How does denervation of skin predispose to ulceration?**
   It predisposes to ulceration because there is atrophy of skin and subcutaneous tissue. Further, the normal protective reflexes are absent.
6. **What are the types of ulcers?**
   The pressure sores are of two types:
   - Acute sores occur in an otherwise healthy person confined to bed following sudden paraplegia, e.g. spinal cord injury
   - Chronic sores develop gradually in patients following prolonged immobilization. These ulcers progress slowly.
7. **What is the earliest sign of pressure ulceration?**
   There is nonblanchable erythema without a break in the epidermis.
8. **What are the grades of pressure sores?**
   The grades of pressure sores are:
   Grade I: Nonblanchable erythema without a breach in epidermis.
   Grade II: Blister, abrasion or a shallow ulcer—epidermal or dermal loss.
   Grade III: Full-thickness skin loss extending into the subcutaneous tissue but not through underlying fascia (Fig. 7).
   Grade IV: Ulcer extending to bone, muscle or joint.
   Grade V: A closed cavity open as a small sinus.

9. **How do you treat a pressure sore?**
It is better to prevent a pressure sore as the prevention is simpler than the treatment.

10. **How do you prevent pressure ulceration?**
The preventive measures are:
- Casts and appliances should be well-padded and the points of pressure and pain are relieved.
- Bed-ridden patients must be turned to a new position at least every 2-hours. A wheel chair-bound patient should lift himself/herself off the seat for 10 seconds every 10 minutes
- Water and air mattresses, sheep skin pads and foam cushions may be used to relieve pressure, but they are not substitutes for frequent turning. Floatation bed system may be employed
- Daily inspection of pressure sore-prone areas must be done.

11. **How much pressure the skin can tolerate without producing ischemic injury?**
The pressure on the skin at any time should be less than the capillary filling pressure that is more than 30 mm Hg, to prevent ischemia.

12. **What is the treatment of a pressure sore?**
The essentials of treatment are:
- Electrical stimulation, biomaterials and growth factors may be used. They may be helpful in healing
- The bed must be kept clean, dry and crease-free. Sometimes, fecal and urinary diversion helps.
- At the local site, the underlying fat and muscle may be more necrotic than the overlying skin. A small ulcer may be hiding a larger area of tissue destruction. An abscess may be present. In such situations the sore needs drainage and debridement
- After debridement, a deeper ulcer needs coverage by a well-vascularized padded tissue, e.g. muscle, musculocutaneous flap or an axial flap.

13. **What is the role of a muscular flap?**
Apart from providing cover to the raw area a muscular flap may even control low-grade infection.

14. **What are the common flaps that are employed?**
The common flaps are:
- Tensor fascia lata flap for covering sores of greater trochanter area
- Gracilis, gluteus maximus or hamstring flap for covering sores of ischial tuberosity
- Gluteus maximus flap for covering sacral sores.

15. **What is an innervated flap?**
It is a flap with sensory supply that is used in paraplegics, for example, a tensor fascia lata flap with supply from lateral cutaneous nerve (L 4-5) to cover an ischial sore.

16. **What is vacuum-assisted closure (VAC)?**
In this method intermittent negative pressure is used to hasten debridement and formation of granulation tissue.

17. **What is the extent of pressure?**
About—25 mm Hg.

DISCUSSION

Pressure sores are the ulcers produced by persistent pressure at a point against an underlying prominent bony point. They occur in 5 percent of all hospitalized patients, with a higher incidence in paraplegics, elderly and severely ill patients who are bed-ridden and unable (because of a cast or appliance) or unwilling to change position (Figs 6 and 7).

Pathogenesis

The persistent or prolonged pressure at a point robs the local tissue of its blood supply that causes ischemic necrosis of affected tissue. Prolonged contact with moisture, urine and feces contribute to ulceration. The predisposing factors are poor nourishment, paraplegia, immobile elderly people after an orthopedic operation, e.g. hip replacement, and drug addicts who take overdoses and then lie immobile for hours. Denervated skin predisposes to pressure breakdown because there is atrophy of skin and subcutaneous tissue. The normal protective reflexes are absent.

Pathology

The ulcer may vary in depth and size and may extend from the skin to the bone responsible for pressure, e.g. greater trochanter, sacrum or the occiput. The sores are of 2 types: acute sores occur in an otherwise healthy person confined to bed following sudden paraplegia, e.g. spinal cord injury; and chronic sores that develop gradually in patients following prolonged immobilization and progress slowly. Initially erythema appears at the pressure site which does not change color on pressure. Later it ulcerates.

Grades of Pressure Sores

I: The skin is intact but has non-blanchable erythema without a breach in epidermis.
II: Epidermal or dermal loss which resembles a blister, abrasion or shallow ulcer.
III: Full-thickness skin loss extending into subcutaneous tissue but not through underlying fascia.
IV: An ulcer extending to bone, muscle, tendon or joint
V: A closed cavity open at a small sinus.

Prevention

It is better to prevent pressure sores, as the prevention is simpler than their treatment. The causative disease must be treated if treatable, as the "bed sores are likely to leave the patient if the patient leaves the bed".

- Casts and appliances should be well-padded and the points of pressure and pain are relieved.
- Bed-ridden patients must be turned to a new position at least every 2 hours. A wheel chair-bound patient should lift himself/herself off the seat for 10 seconds every 10 minutes. The pressure on the skin at any time should be less than the capillary filling pressure (over 30 mm Hg) to prevent ischemia.
- Water and air mattresses, sheep skin pads and foam cushions may be used to relieve pressure, but they are not substitutes for frequent turning. Floatation bed system distributes pressure uniformly over a large surface area. It is another facility which may be employed.
- The pressure sore-prone areas are inspected frequently. Local erythema is the earliest sign of ischemic injury. These areas must be freed of all pressure.

Treatment

- Electrical stimulation, biomaterial and growth factors may be used to expedite wound healing. The results are variable
- The bed must be clean, dry and crease-free. Urinary and fecal diversion may be required
- The area must be examined carefully as the underlying fat and muscle are more likely to become necrotic than the skin. A small skin ulcer may be just the tip of an iceburg as it may have a much larger area of destruction underneath. The small areas of necrosis may be replaced by scar tissue provided continued pressure is avoided. A large area of destruction may form an abscess that needs drainage and debridement
- A small clean pressure sore is treated by drying agents, e.g. silicon spray, and avoidance of all pressure

- An ulcer extending down to bone needs debridement and coverage by well-vascularized padded tissue. The nutritional status and the general condition of the patient must be good for making the wound heal. The coverage is usually done with muscle, musculocutaneous or sometimes an axial flap. A well-vascularized muscle flap may even control low-grade infection. Following muscle flaps are commonly used:

Site of bed sore	Muscle flap
Greater trochanter	Tensor fascia lata
Ischium	Gracilis, gluteus maximus or hamstring
Sacrum	Gluteus maximus

In paraplegics an innervated flap from above the level of paraplegia may be used to provide sensibility, for example a tensor fascia lata flap with the supply from the lateral cutaneous nerve (L 4-5) to cover an ischial pressure sore. Another example is an abdominal flap (with intercostal nerve supply) may be used to cover insensible sacrum. But the results are not good.

In difficult cases tissue expansion techniques may be used where the available tissue is insufficient to close the wound. Postoperatively the donor and recipient areas must be kept pressure free for 2 to 3 weeks till there is complete healing. An air fluidized bed may be used.

Vacuum-assisted closure (VAC): In this method intermittent negative pressure of about 25 mm Hg is used to hasten debridement and formation of granulation tissue. A foam dressing of the size of the ulcer is cut and put on the ulcer. A perforated drain is put over the foam and the wound is closed with transparent adhesive tape and negative pressure is applied to the drain to reduce edema and increase blood flow. It reduces the bacterial count and increases cell proliferation. It prepares the wound for grafting or flap cover.

Results

The overall results are poor. There is a big chance of recurrence. Hence, every effort is made to prevent it.

CASE 4: ULCERS OF LEG AND FOOT

CLINICAL DIAGNOSIS

1. The patient presents with an ulcer on the leg or foot (Figs 8 to 11).
2. A history of its cause may be available, e.g. injury, burn or diabetes mellitus.
3. The ulcer may be purplish, shallow and situated around the ankle, especially near the medial malleolus. It may be associated with varicose veins in the limb (venous ulcer).
4. The patient is a middle-aged or elderly person who presents with a nonhealing ulcer on the lateral ankle or on the borders. The ulcer is pale, punched-out and may be deep. The patient may have intermittent claudication and absence of arterial pulses (arterial ulcer).
5. The patient presents with a non-healing ulcer commonly on the sole or heel. It is pale, deep and punched-out. The patient has signs of neuropathy or some other neurological disorder (neuropathic ulcer).
6. The patient may give history suggestive of infection (cellulitis, abscess) of the foot or leg which gives way to produce an ulcer with signs of inflammation, a sloping edge and slough in the floor of the ulcer (Figs 8 to 10).

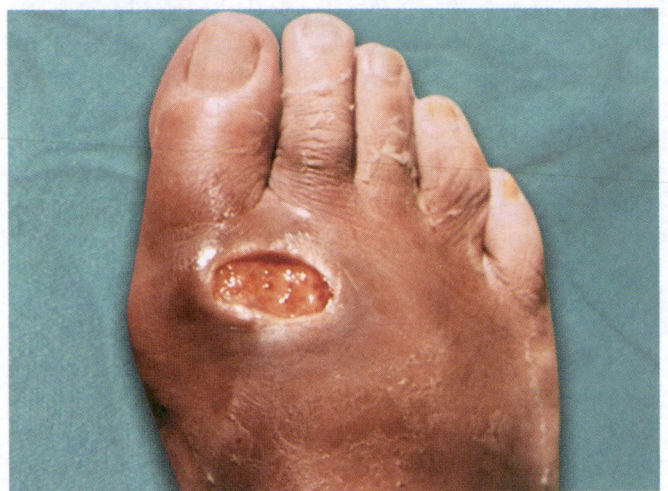

Fig. 8: Nonspecific ulcer of forefoot

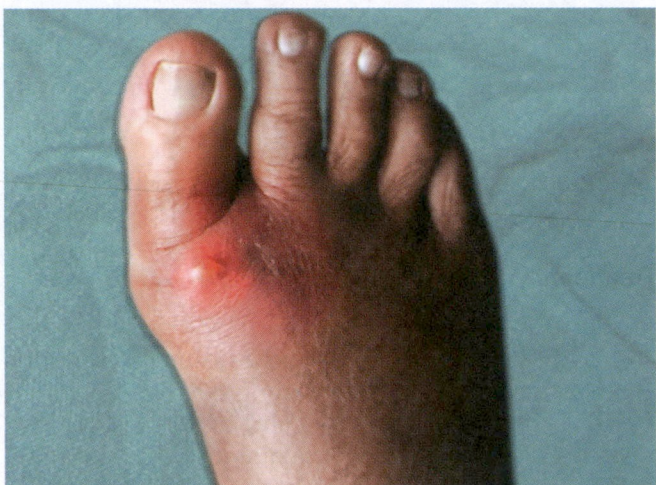

Fig. 10: Cellulitis of forefoot with a purulent blister at the root of great toe (These three pictures (8, 10 and 11) belong to the same patient. The figure 10 shows the start of disease with cellulitis, followed by ulceration)

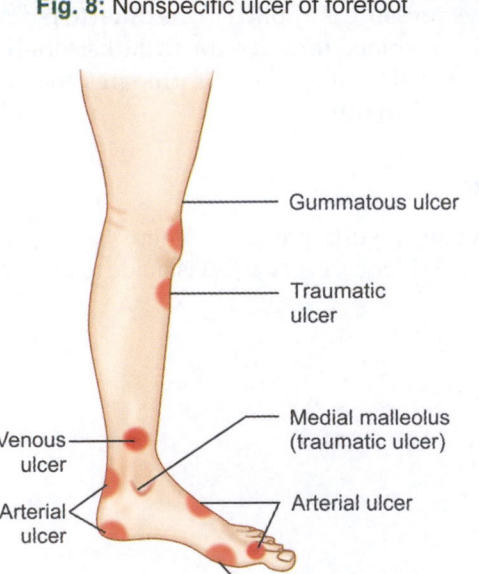

Fig. 9: Sites of common ulcers of leg and foot

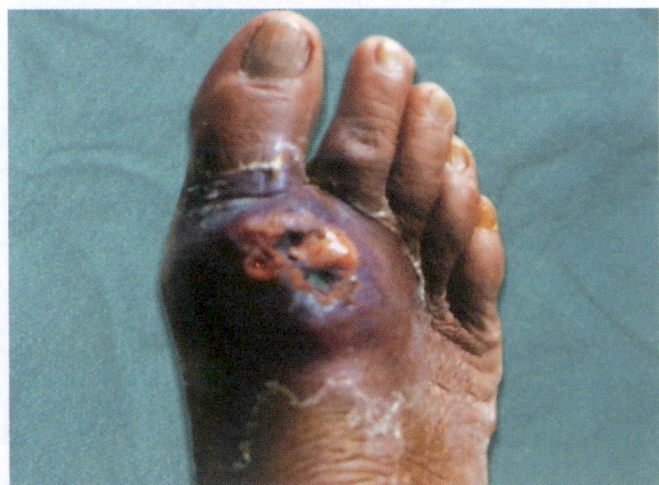

Fig. 11: Non-specific infective ulcer of the dorsum of foot. A lot of slough is visible

7. The patient is a middle-aged or elderly person who presents with a nonhealing ulcer. It is irregular and has a raised (rodent ulcer) or everted edge (carcinomatous ulcer).

Viva Voce

1. **What is an ulcer?**
   An ulcer is an infected raw area of the body which occurs due to gradual loss or molecular death of surface epithelium (Fig. 8).
2. **What is the difference between an ulcer and a wound?**
   - Wound is always caused by trauma, while an ulcer is caused by many other reasons, e.g. infection, malignancy apart from trauma
   - Wound may be sterile or contaminated while the ulcer is always infected.
3. **Why ulceration commonly occurs in the leg and foot?**
   Ulceration is very common in this region because of the following reasons:
   - The leg and foot bear the weight of the body and we move on them. Hence they are more likely to be injured
   - The foot remains in contact with the ground for a significant part of the day. Hence, it is more likely to be infected and bitten by insects. This is especially true for barefoot walkers
   - They are the most peripheral part of the body. Hence, more likely to suffer with insufficiency of supplies, e.g. arterial supply (arterial ulcer), and nerve supply (neurotropic ulcer)
   - They have to pump venous blood and lymph against gravity (mechanical disadvantage). Failure of this mechanism makes these parts prone for ulceration, e.g. venous ulcer in varicose veins and a non-specific ulcer in lymphedematous limb.
4. **What are the special features of these ulcers?**
   - They affect the quality of life because of pain, discharge, odor and reduced mobility
   - They take more time in healing as compared to ulcers of other places
   - They frequently recur with a 26 to 69 percent recurrence rate within a year.
5. **What are causes of ulcers of leg and foot?**
   The causes are (Fig. 9):
   - Venous disease, e.g. venous ulcer of varicose veins
   - Arterial disease (arterial ulcer)
     - Large vessel disease, e.g. atherosclerosis
     - Small vessel disease, e.g. diabetes mellitus, Buerger's disease

- Arteritis associated with autoimmune disease, e.g. lupus
- Trauma—Mechanical, thermal, chemical, electrical, persistent pressure (pressure sores), self-inflicted
- Infection, e.g. nonspecific, tuberculosis, syphilis, tropical ulcer
- Neurotropic ulcer in peripheral neuropathy
- Malignant disease, e.g. squamous cell carcinoma including Marjolin's ulcer, rodent ulcer, melanoma.

6. **Which is the commonest ulcer?**
   The venous ulcer is the commonest ulcer which accounts for 75 percent of cases.
7. **What is a nonspecific ulcer?**
   This ulcer has no special features. It is caused by nonspecific infection or trauma.
8. **What is the pathogenesis of a nonspecific ulcer?**
   Following a puncture or cut the bacteria, e.g. streptococci, staphylococci and others enter the local tissue to produce infection, e.g. cellulitis which is followed by suppuration and ulceration (Fig. 9 and 10).
9. **What are the investigations?**
   There are two main investigations, e.g. bacteriological examination of discharge and biopsy. Depending upon the clinical diagnosis Doppler studies are done in venous and arterial ulcers, blood sugar in a diabetic ulcer, X-ray of the foot to see for involvement of bones.
10. **How will you treat this case (nonspecific infective ulcer)?**
    The treatment is described below:
    - Antimicrobial drugs depending upon the culture and sensitivity.
    - Daily dressing of the ulcer and keeping the limb elevated when the patient is lying down.
    - If slough is present it may be removed chemically or surgically.
    If the ulcer is small it is likely to heal by these measures. In large ulcer resurfacing may be required by grafting.
11. **What are the modern dressing materials?**
    Some of the modern dressing materials are hydrocolloid gels, alginates and microporous polyurethane films.
    - Hydrocolloid gels: On coming in contact with the ulcer exudate they form a gel that expands to fill the ulcer
    - Microporous polyurethane films are good for shallow ulcers. They can be left in place for many days.

DISCUSSION

An ulcer is a breach in the continuity of surface epithelium, skin or mucosa, associated with infection. It may be due to gradual loss (molecular death) of covering epithelium or due to sudden traumatic removal. An ulcer is always infected (primary and, or secondary) (Fig. 8 and 11). The size and depth are such that its floor is visible. The ulcers are very common in the leg and foot because of many reasons.

Etiology

There are many causes of these ulcers, but venous disease accounts for about 75 percent of cases. The causes of leg and foot ulcers are:

- Venous disease resulting in local venous hypertension, e.g. varicose veins (venous ulcers)
- Arterial diseases, e.g. large vessel disease (atherosclerosis), or small vessel disease (diabetes, Buerger's disease)—arterial ulcer
- Arteritis associated with autoimmune diseases, e.g. lupus, rheumatoid arthritis, pyoderma gangrenosum of inflammatory bowel disease
- Trauma: Mechanical, thermal, chemical, electrical, persistent pressure, self-inflicted
- Infection: Tuberculosis, syphilis, staphylococcal ulcer, tropical ulcer
- Neurotropic ulcer due to peripheral neuritis
- Neoplastic diseases, e.g. squamous cell carcinoma including Marjolin's ulcer, rodent ulcer, sarcoma.

Clinical Features

- **Venous ulcer:** The patient, 40 to 60 years of age, more commonly a female presents with a chronic nonhealing ulcer around ankle on its medial side. It is pale, purple-blue in color, shallow, has a sloping edge and with the surrounding skin having pigmentation and induration (lipodermosclerosis). Varicose veins may or may not be present.
- **Arterial ulcer:** The patient is usually an elderly person who presents with a nonhealing ulcer on the lateral ankle or foot. The ulcer is pale, punched-out, deep and may have tendons exposed in the floor. There are symptoms (intermittent claudication) and signs (absence of arterial pulse) of arterial disease.
- **Arteritis-associated ulcer:** The ulcer usually follows breakdown of a nodule (Fig. 12). It is shallow, punched-out, pale and slow to heal. The signs and symptoms of the causative disease, e.g. rheumatoid arthritis may be present.
- **Traumatic ulcer:** They can occur anywhere in the foot and leg. The ulcer is variable in shape, size and depth. A history of trauma is available.

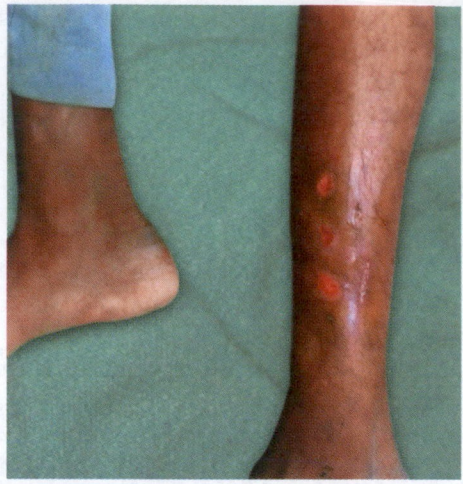

Fig. 12: Multiple small, superficial ulcer of leg (arteritis associated ulcers)

A self-inflicted ulcer commonly occurs on the dorsum of foot. It is superficial and geometric in shape.

- **Tuberculous ulcer:** The patient is usually young and presents with a nonhealing ulcer. It has an undermined pigmented edge and thin syrup-like discharge. The inguinal nodes may be enlarged and matted.
- **Syphilitic ulcer:** The ulcer is now rarely seen. It occurs in tertiary syphilis (gummatous ulcer) in upper outer part of leg. It is characterized by painlessness, punched-out edge and yellowish-gray (wash leather) slough in the floor.
- **Staphylococcal ulcer:** The patient presents with multiple small and red scabbed sores on the leg or ankle
- **Tropical ulcer:** It is due to Vincent's infection. It starts as a papule-pustule with a zone of surrounding redness, induration and pain. It bursts in 2 to 3 days forming an ulcer with undermined and raised edge with copious serosanguineous discharge and pain. The ulcer does not heal for months or even years. When it finally heals it leaves a parchment-like pigmented scar.
- **Squamous cell carcinoma:** It is characterized by a non-healing irregular ulcer with everted edge and indurated base. The inguinal lymph nodes may be enlarged, hard and nontender.
- **Marjolin's ulcer:** Malignant change may occur in a long-standing venous ulcer, in a scar of burn or in a chronic osteomyelitic sinus. This type of cancer is called Marjolin's ulcer. It does not produce metastasis till the cancerous change is confined to the scar as the scar has no lymphatics.
- **Rodent ulcer:** It is the ulcerative form of a basal cell carcinoma. The ulcer scabs in the center and grows at the periphery ('field-fire'). It has a raised edge like motor car tyre. It does not spread to the regional lymph nodes

- **Sarcoma:** A sarcoma may ulcerate and fungate out to present as a progressing ulcer
- **Neuropathic ulcer:** It occurs due to lack of sensation hence the tissues are repeatedly traumatized to produce this ulcer. The ulcer occurs commonly on the sole of foot or heel where it may penetrate to bone or joint level. It is pale, deep and has a punched-out edge (Fig. 13).

Investigations

- **Biopsy:** Biopsy from the edge of the ulcer is the most important diagnostic investigation in most of the ulcers, especially in neoplastic, vasculitic and tuberculous ulcers
- **Smear and culture** of the discharge helps in the diagnosis of infective ulcers
- **Duplex ultrasound** study is the first-line investigation to confirm the diagnosis of venous ulcer
- **Arteriography or MR angiography** may help in the diagnosis of arterial disease
- **Blood** is examined for hemoglobin, counts, ESR, antinuclear antibodies, rheumatoid factor and paraproteins
- **X-ray** of the leg and foot may be done if there is suspicion of bony involvement. It may show calcification of arteries
- **Ankle-brachial pressure index:** Arterial revascularization is indicated if it is less than 0.7, which is indicative of critical ischemia.

Treatment

- **Venous ulcer:** Counteracting venous hypertension is the most important measure and the most effective way of doing this is the elevation of the limb for a good proportion of the day and all through the night.
  The ulcer is cleansed by normal saline and covered with an inert nonadherent, moisture preserving material such as hydrocolloid gel.
  Bandaging: There are many methods of bandaging to counter venous hypertension, e.g. multilayer elastic compression bandaging system (Charing Cross four-layer bandage), rigid multilayered system (Steripaste three-layer bandage), and a low compression regimen for mixed venous-arterial ulcers. A bland absorbent leak-proof dressing beneath a graduated elastic compression stocking is an alternative. The dressing is usually changed weekly.
  Excision and grafting may be required after other factors are controlled. Pinch grafts may be used but meshed skin grafts are better as they allow mobilization and escape of exudates through the mesh.

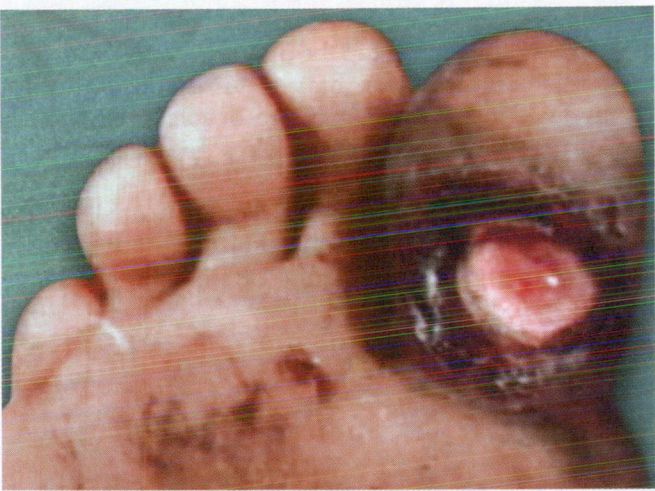

Fig. 13: Callus ulcer of great toe
(*Courtesy:* Deepansh Dalela)

If the deep venous system is normal, the disease of the superficial system is treated by surgery (ligation, excision or stripping) to obliterate any site of saphenous or perforator reflux to prevent ulcer recurrence

- **Arterial ulcer:** The pain is relieved and the infection is controlled.
  Revascularization by percutaneous balloon dilatation or bypass surgery is indicated if ankle-brachial pressure index is less than 0.7.
  Oxygenation of the ulcer can be found by transcutaneous oximetry. Tissues with a low PaO_2 will not heal. If the oxygen tension can be raised into a relatively normal range by oxygen administration the ulcer may heal.
  Hyperbaric oxygenation stimulates angiogenesis, and is an effective though expensive alternative when revascularization is not possible
- **Arteritis associated ulcer:** Here the granulomatous inflammation with or without arteritis kills skin and subcutaneous tissue, may be by excess cytokine release. Corticosteroids may help by reducing inflammation but they cause poor healing, hence not used.
  Topical or systemic vitamin A restores the inflammatory mechanism and may induce healing of the lesions.
  The causative disease is treated
- **Infective ulcers** are treated by appropriate antimicrobial drugs, e.g. antituberculous drugs for a tuberculous ulcer and penicillin for a syphilitic ulcer
- **Neuropathic ulcer:**
  – The cause is treated if possible.
  – Rest and simple dressings.
  – Infection and ischemia are controlled.

- Soft shoes, thick socks and sponge rubber inner soles ('off-loading') may stop the progress of the ulcer. Persistent ulceration may require amputation of involved toe, or excision of heel or sole ulcer together with underlying bony prominences. The defect is closed by skin grafting.
- **Neoplastic ulcers:** If excisable, they are treated by wide excision and skin grafting. Radiotherapy and/or chemotherapy may be required. Rarely, an amputation may be indicated.

- **Self-inflicted ulcer:** It is treated by plastering the affected part to prevent the patient from injuring the part repeatedly, and psychiatric treatment
- **Diabetic ulcer:**
  - The diabetes is kept under control by dietary restriction and injections of insulin.
  - Relief of pressure on the ulcer ('off-loading').
  - Surgical debridement, insulin has been used in dressing.
  - Revascularization.

CASE 5: VENOUS ULCER

CLINICAL DIAGNOSIS

- Varicose ulcer
  1. The patient is usually a young or middle-aged person who presents with a chronic ulcer in the leg associated with varicose veins.
  2. It is usually situated on the medial side of the lower leg and tends to ride a vein.
  3. The ulcer is solitary, shallow and round or oval (Fig. 14).
  4. The edge is irregular but sloping.
  5. The floor is covered by bluish granulation tissue or pale slough.
  6. It is nontender with indurated base. It is mobile on underlying bone.
  7. The surrounding skin is pigmented and slightly swollen (Fig. 14).
- Post-thrombotic ulcer
  1. The patient is usually a young or middle-aged person who presents with a chronic and painful ulcer of lower leg.
  2. The ulcer is deep with variable size.
  3. It is covered by pale slough and it discharges sero-purulent fluid.
  4. The edge is sloping and the base indurated.
  5. The leg may have pitting edema (phlebedema).
  6. Varicose veins may be present.
  7. A history suggestive of deep vein thrombosis may be present.

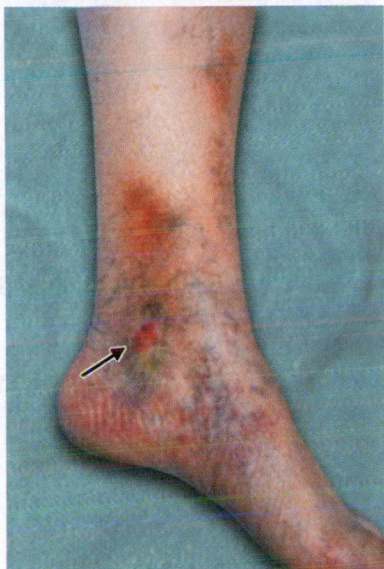

Fig. 14: Venous ulcer with lipodermosclerosis of saphenofemoral incompetence

VIVA VOCE

1. **What is a venous ulcer?**
   It is a chronic ulcer of lower leg due to some venous disease resulting in venous stasis (Fig. 14).
2. **What are the etiological types?**
   Depending upon the cause, it is of two types:
   1. *Varicose ulcer:* This ulcer is associated with varicose veins.
   2. *Post-thrombotic ulcer:* This ulcer occurs following thrombosis and phlebitis in the deep and perforating veins.
3. **How does this ulcer develop?**
   Following deep vein thrombosis when recanalization occurs the valves are destroyed or rendered incompetent resulting in venous stasis and (ambulatory) venous hypertension. Subsequently this venous hypertension is transmitted through the incompetent perforators to the superficial veins.
   In varicose veins there is venous hypertension in the superficial venous system. Due to hypertension fibrinogen escapes through the large pores in the venules resulting in its accumulation in subcutaneous tissue which acts as a barrier ("cuffs") to diffusion of oxygen and other nutrients, resulting in fat necrosis and cutaneous atrophy. A minor trauma breaks the skin resulting in venous ulcer.
   Venous ulcer may be partially attributable to failure of microcirculation of the skin to provide nutrition, but inflammatory mediators and toxic products from inflammatory cells probably play a major part in causing the skin damage.
4. **What is lipodermosclerosis?**
   It is thickening, pigmentation, induration and inflammation of the skin of lower leg. The pigments that are deposited are hemosiderin and melanin (Fig. 14).
   It is produced by persistently high venous pressure in surface veins which distends the capillary bed of skin of the ankle and encourages macromolecules to escape into the tissues. Fibrin, fibrinogen and other large molecules are deposited around the capillaries and prevent diffusion of oxygen and other nutrients into the tissues. Eventually subcutaneous fibrosis produces permanent damage.
5. **What determines the site of venous ulcer?**
   The location of the incompetent perforator determines the site of ulcer, extending from the malleoli upon the lower half of leg.

6. **How much time does it take to develop a venous ulcer?**
   A venous ulcer develops within 10 years of untreated thrombophlebitis in 50 percent of cases.

7. **What are the investigations done in this condition?**
   The investigations are:
   1. Blood—Counts, hemoglobin, ESR, sugar, and autoantibodies.
   2. Biopsy, if indicated.
   3. Discharge from ulcer for culture and sensitivity.
   4. Investigations of venous system, e.g. Duplex ultrasound, bipedal ascending phlebography.

8. **What is the role of phlebography?**
   Usually deep phlebography is done. It is especially indicated in difficult diagnostic problems. It shows the patency and size of the lumen of the deep veins, the presence of valves and high pressure leaks in the calf.

9. **What is functional venography?**
   In this investigation, with X-ray image intensification and TV display, the function of veins, valves, communicating veins and the venous pump are studied by injecting contrast into a superficial vein and observing flow on activating venous pump by standing on the toes.

10. **What is the role of Duplex ultrasound study?**
    This method gives nearly all the information given by venography. Hence, this is the investigation of choice. Further, it is a noninvasive investigation.

11. **How do you treat a venous ulcer?**
    The essentials of treatment are:
    1. Occlusive dressings covered by compression bandage.
    2. Elevation of limb.
    3. Operative treatment, if conservative treatment fails.

12. **What is the technique of dressing?**
    Dry nonadherant multilayered dressings or paste bandages, both covered by elasticated bandages are the most popular methods of achieving compression. The ulcer is gently cleaned once a week and the dressing and bandage are carefully reapplied. The area of ulceration is measured at each attendance, and provided that the ulcer is healing conservative treatment is continued.

13. **What do you use in the dressing of the ulcer?**
    Proprietary zinc and calamine absorbant bandages have proved very effective. 'Calaband' and 'Viscopaste' have their advocates. Hydrocolloid gel is the latest advance in this direction.

14. **How does the compression bandage help?**
    During walking the bandage will relax and stretch alternately helping venous pumping and reducing venous hypertension.

15. **What are the results of this treatment?**
    About 50 to 70 percent of ulcers heal in 3 months and 80 to 90 percent by 12 months.

16. **What is the indication for operative treatment?**
    If the ulcer does not heal or continues to grow operative treatment is indicated.

17. **What is the operative treatment?**
    Excision and skin grafting

18. **Do you know of any pharmacologic agents useful in this ulcer?**
    Many drugs have been used, i.e. stanozolol, oxpentifylline, prostaglandin E_1 and diosmin.

19. **What are the results of pharmacologic treatment?**
    None of these drugs cure the ulcer. They may be of some benefit.

20. **What are the chances of reulceration?**
    If proper precautions are not observed the ulcer can recur.

21. **What will you do to prevent recurrence?**
    1. Venous hypertension should not occur.
    2. The patient should be investigated for the nature of venous abnormality which should be corrected if possible.
    3. Graduated elastic support stockings or pressure garment must be in permanent use.
    4. Trivial trauma or infection of foot or leg must receive immediate attention.

22. **What is the nature of venous surgery?**
    Varicose ulcers are treated by surgery of varicose veins, e.g. Brodie-Trendelenburg's operation for saphenofemoral incompetence.
    Post-thrombotic ulcers in general are not treated by direct venous surgery but by debridement, elevation of limb and pressure dressings.

23. **Do you know of any surgical treatment of thrombosed deep veins?**
    A bypass operation may be performed for thrombosed deep veins. Saphenous vein has been used to bypass segmental venous occlusion of iliofemoral or femoropopliteal vein.
    For iliofemoral occlusion the contralateral saphenous vein is passed suprapubically and anastomosed to the affected side proximal to occlusion.
    For femoropopliteal occlusion the obstructed segment can be bypassed by anastomosis of saphenous vein to the popliteal tibial trunk below the occlusion at the level of knee joint.

DISCUSSION

About 60 to 70 percent of all ulcers of lower leg are due to venous disease. Venous ulcer is a chronic ulcer of lower leg occurring in patients of varicose veins or deep vein thrombosis where recanalization of deep vein has occurred but the venous valves are either destroyed or rendered incompetent due to thrombosis. Both these conditions lead to venous hypertension which if sufficiently severe causes excessive capillary exudation and formation of a fibrin barrier ('cuffs') around capillaries with reduced nutritional exchange between capillary blood and subcutaneous tissues and skin. Also, there is deposition of leukocytes in the capillaries (white cell 'trapping'). Endothelial cells activated by hypoxia cause leukocytes to become sticky and release injurious substances damaging endothelium with consequent migration of leukocytes into surrounding tissue to cause further damage. Probably the leukocytes mistakenly attack impaired capillary walls and neighboring tissue. The destructive effect is aggravated by capillary obstruction due to adherent layer of leukocytes and thrombus resulting from activation of platelets. Edema, induration and fibrosis associated with pigmentation of skin culminate in tissue death and ulceration.

Ulceration is preceded by venotensive changes of local edema, induration (lipodermosclerosis) and brown pigmentation due to extravasated hemosiderin. These changes are always found in the vicinity of ulcer, if not found then the diagnosis is doubtful.

Clinical Features

The patient presents with a chronic nonhealing ulcer in the gaiter region, the area between the muscles of the calf and the ankle. The ulcer usually develops due to minor trauma, infection, and itching which is perhaps associated with mast cell degranulation.

Site—Most of the ulcers occur on the medial side of the calf in the region where many of the Cockett perforators join the posterior tibial vein to the surface vein called posterior arch vein.

Ulcer associated with short saphenous incompetence, usually occur on the lateral side of the leg. In postthrombotic legs, ulcers can occur on any part of calf. Venous ulcers rarely extend on to the foot or into the upper calf.

Type of ulcer—The ulcer is nonspecific having a sloping edge and a floor covered by granulation tissue, slough and exudates.

Skin around the ulcer (ankle and calf) is pigmented, inflamed, thickended and indurated (lipodermosclerosis).

Another cause of ulcer must be considered if there is some elevation in the ulcer edge, if the ulcer is situated at another site, and if there is no evidence of lipodermosclerosis or an ankle flare.

The venous system of lower limb is examined. Venous ulcers are not always associated with varicose veins (Fig. 15).

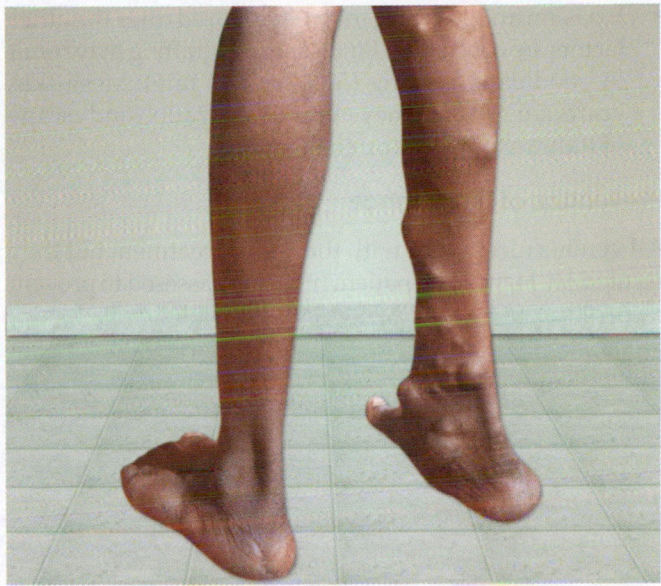

Fig. 15: Varicose veins (Lt) with "blow-outs"

Investigations

- Duplex scan will reveal reflux in the veins
- Bipedal ascending phlebography to detect obstruction and post thrombotic changes missed by duplex scan
- Biopsy to rule out a malignant ulcer
- Other investigations are required depending upon the clinical suspicion to rule out other causes of leg ulceration, e.g. blood counts, ESR, C-reactive protein, sickle cell test, blood sugar, antibody tests and Doppler pressure measurement.

Treatment

- Counteracting venous hypertension is the most important measure and the most effective way of achieving this is elevation of limb for a good proportion of day and all through the night
- The ulcer is cleansed by normal saline and covered with an inert nonadherant, moisture preserving material such as hydrocolloid gel
- Bandaging—There are many methods of bandaging to counter venous hypertension, e.g. multilayered elastic compression bandage system (Charing Cross four-layer bandage), rigid multilayered system (steripaste three-layer bandage), and a low compression regimen for mixed venous-arterial ulcers. A bland absorbent leak proof dressing beneath a graduated elastic compression stocking is an alternative. They are usually changed weekly
- The antibiotics are useless and the ulcer healing drugs, e.g. diosmin have a doubtful role

- Excision and grafting may be required after the other factors are controlled. Pinch or mesh grafting may result in good early healing (50% success rate). Mesh skin grafts are better as they allow mobilization and escape of tissue exudate through the mesh.

Prevention of Recurrence

All venous ulcers heal with the above treatment but they recur soon. Hence, the patient must be reassesed to prevent recurrence.

It is not yet clear whether laser ablation and foam sclerotherapy are as useful as surgery in preventing recurrence of the ulcer.

If the deep venous system is normal, the disease of superficial system must be treated to obliterate any site of saphenous or perforator reflux.

Those who decline this treatment or those having deep venous disease, are advised elastic stockings.

Any type of injury to the leg must be prevented and promptly treated.

CASE 6: PRIMARY CHANCRE (HUNTERIAN CHANCRE)

CLINICAL DIAGNOSIS

1. The patient is an adult who presents with a painless ulcer of glans or prepuce of short duration.
2. A history of sexual exposure is present in the recent past.
3. The ulcer is round or oval, elevated from the surface and has a sharp or clear cut edge.
4. It is hard, and when felt through the prepuce feels like a buried button.
5. It discharges small amount of serosanguineous fluid.
6. The dorsal lymphatics of penis may feel like wire under the skin (wiry lymphatics).
7. The inguinal lymph nodes are mildly enlarged, firm, nontender and mobile (shotty) (Fig. 16).

VIVA VOCE

1. **What is a primary chancre?**
   It is the first lesion of syphilitic infection and commonly occurs on the genitalia at the site of entry of bacteria.
2. **What do you mean by a chancre?**
   Chancre means a destructive sore. The primary chancre does not destroy the tissues but the lesions of the subsequent course of disease are quite damaging.
3. **What is the cause of this lesion?**
   It is caused by a spirochaeta, treponema pallidum.
4. **How is the infection transmitted?**
   The infection is usually transmitted by sexual intercourse with an infected person. Otherwise transmission is by direct contact with a surface lesion containing treponemes which penetrate the skin or mucosa at the point of contact.
5. **Does a person remain communicable after acquiring infection throughout life?**

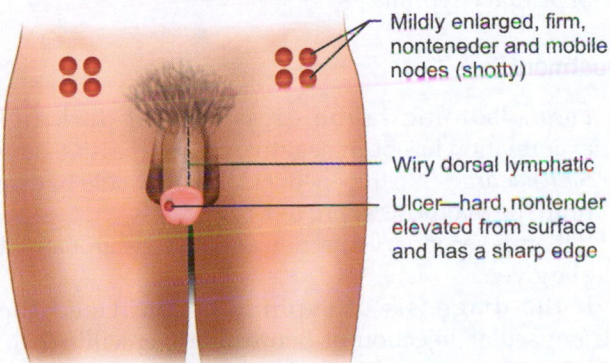

Mildly enlarged, firm, nonteneder and mobile nodes (shotty)

Wiry dorsal lymphatic

Ulcer—hard, nontender elevated from surface and has a sharp edge

Fig. 16: Primary syphilis

No, after 2 years acquired syphilis is rarely communicable and the ulcerative lesions of the skin of tertiary syphilis are not infective as they do not contain or contain very few treponemes.

6. **What are the other sites of a syphilitic chancre?**
   Apart from genitals, it can occur on the lips, tongue and nipple. In a homosexual (passive agent) it can occur in the perianal region or in the rectum.
7. **How will you confirm the diagnosis?**
   - It is done by finding treponema pallidum in the clear exudates from the lesion by dark field microscopy. The same can be done in the aspirate from enlarged lymph nodes
   - Treponema pallidum can be seen in the dried smears of the exudates by immunofluorescence staining.
8. **What is the role of serum tests (STS)?**
   The serum tests have hardly any role in the diagnosis of primary chancre as they are negative for 10 to 40 days after the appearance of primary chancre. Hence, negative serum tests do not rule out primary syphilis.
9. **What is the fate of primary chancre?**
   Even if the disease is not treated the chancre disappears by itself and the patient passes quietly into secondary syphilis the signs of which appear 6 to 12 weeks afterwards.
10. **What are the serological tests for syphilis?**
    - Nontreponemal antibody tests:
      1. Venereal disease research laboratory (VDRL) test.
      2. Rapid plasma reagin (RPR).
    - Treponemal antibody tests:
      1. T pallidum hemagglutination test (TPHA).
      2. T pallidum particle agglutination test (TPPA).
      3. Fluorescent treponemal antibody absorption test (FTA-ABS).
         Out of these tests VDRL and TPPA tests are most popular.
11. **What is the usual order of conversion into positive serum test?**
    In acquired syphilis the usual order of conversion is FTA-ABS and VDRL with rising titer and TPHA. This sequence is not invariable.
12. **How do you treat a primary chancre?**
    The essentials of treatment are:
    1. *Local:* No antiseptic is to be used. The lesion is dressed with normal saline.
    2. *Systemic:* It is treated by one dose of benzathazine penicillin 2 to 4 million units IMI. For penicillin

sensitive individuals tetracycline or ceftriaxone are used as both of them are treponemicidal. The other drugs of choice are doxycycline 100 mg twice daily or erythromycin 500 mg four times daily orally for 14 days.

13. **Do you know of any adverse reaction following injection of penicillin in primary chancre?**
Yes, it is Jarisch-Herxheimer reaction where six hours after the first injection the patient develops pyrexia, malaise and possible rigors lasting a few hours.

14. **What is the incidence of this reaction?**
It occurs in about 60 percent of patients.

15. **Does this reaction occur in late syphilis?**
Yes, this reaction occurs less frequently but is more severe.

16. **What is the prognosis of primary chancre?**
The prognosis is excellent if the patient is treated adequately.

17. **Why is the syphilis called great imitator?**
Because syphilis (late) produces tumor-like swellings called gummas that may involve the gastrointestinal tract, skin, bones, joints, testis, nose or throat. They may invade and destroy tissues such as nasal septum and hard palate.

DISCUSSION

Hunterian chancre is a sore that develops at the site of entry of treponemes in about 2 to 6 weeks of sexual exposure. It is the main manifestation of primary acquired syphilis.

Etiology

Hunterian chancre is a manifestation of venereal infection caused by treponema pallidum which is a delicate spiral organism (spirochaete) 6 to 15 mμ in length. It is transmitted by direct contact with a surface lesion containing treponemes which penetrate the skin or mucosa at the point of contact. Syphilis is only infective in primary, secondary and first 2 years of latency as the causative organisms are present in the surface lesions during that period. The ulcerative cutaneous lesions of tertiary syphilis are noninfective as they contain none or few organisms.

The treponema dies rapidly on drying, hence early infective lesions usually occur on moist areas, i.e. genitalia, perianal area, rectum, pharynx, tongue, lip or elsewhere. Hence, infection is almost always transmitted during sexual intercourse, including orogenital contact and homosexual practices involving anus and rectum.

Pathology

At the site of entry of organisms there occurs first an indurated papule which becomes eroded and soon becomes a shallow indurated sore or ulcer.

Clinical Features

The patient presents with a painless ulcer of glans or prepuce of short duration following sexual contact in the recent past.

The ulcer is round or oval, elevated from the surface and has a sharp or clearcut edge. It is hard and when felt through the prepuce feels like a buried button. It discharges small amount of serosanguineous fluid (Fig. 16).

The dorsal lymphatics of penis may feel like wire under the skin ('wiry lymphatics'). The inguinal lymph nodes are mildly enlarged, firm, nontender and mobile ('shotty'). There are no constitutional symptoms.

In a female the chancre may occur inside the labia, vagina or cervix, and since there are no constitutional symptoms, the patient may not come for treatment and may silently pass into secondary stage of disease.

Extragenital chancres can occur on the lip, tongue, nipple, perianal region or inside the rectum.

Differential diagnosis: In early stage it has to be differentiated from other penile or vulval lesions, traumatic lesions such as splits or tears, chancroid, herpes genitalis, burns, furuncles, carcinoma, balanoposthitis and lymphogranulma venereum.

The anal lesions in homosexuals frequently resemble anal fissures but the pain and anal spasm are less.

Investigations

1. *Dark field microscopy:* The treponemes can be seen in the clear exudate from the lesion in dark field microscopy.
2. *Immunofluorescence staining:* T pallidum can be seen by this method in dried smears of the exudate.
3. *The serologic tests for syphilis:* They are usually negative. They may become positive 3 to 5 weeks after the appearance of the chancre. These tests should be repeated up to 3 months if doubt persists. The tests are VDRL and FTA-ABS, the first one is positive in 75 to 85 percent and the second in 85 to 95 percent of patients of primary syphilis.

Treatment

1. *Local:* Isotonic saline dressings till dark field examination has been negative on 3 successive days.
2. *Systemic drugs:* No treponemicidal drug should be given until the diagnosis is proved.

It there is secondary infection a course of sulfonamides may be given.

If the diagnosis of syphilis is confirmed then intramuscular injection of benzathine penicillin 2 to 4 million units is given (single dose).

In penicillin sensitive cases tetracycline or ceftriaxone can be tried but experience with them is limited. The best drug is doxycycline 100 mg daily for 15 days.

Adverse effects—Sixty percent of patients of early disease develop pyrexia, malaise and possible rigors (lasting a few hours), about 6 hours after the first injection. The patient must be told about this reaction (Jarisch-Herxheimer reaction).

This reaction is less common but more serious in late syphilis and may require help of prednisone.

Prognosis—If the patient of early syphilis is adequately treated the disease is cured completely.

CASE 7: CHANCROID (SOFT SORE)

CLINICAL DIAGNOSIS

1. The patient is an adult who presents with a single or multiple (usually multiple) ulcers on the genitals of short duration.
2. The ulcers are usually present on the prepuce, glans or shaft of penis.
3. They are rounded, shallow, covered by thin slough and have profuse purulent discharge.
4. They are soft, tender, bleed readily and have an undermined and edematous, edge.
5. The inguinal nodes of one or both sides are enlarged, hard and tender. Soon they become matted resulting in a fluctuant swelling with red overlying skin (bubo) (Fig. 17).
6. There is history of sexual exposure 3 to 5 days before the onset of symptoms.

VIVA VOCE

1. **What is chancroid?**
   It is a sexually transmitted disease caused by *Haemophilus ducreii*.
2. **What is incubation period?**
   It is 3 to 5 days.
3. **How do you differentiate this lesion from a syphilitic chancre?**
   The differences are given below:

Features	Soft sore	Syphilitic chancre
Ulcer Number	Usually multiple	Single
Site	Penile shaft may be affected	Shaft is usually not involved
Discharge	Purulent profuse	Serous, slight
Depth	Shallow	Elevated on surface
Edge	Undermined	Sharp, straight
Tenderness	Tender	Nontender
Consistency	Soft	Hard
Inguinal nodes	Enlarged	Enlarged
Tenderness	Present	Absent
Suppuration	Tends to occur	Does not occur

4. **What are the investigations?**
   - Apart from routine investigations, smear and culture of the discharge is required to identify the causative organism.
   - Swab is sent for culture onto a special medium.
   - Dark ground illumination should also to be done to identify concomitant syphilis.
5. **What is the cause of multiple lesions?**
   They are due to autoinoculation.

6. **How do you treat this condition?**
   A single dose of either azithromycin 1 gm orally or ceftriaxone 250 mg IM is the effective treatment.
7. **What are the alternative drugs?**
   The alternative antibiotics are:
   - Erythromycin 500 mg four times daily orally for 7 days, or
   - Ciprofloxacin 500 mg twice daily orally for 3 days.
8. **How do you treat the buboes?**
   Apart from prompt antibiotic therapy, they are treated by needle aspiration.
9. **Why do not you treat them by drainage?**
   Because of the risk of delayed healing.
10. **What are the results of treatment?**
    Prompt treatment results in immediate response.
11. **Do you take any precaution while treating a patient of chancroid?**
    Yes. It is not unusual for two venereal diseases - chancroid and syphilis—to occur together. Hence any antibiotic that may prevent identification of Treponema pallidum must not be given.
12. **What are the complications of chancroid?**
    The complications are – balanitis and phimosis.

DISCUSSION

Chancroid is a sexually transmitted disease caused by the gram-negative bacillus, Hemophilus ducreii. The incubation period is 3 to 5 days.

Clinical Features

The patient usually develops multiple vesicopustules on the genitals which ulcerate resulting in multiple, painful, rounded, soft and readily bleeding ulcers with undermined edge and surrounding erythema.

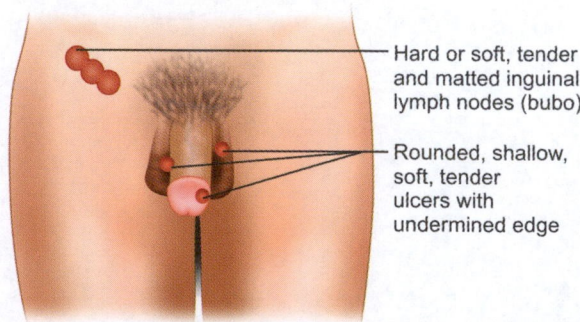

Hard or soft, tender and matted inguinal lymph nodes (bubo)

Rounded, shallow, soft, tender ulcers with undermined edge

Fig. 17: Chancroid (soft sore)

The inguinal lymph nodes are enlarged, hard and tender causing a feeling of stiffness in the groin. Subsequently the lymph nodes may resolve or may suppurate, when they become matted resulting in a unilocular fluctuant swelling (abscess, bubo) with red overlying skin. The nodes of one (usually unilateral) or both groins may be affected (Fig. 17). When the lymph nodes are involved the patient has fever, chills and malaise.

Sometimes the affected tissues are destroyed very rapidly (phagedena).

Investigations

- The swab is cultured onto a special medium for *H. ducreii.*

- Investigations should be done for possible concomitant syphilis (dark field microscopy).

Treatment

1. A single dose of either azithromycin 1 g orally or ceftriaxone 250 mg IM is effective treatment. Other regimens are:
   - Erythromycin 500 mg orally four times daily for 7 days, or
   - Ciprofloxacin 500 gm orally twice daily for 3 days.
2. The sore should be dressed with 0.9 percent saline.
3. The bubo is treated by aspiration and not incision as healing is very slow after incision.

Fistulas

CASE 1: ANORECTAL FISTULA

CLINICAL DIAGNOSIS

1. The patient presents with persistent or recurrent purulent discharge from an abnormal opening around the anus which may be present for months or years.
2. There is usually a single opening situated within one and a half inches of anus, (Figs 1 and 2).
3. It may be flush with the skin level, or it may present as a small elevation with pouting granulation tissue (Fig. 2).
4. The skin and subcutaneous tissue around the opening may be indurated. The fistulous tract may be felt as a cord going from the external opening.
5. The intrarectal palpation may reveal the internal opening as a small nodule or dimple surrounded by an area of induration:
   - The internal opening may be present in the anal canal below the anorectal ring (low level fistula)
   - It may be situated above the anorectal ring (high level fistula)
   - It is situated in the same radial line as the external if the latter is situated in the anterior half of the perianal region and within 1.5 inches of the anal verge
   - It is situated in the posterior midline when the external opening is present in the posterior half of perianal region or in the anterior half beyond 1.5 inches of anal verge (Goodsall's rule) (Fig. 3).

VIVA VOCE

1. **What is anorectal fistula?**
   Anorectal fistula is a narrow track lined by granulation tissue joining two openings, one situated

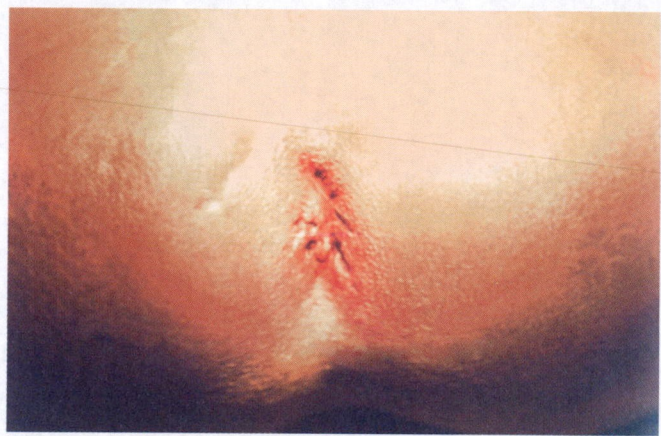

Fig. 1: Anterior anal fistula (direct type)

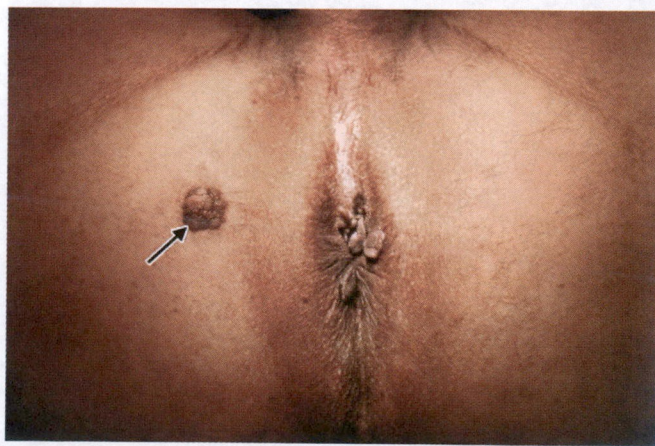

Fig. 2: Old high anorectal fistula with pouting granulation tissue which turned out to be an epidermoid carcinoma in fistula track. Many skin tags are seen around anus

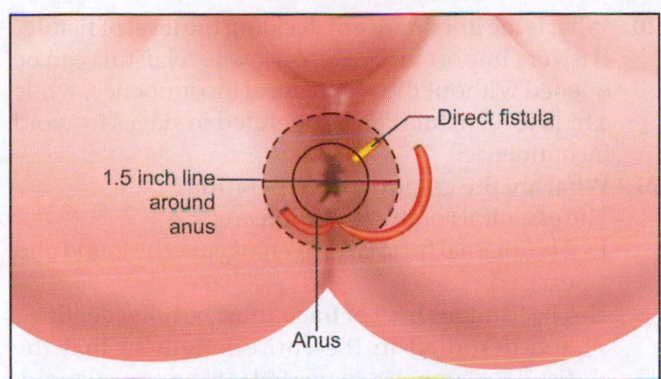

Fig. 3: Goodsall's rule

in the anorectum (primary or internal opening) and the other in the perianal region (secondary or external opening). It discharges a variable amount of pus.

2. **What is Goodsall's rule?**
   Fistulas with an external opening in the anterior half of perianal region tend to be of direct type.
   Those with an external opening or openings in posterior half of perianal region usually have curving tracks which may be the horse-shoe type and have the internal opening in the posterior midline.

3. **What is the pathogenesis of an anal fistula?**
   Most of the anorectal fistulas arise in the anal crypts at the anorectal junction. The crypts are injured or infected (cryptitis) and the infection extends along one of the several well-defined planes resulting in an abscess. When the abscess is drained or ruptures a fistula results.

4. **What are the causes of anorectal fistula?**
   The causes are:
   • Cryptogenic fistula:
     1. Pyogenic infection.
     2. Granulomatous disease of bowel.
     3. Tuberculosis.
   • Noncryptogenic fistula:
     1. Colonic diverticulitis.
     2. Cancer.
     3. Trauma, rectal foreign body.
     4. Congenital – rectal duplication.

5. **What are the types of anorectal fistula?**
   The type of anorectal fistula are:
   1. Subcutaneous.
   2. Submucous.
   3. Low anal.
   4. High anal.
   5. Pelvirectal.

6. **What is Parks' modification in classification?**
   Parks has described four types of fistula:
   1. Intersphincteric (45%).
   2. Trans-sphincteric (high or low) (40%).
   3. Suprasphincteric.
   4. Extrasphincteric.

7. **What is an intersphincteric fistula?**
   The primary track runs directly from the internal to the external opening across the distal internal sphincter. It may extend proximally in the intersphincteric plane to end blindly. It does not cross the external sphincter. It is the commonest fistula.

8. **What is a trans-sphincteric fistula?**
   From the internal opening it passes through both internal and external sphincters and then passes through the ischiorectal fossa to open on the skin of the buttock.

9. **What is low level fistula?**
   It is a fistula the internal opening of which opens below the anorectal ring.

10. **What is a high level fistula?**
    It is a fistula—the internal opening of which opens at or above the anorectal ring.

11. **What are the investigations?**
    The investigations are:
    1. Routine—Hemoglobin, TLC, DLC, ESR, blood sugar, urine examination.
    2. Examination of discharge.
    3. Probing—The internal opening may be probed through a proctoscope with the help of a curved crypt hook (done very gently). It is usually not required.
    4. Fistulography is usually indicated in a complex fistula. The interpretation of this investigation is quite difficult, hence the value is limited.

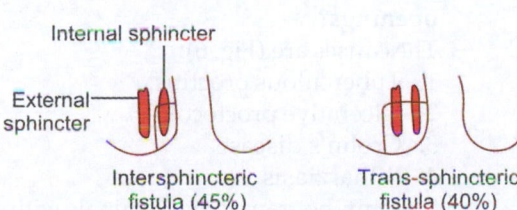
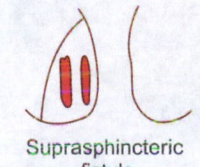
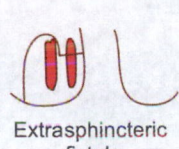

Fig. 4: Parks' classification of anorectal fistula

12. **What is the role of proctosigmoidoscopy?**
It is done to see the internal opening to asses the sphincteric strength and to exclude associated conditions.

13. **What is the role of endoanal ultrasound?**
It gives information about sphincter and fistula.

14. **What is the role of MRI?**
It is the gold standard investigation to see the fistula and its secondary extensions.

15. **How do you treat an anorectal fistula?**
The anorectal fistula is treated by laying open (fistulotomy) along the entire course of fistula. All the ramifications are found and opened (Fig. 5).

16. **What are the contraindications to fistulotomy?**
The contraindications are:
1. Chronic diarrhea.
2. Active ulcerative colitis.
3. Active Crohn's disease.

17. **If the operation is done in these situations what are the disadvantages?**
The disadvantages include:
1. Delayed wound healing.
2. Chances of fecal incontinence.

18. **What should be done in these situations?**
When these problems are associated with an anorectal fistula they must be controlled before the operation is done.

19. **If the fistula is left untreated, what complications can occur?**
The following complications can occur:
1. Systemic infection can occur.
2. Carcinoma may occur in the fistula tract very rarely.

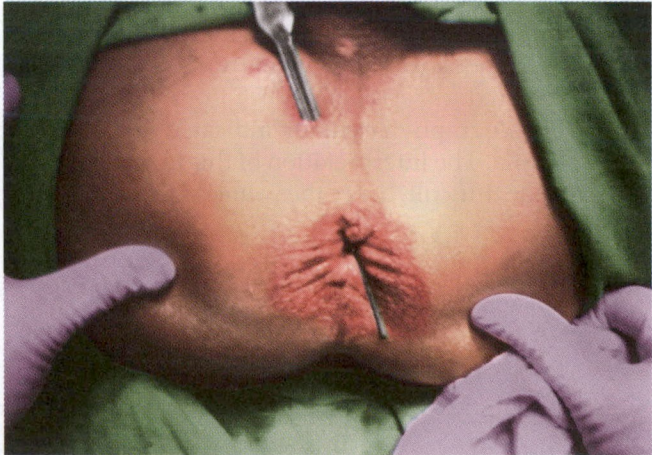

Fig. 5: Anorectal fistula with a grooved director passed into it for fistulotomy

20. **What is the importance of deciding the level of fistula?**
It is very important because a low level fistula can be opened without the fear of fecal incontinence, while a high level fistula can be operated in stages to avoid incontinence.

21. **What are the essentials of operation?**
The essentials of the operation are:
1. The internal (primary) opening must be found and excised.
2. The fistulous tract or tracts must be fully identified and deroofed in the entire length so that the fistulous tunnel is converted into an open wound.
3. The wound must be so constructed that the cavity heals from within outwards.

22. **How do you treat a high level fistula?**
The treatment depends on the further type:
1. Supralevator fistula is treated by removal of its cause. A traumatic fistula may require colostomy. It should never be treated by laying open as it will result in incontinence.
2. Trans-sphincteric fistula may be treated by a staged operation and a covering colostomy.
3. High intersphincteric fistula is treated by dividing the internal sphincter and laying open the whole track.

23. **What are the methods of making the fistula heal quickly?**
- Fibrin glue has been used locally after excision of fistula to plug the tract and permit the ingrowth of healthy tissue
- An advancement skin flap has been used after excision to cover the raw area for early healing and less scarring.

24. **What are the causes of persistence or recurrence?**
The causes of persistence or recurrence are:
1. Failure to excise the internal opening.
2. Missing collateral tracts.
3. Inadequate operation for fear of incontinence.
4. Incomplete diagnosis (cause not identified hence not treated).
5. Inadequate postoperative care (improper dressing).

25. **What are the causes of fistula with many external openings?**
The causes are (Fig. 6):
1. Tuberculous proctitis.
2. Ulcerative proctocolitis.
3. Crohn's disease.
4. Bilharziasis.
5. Lymphogranuloma inguinale with a fibrous rectal stricture.
6. Colloid carcinoma of rectum.

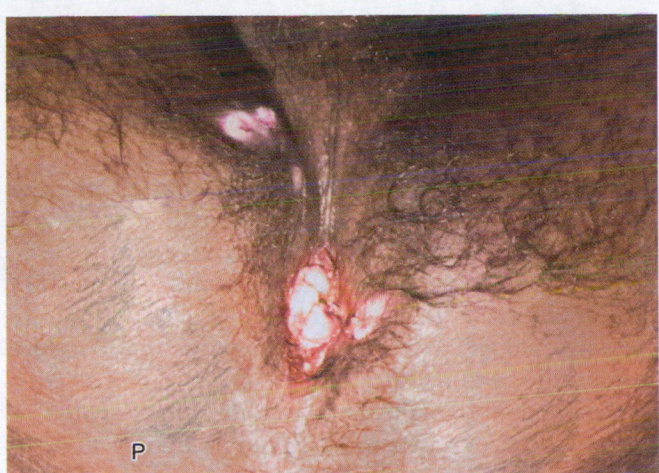

Fig. 6: Multiple anal fistula. Investigations confirmed tuberculous etiology

26. **What are the signs of tuberculous fistula?**
    The signs are:
    1. Lack of induration around fistula.
    2. The opening is ragged and flush with the surface.
    3. The openings are usually multiple.
    4. The surrounding skin is discolored.
    5. Thin syrup-like or watery discharge.
    6. There may be signs of pulmonary tuberculosis.

27. **What are the causes of fistula with internal opening above the anorectal ring?**
    The causes are:
    1. Penetration by an intrarectal foreign body.
    2. Intraluminal incision of a high intermuscular abscess erroneously thought to be submucous.

28. **Do you know of an anal fistula connected with an anal fissure?**
    This fistula is situated close to anal orifice usually posterior midline. The external opening is often hidden by sentinel pile. Pain is the leading symptom, which is due to anal fissure.

29. **What are the causes of supra-levator fistula?**
    The causes are:
    1. Crohn's disease.
    2. Ulcerative colitis.
    3. Carcinoma.
    4. A foreign body perforating the rectal ampulla from above.
    5. Trauma.

DISCUSSION

It is a chronic abnormal communication lined by granulation tissue between the anorectal lumen and the skin of perineum or buttock (or rarely to vagina). It is a common clinical problem, about 9 patients per 1,00,000 population per year occur in western Europe.

Etiology

Most of the fistulas are nonspecific and result from infection of anal gland (cryptoglandular) by the fecal bacteria (mixed infection). These glands are situated at the anorectal junction. From here, the infection (cryptitis) spreads along the ramifications of anal gland and an abscess forms. This abscess may rupture by itself or drained surgically resulting in fistula formation.

Anorectal fistula may occur in association with Crohn's disease, tuberculosis, lymphogranuloma venereum, actinomycosis, rectal duplication, foreign body (rectal foreign body penetrating the rectal wall), colonic diverticulitis and malignancy.

Clinical Features

- Most of the patients are in their third, fourth and fifth decades of life
- The patient usually presents with intermittent purulent discharge which may be bloody, and pain which may be relieved intermittently with more pus discharge
- The passage of flatus or feces through the external opening is a sign of rectal rather than an anal internal opening
- Perineal examination—The site and its distance from the anal opening is seen. Its mouth may be flush with the skin level or may have pouting granulation tissue (proud flesh) which is indicative of a foreign body in the fistula track. If the opening is lifted the fistulous tract may be seen or felt as a cord.
- Intra-anorectal palpation may reveal the internal opening as a small nodule or dimple surrounded by an area of induration.

Salmon-Goodsall's Rule

Cryptoglandular fistulas having their external opening posterior to the imaginary line passing transversely through the center of anal canal usually have their internal opening in a crypt in the posterior midline.

If the external opening is anterior to the transverse line, the internal opening is usually in a crypt immediately opposite the external opening (direct-fistula) (Fig. 3).

Investigations

Proctosigmoidoscopy is done to see the internal opening, to gain information about sphincter strength and to exclude associated conditions. The sphincters may be more objectively assessed by manometry.

Endoanal ultrasound gives useful information about sphincter integrity. When done with dilute hydrogen peroxide injection into the fistula, it is useful to delineate the fistula. Ultrasound is useful to find whether the fistula is relatively straight forward or not.

MRI – It is the gold standard to reveal the fistula and its secondary extensions.

Fistulography and CT scan are useful if an extrasphincteric fistula is suspected.

Classification

Depending upon the length of the tract the site of fistulous opening the fistula can be subcutaneous, submucous, low anal, high anal (ano-rectal) or pelvi-rectal. In the first three types, the internal opening is situated below the ano-rectal ring while in the last two types it is above the ano-rectal ring usually in posterior midline. Parks has classified the fistulae into four types:

1. **Intersphincteric fistula (45%)**—It runs directly from the internal to the external opening across the distal internal sphincter. It may extend proximally in the intersphincteric plane to end blindly with or without an abscess. It does not cross the external sphincter.
2. **Trans-sphincteric fistula (40%)**—From the internal opening it passes through both internal and external sphincters and then passes through the ischiorectal fossa to open on the skin of the buttock.
   Secondary tracks may arise from the primary track and may reach the roof of ischiorectal fossa, and from there through the levator may reach the pelvis rarely.
   The infection may spread circumferentially in the pelvic, intersphincteric, pararectal planes or a ischiorectal plane to produce a horse-shoe fistula.
3. **Suprasphincteric fistula**—The internal opening is above the anorectal ring and from there the track crosses both the sphincters and opens in the ischiorectal fossa. This fistula is very rare.
4. **Extrasphincteric**—It results from pelvic disease or trauma. The track passes without any specific relationship with the sphincters.

Complex fistula—It is a fistula in which the primary track crosses the sphincters and secondary extensions are present or there occur difficulties during treatment. Fistula with multiple openings is due to tuberculosis, inflammatory bowel disease, lymphogranuloma venereum, actinomycosis, foreign body and malignancy. It may have symptoms and signs of associated condition, e.g. diarrhea in inflammatory bowel disease.

Treatment

- A small acute fistula may heal with antibiotic treatment
- Majority of fistulas require surgery for eradication of sepsis and most of them are simple to treat

- **Fistulotomy or laying open (Fig. 5)**—After a thorough examination under general anesthsia, a grooved fistula probe is passed from the external to the internal opening. The thickness of the sphincter below and above the track is assessed and if indicated the track is laid open. The granulation tissue is curetted and sent for histology. The track is deroofed in its entire length so that it is converted into an open wound.

The secondary tracks are detected by the persistence of the granulation tissue despite curettage.

Marsupialization of the wound may be done to reduce its size and speed up healing.

If more than 30 percent of the sphincter is elevated by the grooved probe a staged fistulotomy may be done in which the secondary tracks are laid open and a part of the sphincter is divided and the rest is encircled by a loose seton which is divided after adequate fibrosis in the wound at a second stage.

This operation is not done in the presence of diarrhea or active inflammatory bowel disease. These problems must be controlled before surgery is attempted.

Fistulectomy—It is the dissection and excision of the fistula tract. Sometimes, it may be possible to repair the divided sphincter and anorectum after complete excision of the fistula.

Seton method of fistulotomy—A nonabsorbable, nondegenerative and comfortable suture is passed through the left over primary track related to the sphincter and tied loosely. The wound is managed by dressing. After 3 months, if there is evidence of good healing, the seaton is simply removed. The healing rate of this technique is 50 to 60 percent.

Cutting seton—The encircled sphincter is gradually divided (cheese wiring through ice) in such a manner that divided muscle does not spring apart and the fistula track heals down in a thin line as the seton is brought down.

Ayurveda describes Kshar sutra, which burns through the encircled tissue.

Fibrin glue has been used locally after excision of fistula to plug the track and permit ingrowth of healthy tissue to replace it. Still the results are being studied.

Advancement flap has been used after excision to cover the raw area for early healing and less scarring.

Follow-up and Results

After the operation regular examination is done to make sure that bridging and reformation of fistula does not occur. The overall results are good. Rarely, a fistula may persist for the following reasons:

1. Failure to excise the internal opening.
2. Missing a secondary fistula.
3. Inadequate operation for fear of incontinence.
4. Poor postoperative wound care.

CASE 2: BRANCHIAL FISTULA

CLINICAL DIAGNOSIS

1. The patient is usually a young person who presents with an abnormal opening in the neck discharging a small amount of mucus or mucopus.
2. It may be unilateral or bilateral.
3. It is situated in lower third of neck near the anterior border of sternomastoid (congenital type, usual) (Figs 7 and 8).
4. It may be situated higher up in the neck near the angle of jaw when it follows rupture or drainage of an infected branchial cyst (acquired type).
5. The opening is usually very small or like a small dimple.
6. A cord-like structure going up in the neck from this opening may be palpable.

VIVA VOCE

1. **What is a branchial fistula?**
   It is a long and narrow track going from the skin of the neck to the pharynx in the tonsillar fossa.
2. **What is the cause of this condition?**
   - In most of the cases it is a developmental defect which represents a persistent second branchial cleft, the occluding membrane of which has broken down
   - Rarely, it may be acquired following rupture or incision into an infected cyst.

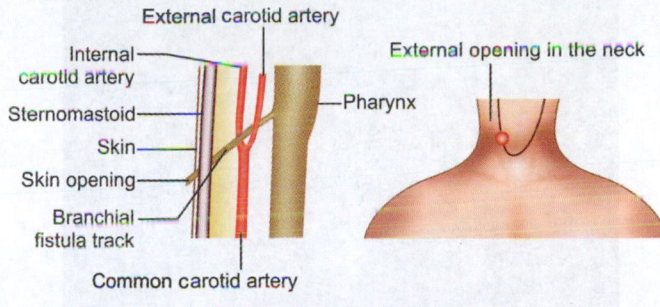

Fig. 8: Branchial fistula

3. **What is the course of the tract of fistula?**
   From the skin opening, it passes upwards and backwards through the fork of carotids upto the pharynx.
4. **Where is the internal opening?**
   The internal opening is situated on the anterior aspect of posterior pillar of fauces just behind the tonsil.
5. **Is it always a fistula?**
   Sometimes the internal opening may end blindly on the lateral pharyngeal wall. Then it is a sinus and not a fistula.
6. **What lines the fistulous tract?**
   It is clothed with muscle and lined by ciliated columnar epithelium.
7. **What are the relations of the fistulous tract?**
   It pierces the deep fascia at the upper border of thyroid cartilage and passes through the fork of carotids lying superficial to internal carotid artery and deep to external carotid artery and its branches. Further up, it lies superficial to stylopharyngeus muscle and glossopharyngeal nerve, and deep to hypoglossal nerve and stylomandibular ligament.
8. **What are the investigations?**
   The investigations are:
   1. Examination of discharge.
   2. Sinography to see the direction and depth of fistula (Fig. 9). MRI may be done with sinography (MR sinography).
9. **How do you treat this condition?**
   The whole of the fistulous tract should be excised.
10. **What is the technique of excision?**
    A ureteric catheter or a probe is passed into the track to facilitate dissection and identification during operation. A transverse incision in one of the creases of neck is given above the external opening and the track is dissected as it passes through the fork of carotids. After completing dissection of the upper end the lower orifice is excised by a small elliptical incision and the whole fistula is dissected out. The wound is closed around a small drain.

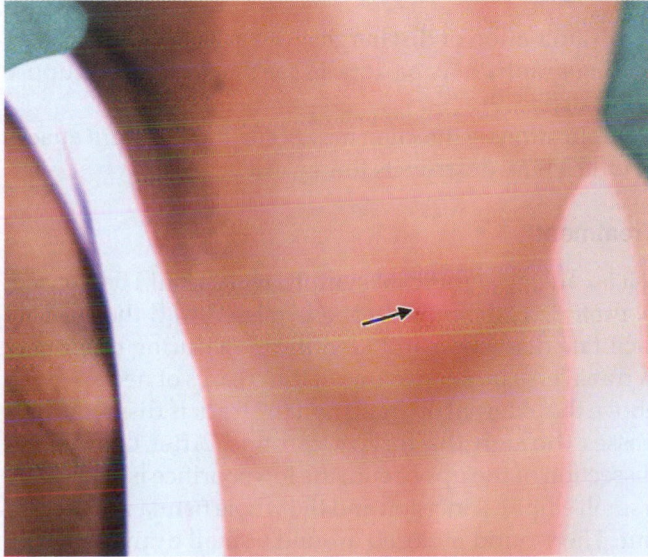

Fig. 7: Branchial fistula (right)

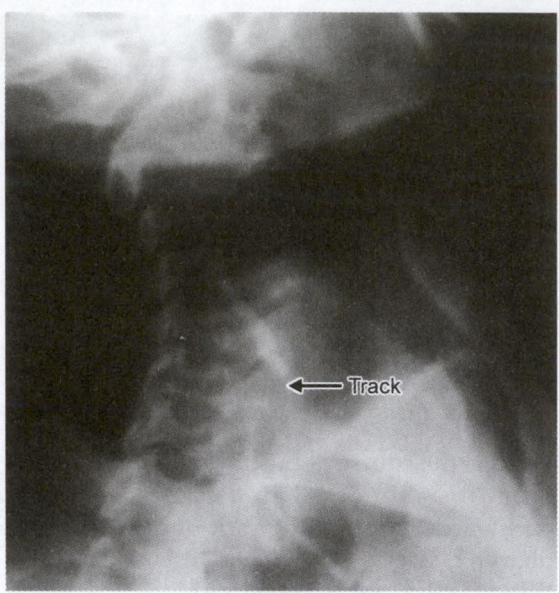

Fig. 9: Branchial fistula as seen on a fistulogram. The arrow is pointing at its cervical opening

11. **What is step ladder operation?**

The external opening of the fistula is lower down in neck while the internal opening is near the tonsillar region hence the course of track is long and oblique. Thus, it is often not possible to remove the complete track by one incision.

Therefore, a second incision is required above and parallel to the first incision. Now, the dissected tract is delivered out through the second incision, and the dissection continues further upwards. More such parallel incisions may be required further up till dissection is complete. This pattern of incision and dissection is known as step ladder operation.

12. **What are the precautions you will take during dissection?**

As the track passes through the fork of carotids and in close proximity to hypoglossal nerve, these structures must be protected from injury.

The dissection of the track is effort and time consuming, a little laxity may result in incomplete excision and recurrence.

13. **What is branchiogenic carcinoma? Is it related to bronchogenic carcinoma?**

- It is a very rare tumor and arises from the remnants of branchial clefts
- It is nothing to do with bronchogenic carcinoma which is a malignant lesion of lungs and quite common.

DISCUSSION

Branchial fistula is a congenital anomaly of neck which represents a persistent second branchial cleft, the occluding membrane of which has broken down.

Etiology

It is usually a developmental defect but it may also be secondary to an incision into or rupture of an infected branchial cyst.

Pathology

The external orifice of the fistula is nearly always situated in the lower third of neck at the anterior border of sternomastoid muscle.

The internal opening is situated on the anterior aspect of posterior pillar of fauces just behind the tonsil. The internal opening may end blindly on the lateral pharyngeal wall. It is then a sinus and not a fistula.

The track is usually long and narrow and passes through the fork of carotids. It is clothed with muscle and lined by ciliated columnar epithelium.

Clinical Features

- The patient is usually a young person who presents with an abnormal opening in the neck discharging a small amount of mucus or mucopus.
- It may be unilateral or bilateral.
- It is situated in lower third of neck near the anterior border of sternomastoid (congenital type, usual type).
- It may be situated higher up in the neck near the angle of mandible when it follows rupture or drainage of an infected branchial cyst (acquired type).
- The opening is usually very small or like a small dimple.
- A cord-like structure going up in the neck from this opening may be palpable.

Investigations

1. Examination of discharge.
2. Sinography may be done to see the track and its upper limit (Fig. 9).

Complications—Infection may occur, the recurrent attacks of which may destroy its lining.

Treatment

If it is causing significant symptoms, it should be excised. A ureteric catheter or probe is passed into the track to facilitate dissection and identification during operation. A transverse incision in one of the creases of neck is given above the external opening and the track is dissected as it passes through the fork of carotids. After completing dissection of the upper end, the lower orifice is excised by a small elliptical incision and the whole fistula is dissected out. The wound is closed around a small drain.

CASE 3: THYROGLOSSAL FISTULA

CLINICAL DIAGNOSIS

1. The patient is usually a child or young adult who presents with an abnormal opening in the neck in the anterior midline a little to the left.
2. It is usually situated below the hyoid bone (Figs 10 and 11).
3. It discharges a small amount of mucus or mucopus.
4. There is a semilunar hood of skin at the upper edge with concavity downwards. The hooding of the skin becomes more prominent on protrusion of tongue.
5. The opening moves up with deglutition and protrusion of tongue.

VIVA VOCE

1. **What is a thyroglossal fistula?**
   It is a fistula connected to thyroglossal tract.
2. **What are the causes of this disease?**
   The causes of a thyroglossal fistula are:
   - Rupture or drainage of an infected thyroglossal cyst.

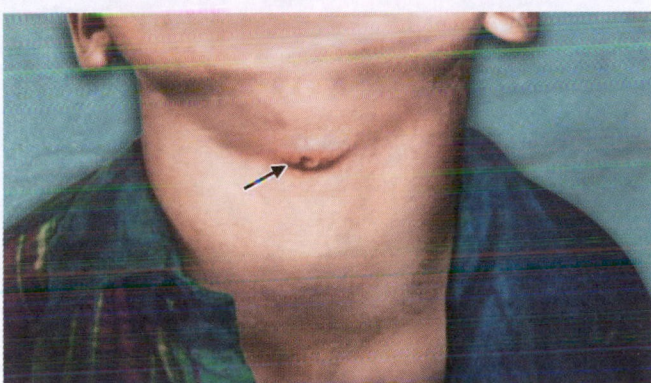

Fig. 10: Thyroglossal fistula

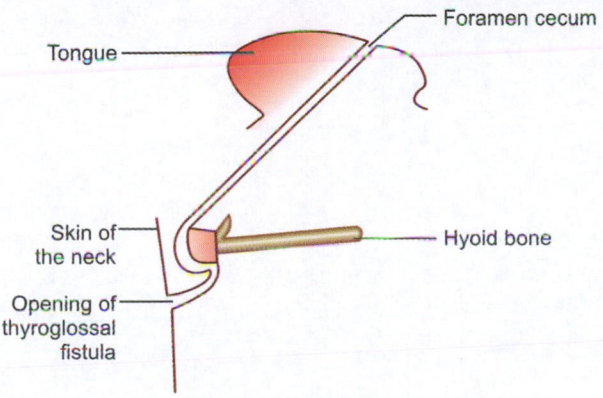

Tongue —
Foramen cecum —
Skin of the neck —
Hyoid bone —
Opening of thyroglossal fistula —

Fig. 11: Thyroglossal fistula

- Incomplete removal of a thyroglossal cyst.
- Congenital (extremely rare). It occurs when the cellular median thyroid diverticulum communicates with the skin of neck. Some authors deny its existence.

3. **What is the extent of fistulous tract?**
   It extends from the foramen cecum of tongue to skin of the neck near the midline in the upper part of neck (Fig. 11).
4. **What is the nature of its lining?**
   The tract is usually lined by squamous epithelium.
5. **What are the investigations?**
   The investigations are:
   - Routine—Hgb, TLC, DLC, blood sugar, urine, etc.
   - Examination of discharge by smear and culture
   - Fistulogram—It may show the extent of the tract.
6. **What are the complications?**
   Complications are uncommon. Secondary infection can occur.
7. **How do you treat this lesion?**
   It is treated by excision of the whole tract.
8. **What is the essential step of excision?**
   Apart from the excision of complete fistulous tract, the body of the hyoid bone should also be excised.
9. **What do you do to facilitate better visualization of fistulous tract?**
   For better visualization of the tract methylene blue is injected through the opening of fistula on the night before operation and the opening is closed by a purse string suture.
10. **What are the complications of operation?**
    The complications include:
    1. Wound infection.
    2. Hemorrhage.
    3. Perforation of larynx.
    4. Recurrence.

DISCUSSION

Thyroglossal fistula is a fistula connected with thyroglossal tract.

Etiology

The causes of this fistula are:
1. Spontaneous rupture or drainage of an infected thyroglossal cyst.
2. Incomplete removal of a thyroglossal cyst.
3. Congenital—It is extremely rare. It occurs when the cellular median thyroid diverticulum communicates with the skin of neck. Some authors deny its existence.

Pathology

The fistulous tract extends from the foramen cecum of tongue to the skin of neck near the midline in the upper part of the neck. It is closely related to the body of hyoid bone. It is usually lined by squamous epithelium and discharges a small amount of serous, mucoid or purulent fluid.

Clinical Features

- The patient is usually a child or young adult who presents with an abnormal opening in the neck in the anterior midline a little to the left (Fig. 10).
- It is usually situated below the hyoid bone.
- It discharges a small amount of serous, mucoid or purulent fluid.
- There is a semilunar hood of skin at the upper edge with concavity downwards. The hooding becomes more prominent on protrusion of tongue.
- The opening moves up with deglutition and protrusion of tongue.

Investigations

- Routine—Hgb, blood counts, blood sugar, urine.
- Examination of discharge by smear and culture.
- Fistulography to see the direction and extent of the fistulous tract.

Complications

- Secondary infection can occur repeatedly.
- Dysgenetic thyroid tissue may be present in the thyroglossal tract. It has a malignant potential more than normal thyroid tissue.

Treatment

The whole of the fistulous tract upto the foramen cecum of tongue should be excised. The body of hyoid bone should also be removed to prevent recurrence (Sistrunk's operation).

CASE 4: PAROTID SALIVARY FISTULA

CLINICAL DIAGNOSIS

1. The patient presents with excessive moisture or watery discharge at the parotid region.
2. The discharge increases during meals, or even thinking or imagination of delicious foods.
3. There is a small orifice in the parotid region which discharges the fluid.
4. In long-standing disease, the skin around the opening may be inflamed or excoriated (Fig. 12).

VIVA VOCE

1. **What is a salivary fistula?**
   It is an abnormal communication of salivary ductal system with the skin which results in leakage of saliva on the skin (Fig. 12).
2. **What are the causes of parotid salivary fistula?**
   The causes of a parotid salivary fistula are:
   - Postoperative parotid fistula:
     - Badly placed incision for draining a parotid abscess.
     - Superficial parotidectomy.
   - Post-traumatic fistula following penetrating injury in the parotid region.
3. **What are the types of parotid salivary fistula?**
   They are of two types (Fig. 13):
   - Gland fistula.
   - Duct fistula.
4. **What are the features of a gland fistula?**
   It is the cutaneous communication of glandular acini. The opening is situated at the periphery of the parotid

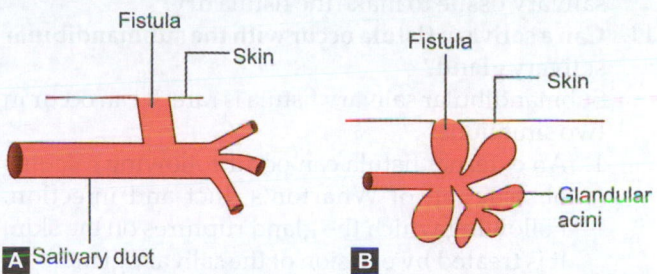

Fig. 13: Types of parotid salivary fistula; A, Dust fistula, B, Gland fistula

region which discharges very small amount of saliva (just moisture in the parotid region).

5. **What are the features of a duct fistula?**
   It is the cutaneous communication of the salivary duct. The opening is usually situated in the central and anterior part of parotid region. It discharges significant amount of saliva, especially during meals.
6. **What are the investigations?**
   Sialography may be done to see the communicating ductal system.
7. **What will you see in the sialogram?**
   The things to be noted are:
   - Site of internal communication of fistula.
   - Presence of a stricture or a filling defect in the ducts.
8. **How do you treat a parotid salivary fistula?**
   - A small fistula may disappear spontaneously with passage of time. Probanthine 50 mg four times daily may be of help
   - A large fistula is treated by Newman and Seabrook's operation in which the fistula is excised and the ends of the duct are anastomosed over a splint (Fig. 14).
9. **What are the results of treatment?**
   Overall results are good, but recurrence can occur rarely.

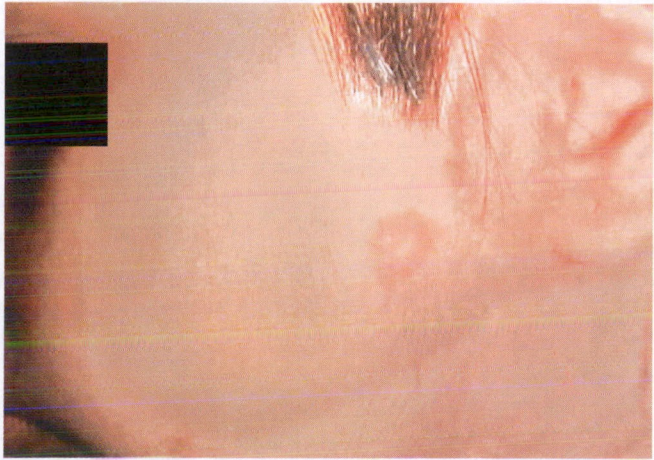

Fig. 12: Traumatic parotid salivary fistula. Note the redness around the fistula opening. (*Courtesy:* Professor Sandeep Kumar)

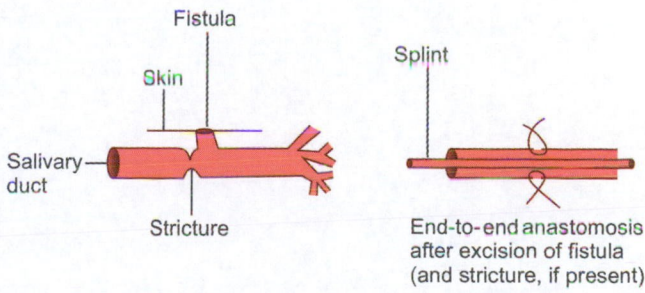

Fig. 14: Newman and Seabrook's operation

10. **How do you treat recurrence?**

It is treated by radiotherapy which destroys the salivary tissue to make the fistula dry.

11. **Can a salivary fistula occur with the submandibular salivary gland?**

Submandibular salivary fistula is rare. It can occur in two situations:

1. An external fistula can occur following calculus obstruction of Wharton's duct and infection. Following which the gland ruptures on the skin. It is treated by excision of the salivary gland.
2. An internal fistula into the mouth following lithotomy of a ductal stone—It is of no clinical consequence as the saliva is draining into the oral cavity.

DISCUSSION

It is an abnormal opening in the parotid region discharging saliva. It is an uncommon problem (Fig. 12).

Etiology

- Postoperative parotid fistula:
  1. Badly placed incision for draining a parotid abscess.
  2. Superficial parotidectomy.
- Post-traumatic fistula following penetrating injuries of parotid region.

Clinical Features

- Depending upon the site of internal communication parotid fistulae are of two types—gland fistula and duct fistula
- A gland fistula produces some moisture on the skin of the parotid region which increases during meals. It causes very little inconvenience to the patient
- A duct fistula causes free flow of saliva on the skin especially during meals or when the patient smells or even think of food. In long-standing leak, the skin around the opening may be inflamed or excoriated (Fig. 12).

The communication of the fistula with the main duct or a ductule can be seen by sialography done through the fistula. It will also show if the salivary ductal system is obstructed (stricture or a stone).

Treatment

- A small fistula may disappear spontaneously with passage of time. Probanthine 50 mg four times daily may be of help
- A large fistula is repaired by Newman and Seabrook's operation where the fistula is excised alongwith the stricture (if present), and the ends of the duct are anastomosed over a splint passed through the duct orifice
- If the fistula persists the salivary tissue is destroyed by radiotherapy to dry up the fistula.

CASE 5: URACHAL FISTULA

CLINICAL DIAGNOSIS

- The patient is usually an adult or elderly person who presents with discharge of watery fluid from the umbilicus (Fig. 15).
- The umbilicus is wet and smells of urine.
- The patient has obstructive urinary symptoms—difficulty in micturition, thin stream and dribbling.
- An induration may be palpable in the urethra.
- The prostate may be enlarged on digital rectal examination.

VIVA VOCE

1. **What is urachal fistula?**
   In this condition, the urachus is open at umbilicus (Fig. 15).
2. **What is urachus?**
   It is an embryological structure which is attached to the apex of bladder and the other end is attached at the umbilicus. In a normal person, it gets obliterated.
3. **What is the pathogenesis of a urachal fistula?**
   In a normal person as the contractions start at the apex of bladder and then pass downwards even the patent, urachus is closed during micturition. If there is lower urinary tract obstruction due to any cause (stricture of urethra, enlarged prostate), the bladder remains overfull resulting in urinary leakage from umbilicus.

4. **How will you confirm the diagnosis?**
   Fistulography done through the umbilical opening will show the dye entering into the bladder. It may show the intravesical enlargement of the prostate (Fig. 16).
5. **What are the other investigations?**
   The whole of lower urinary tract must be visualized, e.g. by cystoscopy and urethrocytography to rule out other causes of BOO.
6. **How do you treat this condition?**
   The obstruction of the lower urinary tract is removed, e.g. TURP for BHP or optical urethrotomy for stricture of urethra. The urinary leak may stop.
7. **If it does not stop, what will you do?**
   The urachus is excised completely by an extraperitoneal approach, and the bladder wall is closed in two layers with an indwelling catheter for 7 to 10 days.
8. **What is TURP?**
   It is endoscopic piece-meal removal of enlarged prostate through the urethra.
9. **What is optical urethrotomy?**
   It is endoscopic division of the stricture ring by a very fine knife to increase the urethral lumen at the site of stricture.

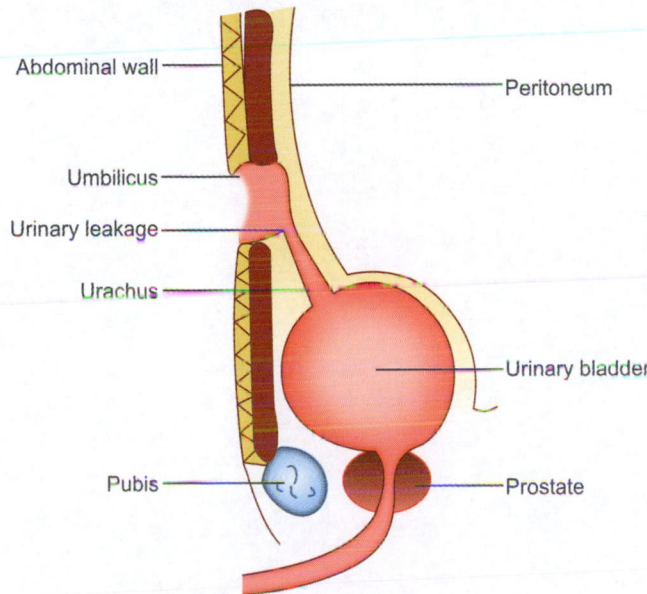

Fig. 15: Urachal fistula

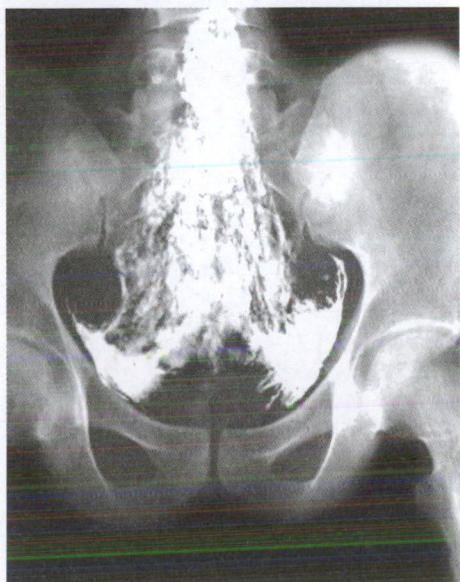

Fig. 16: Urachal umbilical fistula showing a negative convex shadow in the lower part due to enlarged prostate. The bladder is enlarged due to chronic obstruction caused by BPH, and tethered at umbilicus due to fistula. Hence this shape.
Note: This fistulogram was done in year 1938 by lipoidol injection (oily medium hence this texture). (From the collection of late Professor SC Misra, senior author's teacher)

10. **What is a urachal cyst?**

It is a tubulodermoid occurring in the urachus.

11. **What are the symptoms?**

Usually, it is asymptomatic till some complication occurs in it, e.g. infection with abscess formation.

12. **How will you confirm the diagnosis?**

It can be seen by ultrasound or CT scan.

13. **How do you treat it?**

It is treated by excision of cyst with the urachus.

DISCUSSION

Urachus is an embryological tubular structure which joins the urinary bladder with the umbilicus. It gets obliterated normally at the time of birth. Even if it is not obliterated it does not leak urine as the contraction of bladder for micturition starts at the apex and passes downward. Thus, it keeps the urachus closed during micturition.

If there occurs lower urinary tract obstruction, e.g. due to enlarged prostate or stricture of urethra the bladder remains overfull causing leakage of urine through the urachal fistula (Figs 15 and 16).

The patient, usually a middle-aged or elderly person presents with leakage of urine from the umbilicus.

The diagnosis can be confirmed by fistulography which shows the communication with the apex of bladder. The cause of fistula is detected by cystoscopy or urethrocystography.

The leakage may stop after the cause of lower urinary obstruction is removed. If it does not, the urachus is excised completely and the bladder wound is closed with an indwelling catheter in the bladder for 7 to 10 days.

Sinuses

CASE 1: CHRONIC OSTEOMYELITIS OF FEMUR

CLINICAL DIAGNOSIS

1. The patient is usually a young person who presents with a sinus (or sinuses) in the thigh of long duration.
2. It is usually situated on the posteromedial aspect of the thigh lower down.
3. It discharges pus continuously or intermittently. It may at times discharge bone chips.
4. It is fixed to the underlying bone which is thickened and tender on deep pressure (Fig. 1).
5. Pouting granulation tissue ('proud flesh') may be present at the mouth of the sinus.

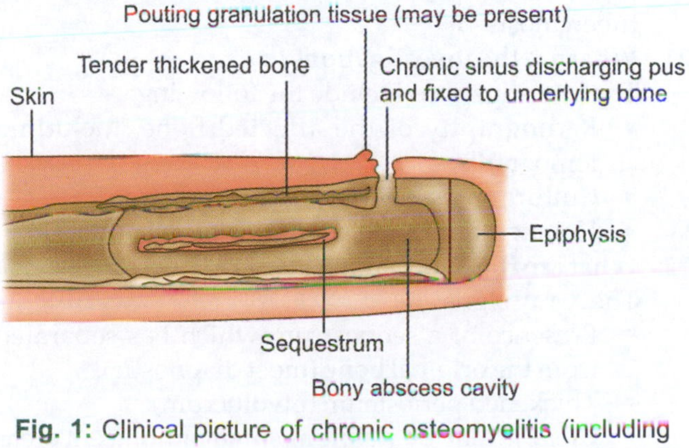

Fig. 1: Clinical picture of chronic osteomyelitis (including pathology)

VIVA VOCE

1. **What is chronic osteomyelitis?**
   It is chronic pyogenic infection of bone characterized by inflammation of bone including the bone marrow.
2. **What is the cause of chronic osteomyelitis?**
   It is the acute osteomyelitis which may pass into chronic osteomyelitis due to the following reasons:
   1. Failure to treat the patient early.
   2. Inadequate treatment so that infected bone dies to form a sequestrum and cavity.
3. **What is the cause of acute osteomyelitis?**
   It is the acute infection of bone caused by pyogenic bacteria, Staphylococcus aureus being the commonest, reaching the site of infection usually by hematogenous route.
4. **What is the commonest site of involvement in femur?**
   Lower metaphyseal region.
5. **What are the anatomical types of chronic osteomyelitis?**
   It is of two types:
   1. Osteomyelitis affecting a large volume of bone
   2. Intraosseous abscess - Brodie's abscess
6. **What is a Brodie's abscess?**
   It is a localized type of abscess in the end of a bone having pus or jelly-like granulation tissue surrounded by sclerotic bone (Fig. 2).

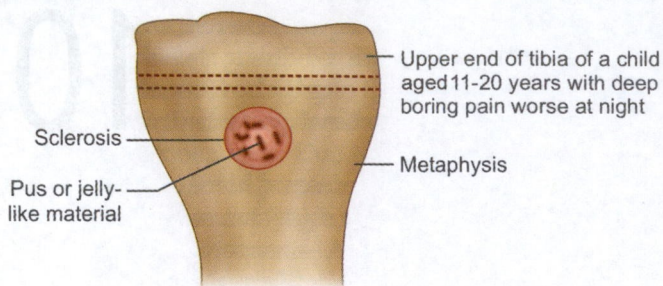

Upper end of tibia of a child aged 11-20 years with deep boring pain worse at night

Sclerosis

Metaphysis

Pus or jelly-like material

Fig. 2: Brodie's abscess upper end of tibia

7. **What is the cause of a Brodie's abscess?**
The causes of a Brodie's abscess are:
• Pyogenic septicemia from which the patient has recovered leaving a focus of infection (abscess) in the bone which may remain dormant for years.
• Osteomyelitis (but not septicemia) affecting the bone other than the one in which the Brodie's abscess is discovered.

8. **What are the clinical signs of a Brodie's abscess?**
The signs of a Brodie's abscess are:
• The patient is usually in second decade of life and presents with recurrent attacks of pain near the end of a long bone which is worse at night.
• It commonly occurs in the lower end of tibia, upper end of tibia, lower end of femur or upper end of humerus - in that order.
• The joint in the vicinity may have transitory effusion but permits every movement and apparently normal.
• There is localized thickening and tenderness on deep pressure near the end of a bone.

9. **How do you confirm the diagnosis of a Brodie's abscess?**
By radiography.

10. **What are the X-ray signs of a Brodie's abscess?**
The X-ray signs are:
• Localized area of radiolucency near the end of a long bone.
• Bony sclerosis of the wall of cavity.

11. **What are the causes of chronicity in a Brodie's abscess?**
The causes of chronicity are:
• Failure of closure of abscess cavity by collapse of its walls as happens in the abscess cavity in soft tissues.
• The dense sclerotic bone of the wall of the cavity prevents leukocytes, antibodies and antibiotics to reach the contents of the cavity.

12. **What is a sequestrum?**
It is a dead piece of bone lying in an osteomyelitic cavity.

13. **How do you visualize a sequestrum?**
It can be seen by radiography, including tomography.

14. **How does it look like radiographically?**
It is a loose piece of bone lying in a cavity inside the bone and is usually denser than the surrounding bone.

15. **What is involucrum?**
It is a sheath of new bone laid down by elevated periosteum that surrounds the dead bone within.

16. **How does it look like radiographically?**
It is the radiopaque sheath of new bone around the original bone commonly described as thickened periosteum.

17. **What are cloacae?**
These are the holes in the involucrum through which pus comes out to be discharged on the skin through the sinus or sinuses.

18. **Why are they called cloacae?**
Because they discharge pus (liquid) and pieces of dead bone (solid) similar to cloaca of a frog which discharges both urine (liquid) and feces (solid).

19. **What are the causes of chronicity in osteomyelitis?**
The causes of chronicity are:
• The presence of sequestrum inside the bone which cannot be resorbed.
• Intraosseous infected bony cavity which cannot collapse.

20. **How do you differentiate it from tuberculous osteomyelitis (tuberculosis of bone)?**
In tuberculous disease the discharge is often thin and watery. The sinus may be single or multiple (commonly multiple) and have an undermined and pigmented edge. There may be other signs of tuberculosis.

21. **What are the investigations?**
The investigations include the following:
• Radiography of the affected bone, including tomography.
• Culture and sensitivity of the discharge.
• Hemoglobin, blood counts, urine examination.

22. **What are the X-ray signs?**
The X-ray signs are:
• Presence of a sequestrum which has separated from the original bone (most diagnostic).
• Thickened periosteum (involucrum).
• Cloacae may be visible as small radiolucent areas in the thickened periosteum.
• Presence of a cavity in the bone (Fig. 3).

23. **How will you measure the size of the cavity?**
• A plain radiograph done in two planes gives the approximate size of the cavity.
• The cavity can be exactly measured by sinography or CT scan.

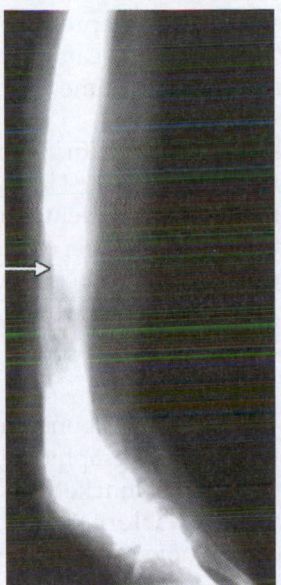

Fig. 3: Chronic osteomyelitis of femur showing a large sequestrum (original bone) in the sheath of thickened periosteum (involucrum)

24. **What are the complications of chronic osteomyelitis?**
    The complications are:
    - Spread of infection into the neighboring joint resulting in suppurative arthritis.
    - Metastatic infection.
    - Growth abnormalities if the growth plate is involved.
    - Pathological fracture.
    - Soft tissue contracture in long standing patients.
    - Amyloidosis if there is significant pus discharge for many years.

25. **How do you treat chronic osteomyelitis?**
    The patient is usually treated by an operation with the twin objectives of removal of sequestrum and obliteration of cavity or dead space (Fig. 4).

26. **How do you remove the sequestrum?**
    The bone is exposed through the previous scar, the soft tissues are stripped and the involucrum is cut to reach the sequestrum. The overhanging walls of the cavity are excised and the sequestrum is pulled out and removed en bloc.

27. **How do you obliterate the cavity?**
    The overhanging edge of the cavity is excised with osteotome or nibbled to saucerize the bony cavity so as to obliterate it by soft tissues.

28. **Do you know of any other method of obliterating the bony cavity?**
    Gentamicin impregnated beads may be implanted in the wound following surgery, which are removed 14 days later and the dead space is filled with cancellous bone chips or local muscle flap.

29. **What are the results of surgical treatment?**
    - If a sequestrum is present and is removed, the sinuses usually heal and the disease is cured.
    - If only a cavity or sclerosis is present without a sequestrum, the disease may heal or the saucerization may fail and the sinuses may persist.

30. **What will you do if a sinus persists after surgery?**
    - The case should be reviewed to find the cause of sinus which should be eliminated.
    - If the sinus persists and the discharge is slight it can be managed by daily dressing, rather, the patient should learn to live with it.

31. **How do you treat a Brodie's abscess?**
    It is treated by evacuation and curettage of the cavity under antibiotic cover. If the cavity is of moderate size it is filled with cancellous bone chips.

32. **Is there any indication for amputation in this disease?**
    It is very rarely required. It is indicated if there are frequent or prolonged exacerbations with painful disability and risk of amyloidosis.

33. **How do you treat exacerbations of disease?**
    The exacerbations are treated by:
    - Immobilization of limb.
    - Appropriate antibiotic treatment.
    - Analgesics for pain.

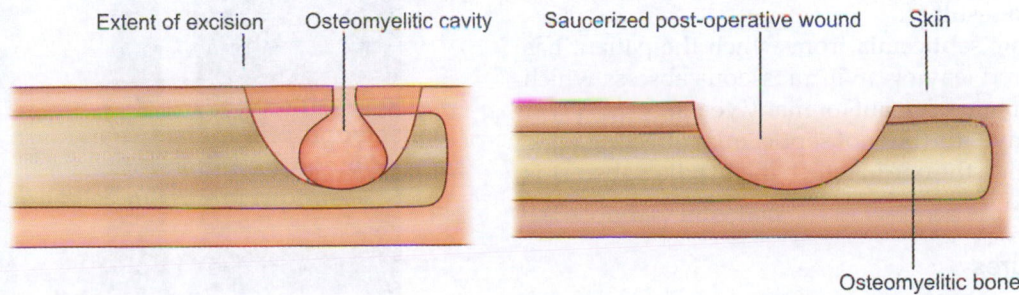

Fig. 4: Saucerization

DISCUSSION

Chronic osteomyelitis is a chronic infective disease of bone including marrow cavity.

Etiology

It is usually conversion of acute hematogenous osteomyelitis into chronic due to the following causes:
- Failure to treat the disease in early stage.
- Inadequate or inappropriate treatment.

The result of these two factors is death of infected bone with formation of a sequestrum which cannot be discharged like pus resulting in persistence of infection inside the bone.

Pathology

There is chronic inflammation of the bone with osteitis, periosteitis and endosteitis. Due to tissue necrosis and liquefaction there occurs pus formation which comes out through the sinus. Surrounding the sequestrum the elevated periosteum lays down new bone which entombs the dead bone lying inside. This ensheathing mass of new bone is called as involucrum. At the points where the pus has broken through the periosteum sinuses form which are represented in the involucrum by holes known as cloacae. The chronicity of the disease is because of the following reasons:
- The presence of sequestrum which is dead and infected bone and cannot be resorbed.
- Intraosseous abscess cavity which does not get obliterated because of rigid bony wall. Thus, the body's normal defence mechanism together with the antibiotics cannot reach to kill the bacteria in the bone. Pathologically it is of two types—osteomyelitis involving a large volume of bone and Brodie's abscess.
- Osteomyelitis involving a large volume of bone—It is the common type of osteomyelitis where the inflammation involves a significant portion of bone.
- Brodie's abscess is the uncommon form where there is a chronic intraosseous abscess containing pus or jelly-like granulation tissue surrounded by sclerotic bone. It is usually a result of:
  - Pyogenic septicemia from which the patient has recovered leaving an intraosseous abscess which may remain dormant for many years.
  - Osteomyelitis (but not septicemia) affecting bone other than the one in which the Brodie's abscess is detected.

Clinical Features

This disease usually presents with a chronically or intermittently discharging sinus fixed to a bone which is thickened and tender on deep pressure (Fig. 5). It may remain quiescent for months or years but acute or subacute exacerbations may occur from time to time. The adjacent joint may be stiff.

A Brodie's abscess presents with intermittent local pain and sometimes transient effusion in the adjacent joint during an exacerbation. The patient is 11 to 20 years of age. The common sites are the upper end of tibia and lower end of femur in the metaphysis of bone. On palpation there is tenderness and thickening of the bone.

Investigations

1. **Radiography**—The affected bone is radiographed in both the planes. The radiographic signs are:
   - The periosteum is markedly thickened with irregularity and sclerosis to honey-combed appearance. It is now called involucrum
   - The involucrum may have a single or multiple holes (cloacae)
   - There is a cavity in the bone seen as an area of rarefaction
   - There is sequestrum inside the cavity which is irregular, variable in size and denser than surrounding bone. The granulation tissue around the sequestrum gives rise to a radiolucent zone around it.

The signs of a Brodie's abscess are:
   - A rounded radiolucent area in the end of a long bone.
   - Sclerosis of the wall of radiolucency varying from dense sclerosis extending a considerable distance

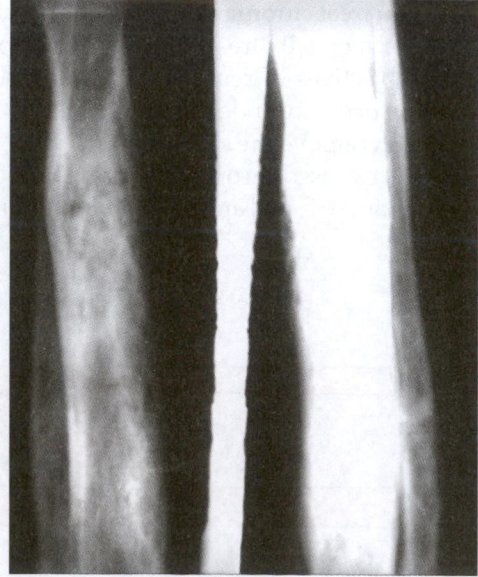

Fig. 5: Garre's osteomyelitis affecting both the bones of leg. (*Courtesy:* Late Professor SC Misra's case)

round the cavity to a faint line of sclerosis at the junction of the abscess with the cancellous bone.

2. Probing of the sinus may be done to detect sequestrum.
3. Sinogram—It may delineate the abscess cavity inside the bone.
4. Pus culture and sensitivity.

Complications

- Recurrent acute exacerbations or flare-up of infection
- Growth abnormalities if the growth plate is affected—Shortening, lengthening due to increased vascularity of growth plate, and deformities
- Pathological fracture
- Joint-stiffness
- Malignancy in the sinus tract
- Amyloidosis where there is long-standing suppuration. It is a late complication.

Treatment

a. *During exacerbation*—The affected limb is immobilized and appropriate antibiotics are given. The disease is not cured, only the exacerbation is controlled.

b. *Quiescent phase*—The patient is treated surgically with the objectives of removal of dead bone and the elimination of dead space. According to sensitivity report an appropriate antibiotic is given for some days prior to the operation. The bone is exposed through the previous scar, the soft tissues are stripped and the involucrum is cut to reach the sequestrum. The overhanging walls of the cavity are excised with an osteotome or nibbled to saucerize the bony cavity. The sequestrum is removed en bloc. One must be careful as the bone may fracture during saucerization.

The wound is drained and closed in a manner to obliterate the dead space as much as possible.

Gentamicin—impregnated beads may be implanted in the wound following surgery, which are removed 14 days later and the dead space is filled with cancellous bone chips or local muscle flap.

Brodie's abscess—It is treated by evacuation and curettage of the cavity under antibiotic umbrella. If the cavity is of moderate size it is filled with cancellous bone chips.

Amputation—It is indicated if there are frequent or prolonged exacerbations with painful disability and risk of amyloidosis.

Prognosis

If a sequestrum is present and is removed the sinuses usually heal and the disease is cured.

If only a cavity or sclerosis is present without a sequestrum the saucerization may fail and the sinus may persist. Hence, if the discharge is slight and can be managed by daily dressing, it is better to live with it. Amyloid disease need not be feared as it takes many years to develop provided there is copious pus discharge.

Garre's Osteomyelitis

It is a sclerosing nonsuppurative chronic osteomyelitis which is now rare. It may begin like acute osteomyelitis with pain, fever and swelling. As time passes, the pain and fever disappear but the swelling of the bone continues. There is no pus and no discharging sinus. The femoral and tibial shafts are most commonly involved (Fig. 5). It has to be differentiated from bone tumors (Ewing's tumor or osteosarcoma) for which biopsy is required.

Treatment—Acute symptoms are treated with analgesics and broad-spectrum antibiotics. For permanent pain relief making a gutter or holes in the bone may be required.

CASE 2: PILONIDAL SINUS

CLINICAL DIAGNOSIS

1. The patient is usually young, may be a driver by profession, who is exceptionally hairly and often obese, and presents with a discharging sinus in the sacrococcygeal region of insidious onset.
2. The discharge is foul-smelling, blood-stained purulent fluid.
3. The sinus is present in the midline 5 cm behind the anus near the tip of coccyx.
4. A tuft of hair may project from its mouth (Fig. 6).
5. There may be excessive granulation tissue at the opening.

VIVA VOCE

1. **What is a pilonidal sinus?**
   It is a chronic discharging sinus in the natal cleft in the midline about 5 cm behind the anus usually with a tuft of hair projecting from its mouth.
2. **What is pilonidal disease?**
   The pilonidal disease consists of a draining sinus or an acute abscess in the sacrococcygeal area. Also, there may be an underlying cyst associated with granulation tissue, fibrosis, and frequently a tuft of hair (Figs 6 to 8).
3. **What is the etiology of the condition?**
   - This disease is now accepted as an acquired disease, although theories of congenital origin were once popular.

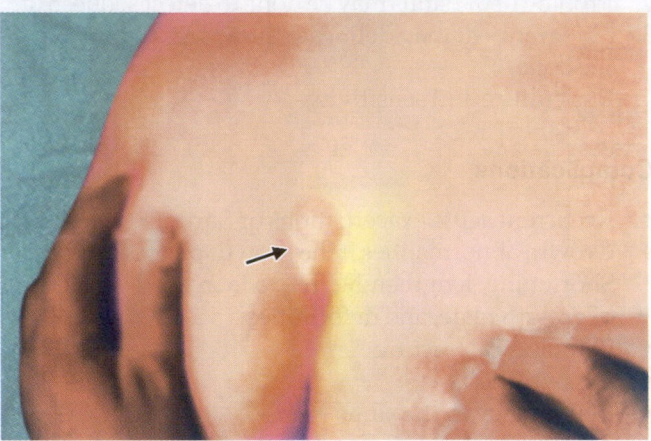

Fig. 7: Pilonidal abscess

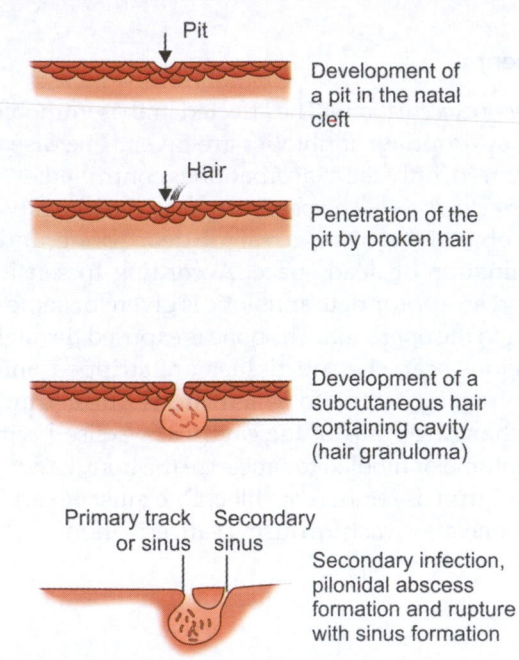

Fig. 8: Pathogenesis of a pilonidal sinus

   - The cause in most cases is probably infection, irritation and trapping of hair in the sacrococcygeal area.
4. **What is the pathogenesis of this disease?**
   The broken collected hair are drilled or sucked into the cavity owing to friction with movement of the buttocks. Barbs on the hair prevent their expulsion, so they become trapped provoking a foreign body type reaction and infection (Fig. 8).
5. **What are the complications of this disease?**
   It may result in an acute abscess formation. Very rarely, malignancy can occur.

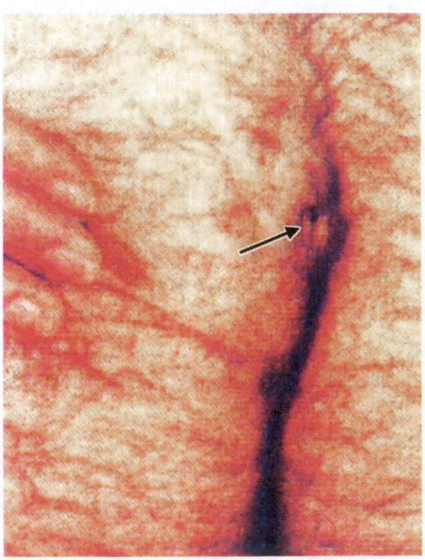

Fig. 6: Pilonidal sinus of a hirsute

6. **How do you treat this condition?**
The principles of treatment are:
- Noninfected sinus
  1. Excision with primary closure by Z-plasty.
  2. Excision and laying open.
- Infected sinus or abscess—It is treated by drainage and excision so that it heals by secondary intention. The wound must drain adequately, and pocketing and bridging must be prevented.

7. **What are the advantages/disadvantages of excision with primary closure versus laying open?**
They are given in the following table:

Feature	Excision with primary closure	Laying open
Healing time	Less	More
Operating skill	More skill is required	Less skill will do
Return to work	Early	Delayed
Hospital stay	More	Less
Wound care required	Minimal	Active wound care and dressing

8. **Can this disease recur, if so what are the causes of recurrence?**
This disease can recur, and the causes of recurrence are:
- Inadequate wound care
- Poorly drained tracks (early recurrence)
- Recurrent infection due to further entry of broken hair
- Midline scars.

9. **How do you prevent recurrence?**
The recurrence is prevented by the following measures:
1. Sometimes sinus pits are missed at the time of primary surgery due to edema, but they can be easily distinguished and excised a week after primary operation.
2. The patient is advised to keep the area clean and dry, to avoid direct trauma, and to shave the skin or apply a depilatory cream regularly to prevent further entrapment of hair.
3. The procedures which leave a midline scar are most susceptible to further hair penetration, hence should be avoided.
4. In persons with a deep natal cleft, the depth of the natal cleft, may be reduced by debulking both the buttocks. This step will prevent entrapment of hair, avoid the friction of buttocks and prevent injury of the skin by broken hair.

10. **How do you treat a pilonidal abscess?**
A pilonidal abscess is incised, drained and curetted free of hair and granulation tissue.

Some residual pits may be left over which will cause recurrence as they may not be recognized at the time of drainage. They are more easily identified and excised a week after primary drainage, when the edema has resolved.

PILONIDAL SINUS

Pilonidal disease consists of a hair containing sinus or abscess which involves the skin and subcutaneous tissues in the postcoccygeal intergluteal region. It is a common disease among the military. Hence, also known as jeep disease.

Etiology

Initially, it was thought to be a congenital (or developmental) disease but now the acquired theory of occurrence has been accepted. The reasons are given below:
1. This disease usually manifests at 20 to 29 years of age while most of the congenital diseases are present since birth.
2. Histology of sinus has never shown hair follicles in the wall of the sinus.
3. The hairs in the sinus are dead hairs and their pointed ends are directed towards the floor of sinus.
4. Pilonidal sinus can occur in the interdigital clefts of hair dressers, and the hair present in the sinus are of customers.

Pathogenesis

This disease is commonly seen in hairy men (dark hard hair) with a deep natal cleft and closely approximated buttocks. The broken or shed hair are trapped in the cleft. The movement of the buttocks result in drilling of the skin by the collected hair, allowing them to enter the skin by the suction created during movements. It produces skin and subcutaneous infection with formation of sinus and its tract or tracts containing broken hair. The sinus tract usually runs cephalad (Fig. 8).

Clinical Features

Age and sex—This disease is more commonly seen in males than females between 20 to 29 years of age.

It commonly occurs in dark haired persons and uncommon in those with soft and blond hair.

There is pain, swelling and discharge which occurs intermittently in the posterior part of the natal cleft (Figs 6 and 7).

A past history of repeated abscess formation and rupture in this region may be available.

There is one or more sinuses in the midline in the retrococcygeal region. The hair may be visible in the mouth of the sinus.

Investigations

Usually the diagnosis is obvious hence no investigations are required. The pus may be sent for culture. X-ray shows local bones to be normal. Sinogram reveals a subcutaneous sinus which may have multiple tracks or branches.

Treatment

When the patient comes for the first episode or in early disease the area is cleaned, shaved and dressed daily. With this treatment the disease may heal.

Pilonidal abscess—The abscess is drained with a midline incision with cleaning the cavity of pus, necrotic tissue, hair and granulation tissue. It may result in healing of the disease (Fig. 7).

Chronic pilonidal sinus—Many operative procedures are described which include laying open of all tracks with or without marsupialization, excision of all tracks and closure with a method avoiding a midline scar (Z-plasty, Karydakis procedure, and Bascom procedure). If both the buttocks are debulked to avoid their friction and to make the natal cleft shallow—the chances of recurrence are markedly reduced.

Karydakis procedure—The diseased tissues are excised with a semilunar incision and the flaps are mobilized to allow a tension free closure a little away from the midline.

Bascom technique—The sinus cavity is entered by a paramedian incision and cleared of the hair and the granulation tissue. The midline pits are excised and closed while the lateral wound is left open.

CASE 3: ACTINOMYCOSIS

CLINICAL DIAGNOSIS

1. The patient is usually a man between 15 and 30 years of age who presents with a swelling with multiple sinuses in the cervicofacial region, chest wall or right lower abdomen of insidious onset (Figs 9 and 10).
2. The swelling is hard, ill-defined and painless.
3. The skin is bluish or violaceous in color.
4. The sinuses are hard and fixed and may feel like a strand or strands of a whipchord.
5. The discharge is thin watery pus containing yellow or 'sulfur' granules.
6. The regional lymph nodes are not enlarged.

VIVA VOCE

1. **What is actinomycosis?**
   It is a chronic infection caused by Actinomyces israeli that may involve almost any site in the body the commonest being faciocervical (accounting for about half the cases) region.
2. **What are the other clinical types?**
   The other clinical types are:
   - Right iliac fossa (Fig. 12)
   - Thoracic type
   - Hepatic type
   - Female genital tract disease.
3. **What are the morphological features of this organism?**
   It is a gram-positive, branching, filamentous and microaerophilic organism which sometimes lives as a harmless commensal in the normal mouth.

4. **Is it a bacteria or fungus?**
   It is a bacteria, often inaccurately described as fungus (Fig. 1).
5. **Is this disease caused by *Actinomyces israelii* alone?**
   No, sometimes other actinomyces such as *Arachnia proprionica* are responsible, and very frequently other organisms, both aerobes and anerobes are found.
6. **What are 'sulfur granules'?**
   These are yellowish granules found in the discharge. Microscopically, a granule consists of gram-positive mycelia (Fig. 12).
7. **What is 'ray' fungus?**
   It is the other name of the causative organism as the peripheral filaments radiate from the central part of the granule.
8. **Is it an exogenous infection?**
   No, it is an endogenous infection as actinomyces form part of the normal flora of oral cavity, gastrointestinal tract and female genital tract
9. **What is the source of infection in faciocervical actinomycosis?**
   In most of the patients there is obvious dental disease which is the usual source of infection.
10. **How does the disease present before the development of sinuses?**
    This disease presents as a gradually enlarging, generally painless and indurated swelling of the gum or near the angle of the mandible.
11. **How does the infection spread?**
    The infection spreads by:
    - Local extension by anatomical continuity and contiguity

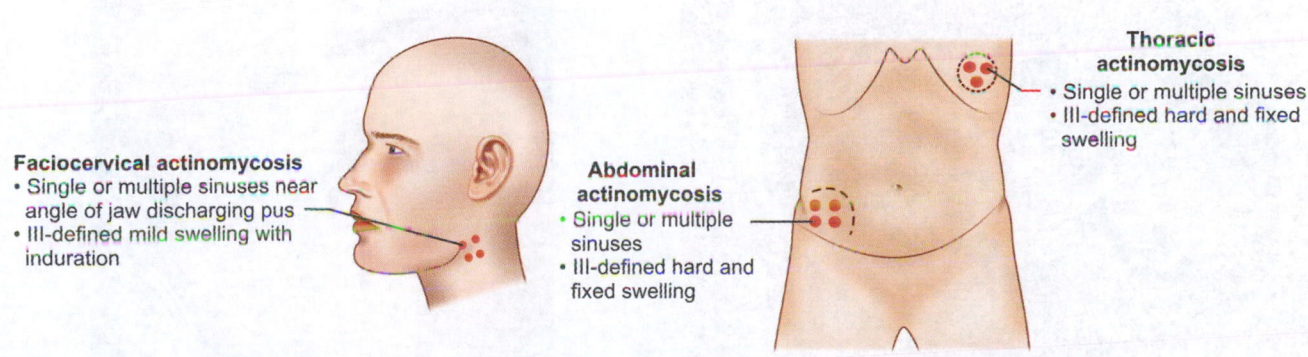

Faciocervical actinomycosis
- Single or multiple sinuses near angle of jaw discharging pus
- Ill-defined mild swelling with induration

Abdominal actinomycosis
- Single or multiple sinuses
- Ill-defined hard and fixed swelling

Thoracic actinomycosis
- Single or multiple sinuses
- Ill-defined hard and fixed swelling

Fig. 9: Clinical actinomycosis

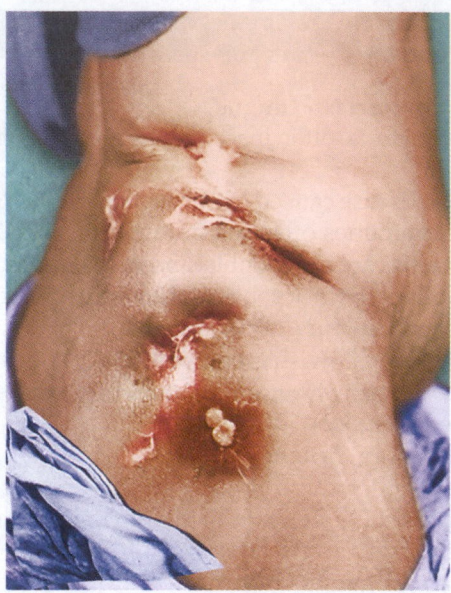

Fig. 10: Actinomycosis of ileocecal region which has made many sinuses at the back and even by perforating the ilium bone

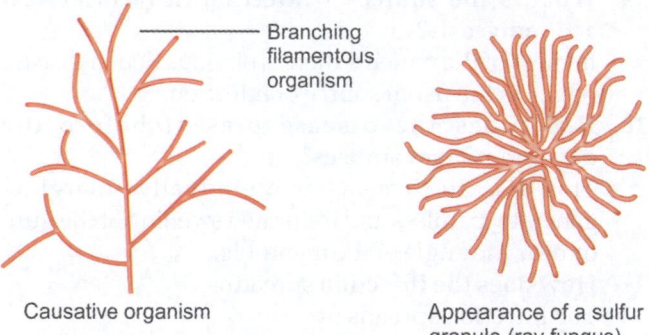

Branching filamentous organism

Causative organism

Appearance of a sulfur granule (ray fungus)

Fig. 11: Causative organism of actinomycosis

- Hematogenous spread due to invasion of a vein
- Aspiration, i.e. aspiration from the oral cavity or pharynx into the lungs.

12. **Why does this infection not spread by lymphatics?**
    Probably this organism is too big for the lymphatics to carry to lymph nodes.

13. **How do you confirm the diagnosis?**
    The diagnosis is confirmed by finding the causative organism in the pus or tissue sections (biopsy).

14. **What about culture of pus?**
    The culture of the pus is made difficult by the presence of secondary infection.

15. **How do you collect pus?**
    The pus should be collected in a sterile tube; a swab is usually insufficient.

16. **How do you treat this disease?**
    This organism is sensitive to many antibiotics such as penicillin, tetracycline, lincomycin, etc. Penicillin is the drug of choice. A prolonged intensive course of penicillin (10 mega units reducing to 4 mega units) is administered till all the signs of disease have disappeared.

17. **What is the role of surgery?**
    It may be required for drainage of pus, debridement or subsequent repair of defects (Fig. 13).

DISCUSSION

Actinomycosis is a chronic infective granuloma caused by *Actinomyces israelii* that may involve almost any site in the body, the commonest being the faciocervical region.

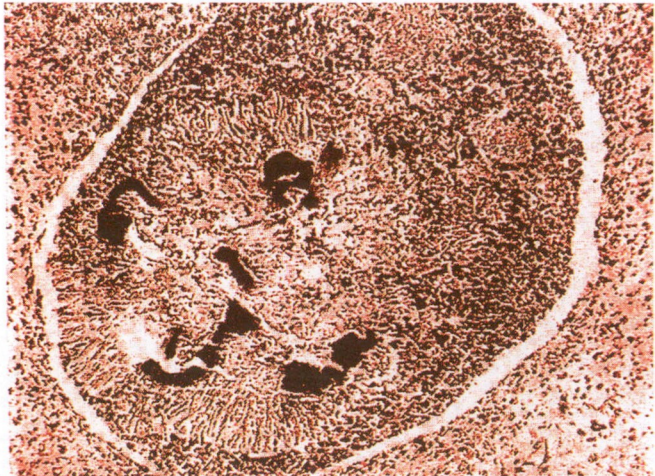

Fig. 12: Structure of a sulfur granule of actinomycosis

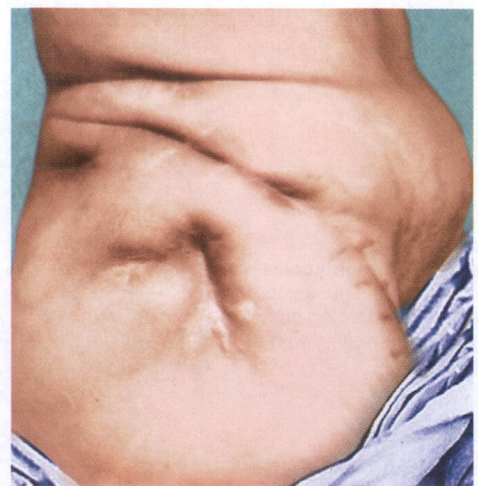

Fig. 13: Post-treatment picture of the patient shown previously after right ileocecal resection along with the sinuses. The patient was given antibiotics for 6 weeks postoperatively. There was complete healing of the disease

Etiology

Actinomyces israeli is an anaerobic, gram-positive and branching filamentous organism that may sometimes be found in tonsillar crypts and dental cavities of otherwise healthy oral cavity. The organism which is present in corn and grasses is not pathogenic. When introduced into traumatized tissues and associated with other anaerobic bacteria, these organisms become pathogenic.

Pathology

This organism invades the tissues directly. Trauma and dental caries are important predisposing factors in faciocervical actinomycosis. After the invasion, it causes subacute pyogenic inflammation with much induration and sinus formation.

Clinical Features

This disease is characterized by the formation of a firm, indurated mass the edges of which are indefinite. The lymph nodes are not enlarged. A vein may be invaded resulting in pyemia. Actinomycosis is of four main clinical types (Figs 9 and 10):

1. *Faciocervical actinomycosis:* This is the commonest type. The lower jaw adjacent to a carious tooth is frequently affected. The gum swells and becomes indurated. Subsequently nodules appear and burst discharging pus, containing sulfur granules. The skin overlying the affected lower jaw also swells, becomes indurated and bluish in color. Subsequently abscesses develop and rupture resulting in multiple sinuses.
2. *Thoracic disease:* The infection enters the lungs and pleura either by aspiration of organism or by direct spread from the pharynx or neck or even upwards through the diaphragm. Empyema can occur. Finally it invades the chest wall resulting in many sinuses. The infection may spread through the diaphragm to subphrenic spaces and liver.
3. *Right iliac fossa disease:* This disease is rare. The patient presents with a discharging wound or multiple sinuses

in right iliac fossa following appendicectomy three weeks earlier. At first the discharge is thin and watery and later on it becomes thick and malodorous. There is no obstruction but a fecal fistula may occur (Fig. 12).
4. *Hepatic actinomycosis:* The infection can reach the liver via the portal vein from right iliac fossa disease, via the hepatic artery from faciocervical disease or from contiguous viscera, e.g. penetrating peptic ulcer into the liver. It slowly destroys the liver with multiple abscesses (honeycomb liver).

Investigations

1. Examination of pus: The pus is collected in a sterile tube (swab is not good) and inspected in good light for pinhead sized 'sulfur granules'. Microscopically, a granule consists of gram positive mycelia. The peripheral filaments radiate (ray fungus) from the central part of the granule and may be surrounded by gram-negative tissue clubs. The culture of the organism is made difficult by the presence of secondary invaders.
2. Biopsy: This organism is visible in the tissue sections.
3. Radiography of the affected part (e.g. lower jaw, thorax) may be required.
4. CT scan or MRI reveals the extent of the mass extending to involve local bone/bones.

Treatment

Penicillin G is the antibiotic of choice. Ten to 20 million units are given daily by intramuscular injection for 4 to 6 weeks, followed by oral penicillin V 500 mg four times daily till healing occurs. Alternatives include ampicillin 12 g/day intravenously for 4 to 6 weeks followed by oral amoxicillin 500 mg thrice daily, or doxycycline 100 mg twice daily intravenously or orally till healing occurs.

Surgery is required for drainage of pus, excision of necrotic tissue and resection of destroyed organs or parts (Figs 10 and 13).

The prognosis of this disease is good.

CASE 4: MADURA FOOT (MYCETOMA PEDIS)

CLINICAL DIAGNOSIS

1. The patient, usually living in a tropical country and a bare foot walker, presents with single or multiple nodules or sinuses around the foot (Fig. 14).
2. The sinuses discharge watery fluid, which may have black, yellow or red granules.
3. There is a diffuse swelling of the foot with bluish black hue.
4. The instep of the foot is flattened or swollen.
5. The skin of the sole escapes.
6. The regional lymph nodes are not enlarged.

VIVA VOCE

1. **What is Madura foot?**
   It is a chronic granulomatous infection with suppuration and extensive bone destruction affecting the foot with hardly any systemic illness.
2. **What is the causative organism?**
   Two conditions come under Madura foot:
   - Maduromycosis (eumycetoma) is caused by true fungi and by phylogenetically diverse organisms.
   - Actinomycotic mycetoma is caused by Nocardia and Actinomadura species.
3. **What is the habitat of this organism?**
   It is available in plenty in road dust.
4. **What is the mode of infection?**
   This organism usually enters the tissues through a prick. Hence, this disease is commonly seen in barefoot walkers.

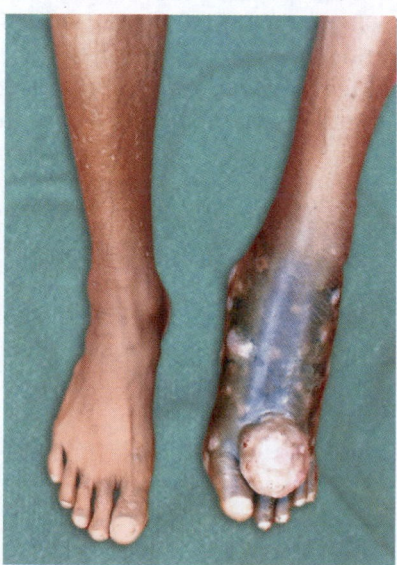

Fig. 14: Madura foot (left)

5. **What is the clinical presentation of this disease?**
   The patient presents with multiple nodules or discharging sinuses around the foot (Fig. 14).
6. **What is the nature of the discharge?**
   The discharge is watery and may have black, yellow or red granules.
7. **What is the clinical significance of the color of the granules?**
   In 'black' Madura foot, the spread of disease is mainly in the subcutaneous plane.
   In 'yellow' and 'red' varieties, the infection burrows deeply resulting in necrosis of bones.
8. **What are the investigations?**
   The investigations are:
   - Bacteriological examination of discharge by smear and culture.
   - Radiography of foot to see for any changes in the bones.
   - Biopsy of one of the nodule may be done.
9. **What do you find on biopsy?**
   The tissue gram stain reveals fine branching hyphae in actinomycotic mycetoma. Larger hyphae are present in fungal mycetoma. The causative species can be idenfied by the color of grains in the tissues.
10. **How do you treat this condition?**
    - Maduromycosis is treated by terbinafine or itraconazole for a prolonged period combined with surgical debridement.
    - Actinomycetoma is treated by sulfonamides and sulfones. Other drugs are TMP+SMZ or dapsone and streptomycin.
11. **Is there any indication for surgery?**
    The indications for operation are:
    - When the patient does not improve on medical treatment and continues to discharge.
    - In late disease with extensive tissue destruction and necrosis of bones.
12. **What is the nature of surgery?**
    Early cases require drainage of abscesses, and excision of necrotic tissue and sinus tracts. Late cases may require amputation.
13. **Can this disease occur in the hand?**
    Yes, involvement of the hand can occur rarely.
14. **Why are the lymph nodes not enlarged?**
    Because like actinomyces these organisms do not spread through lymphatics.
15. **What is the prognosis?**
    The prognosis is poor in maduromycosis and good in actinomycetoma.

DISCUSSION

Mycetoma pedis or Madura foot is a chronic slowly progressive destructive infection with suppuration with extensive bone destruction of foot with little systemic illness.

Etiology

Two conditions come under this heading:
1. Maduromycosis (eumycetoma) is caused by true fungi and by phylogenetically diverse organisms.
2. Actinomycotic mycetoma is caused by *Nocardia* and *Actinomadura* species.

They enter the tissues through a prick in those who go about barefooted.

Clinical Features

This disease is commonly seen in tropical countries notably India and Africa. The first manifestation is a papule, nodule or abscess, that over months to years progress gradually to develop multiple abscesses and sinuses (Fig. 14). Secondary infection may occur to cause ulceration. The discharge is watery and may have yellow, red or black granules. The foot is swollen and the concavity of the instep is lost, or it may become convex. The skin of the sole is otherwise normal. There is no lymphatic involvement and dissemination to other parts of the body does not occur.

Investigations

- The discharge is sent for bacteriological examination.
- X-ray of the foot may show destructive changes in the bones of the foot.
- Biopsy: The tissue gram stain reveals fine branching hyphae in actinomycotic mycetoma. Larger hyphae are present in fungal mycetoma. The causative species can be detected by the color of the grains in the tissues.

Treatment

- Maduromycosis: Surgical debridement along with prolonged terbinafine or itraconazole therapy may result in a response in 70 percent of cases. Amputation is indicated in advanced disease.
- Actinomycetoma: It responds well to sulphonamides and sulfones, especially if treated early. Trimethoprim-sulfamethoxazole, 160/800 mg twice daily orally, or dapsone 100 mg twice daily after meals is also effective. Streptomycin 14 mg/kg/day IMI may be useful in the first month of treatment. The drug treatment has to be given for months for cure, and then continued for months to prevent relapse. Debridement of necrotic tissue helps in healing.

Prognosis

- Maduromycosis: poor
- Actinomycetoma: good

Bleedings

CASE 1: HEMORRHOIDS

CLINICAL DIAGNOSIS

1. The patient is usually a middle-aged or elderly person who presents with painless and fresh bleeding per rectum of insidious onset.
2. The bleeding occurs during and immediately after defecation.
3. The blood is not mixed with stool. It may be streaked on the bed pan.
4. Pinkish blue, soft and non-tender mass or masses are present in the anal canal at 3, 7 and 11 o'clock positions (on proctoscopy) (Fig. 1).
   - The mass or masses are small and remain in the anal canal all the time (first degree).
   - The masses are that large that they prolapse during defecation only (second degree).
   - The masses are large and prolapse at least provocation, for example during laughing (third degree) (Figs 2 and 3).

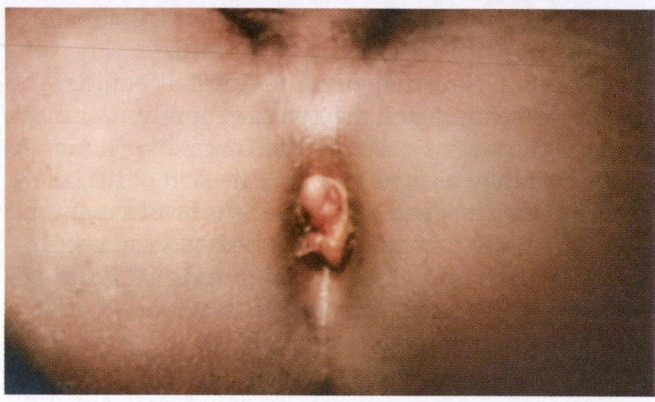

Fig. 2: Grade III hemorrhoids. The one at the 11 o'clock position is the largest and that at 7 o'clock position is the smallest

- The masses may remain permanently prolapsed and if all the three hemorrhoids are present, there may be a circumanal collar of piles (fourth degree) (Fig. 4).

VIVA VOCE

1. **What are hemorrhoids?**
   Hemorrhoids are displaced anal cushions having a rich arterial supply with distended venous spaces that bleed during defecation.
2. **Why do hemorrhoids occur at 3, 7 and 11 o'clock positions?**
   They occur at these positions because these are the areas of three terminal branches of superior hemorrhoidal artery.
3. **What are the etiological types of hemorrhoids?**
   Etiologically hemorrhoids are of two types:
   - Primary hemorrhoids
   - Symptomatic or secondary hemorrhoids

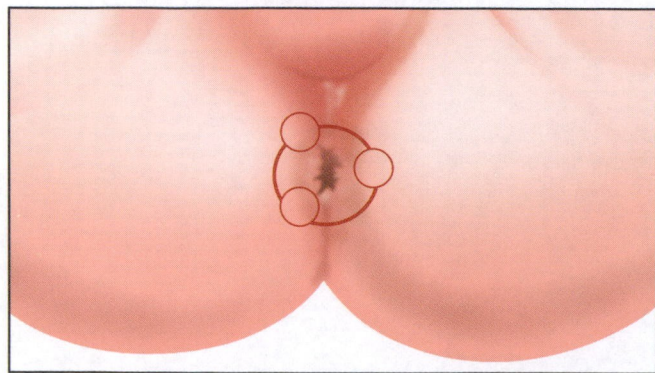

Fig. 1: Primary hemorrhoids at 3, 7 and 11 o'clock position

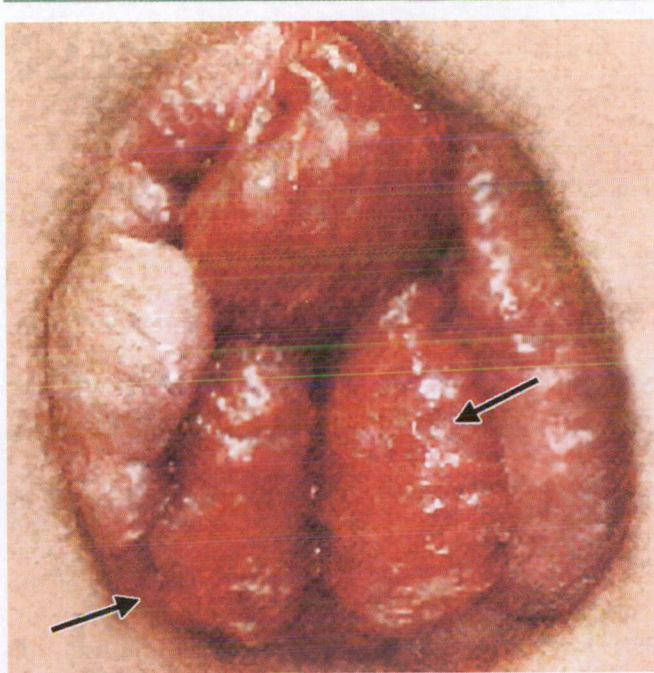

Fig. 3: Prolapsing hemorrhoids

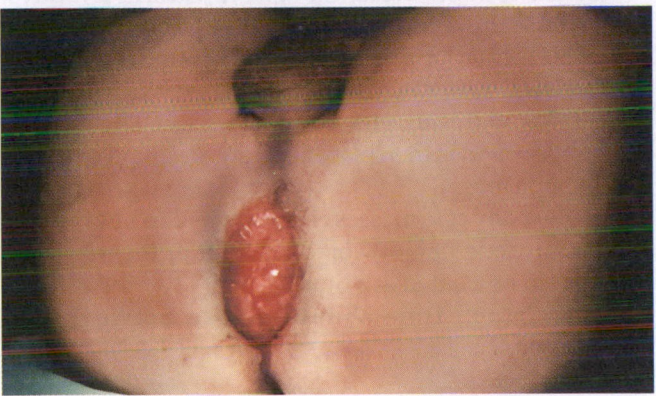

Fig. 4: Prolapsing hemorrhoids (circumanal collar). They are permanently prolapsed out (fourth degree hemorrhoids)

4. **What are the causes of primary hemorrhoids?**
   The exact cause is not known. The current view is as follows:
   - Caudal displacement of anal cushions and mucosal trauma due to shearing forces
   - Loss of elasticity of anal cushions that they do not retract following defecation due to fragmentation of supporting structures.

5. **What are anal cushions?**
   The anal cushions are vascular tissue masses underlying the mucosa of upper third of anal canal consisting of vascular spaces in a fibrous stroma. This tissue hypertrophies when the internal hemorrhoids develop.

6. **What do you mean by symptomatic hemorrhoids?**
   When the hemorrhoids are a symptom of some other disease they are called symptomatic hemorrhoids.

7. **What are the causes of symptomatic hemorrhoids?**
   The causes of symptomatic hemorrhoids are:
   - Anorectal carcinoma
   - Anorectal deformity, hypertonic anal sphincter
   - Persistently raised intraabdominal pressure, e.g. ascites
   - Pelvic problems, e.g. pregnancy, large uterine or ovarian tumors, cancer of urinary bladder
   - Neurological disorders, e.g. paraplegia, multiple sclerosis

8. **How does a carcinoma of rectum produce hemorrhoids?**
   The carcinoma of rectum produces hemorrhoids by compression or thrombosis of superior hemorrhoidal vein.

9. **What is the cause of hemorrhoids of pregnancy?**
   The hemorrhoids of pregnancy are due to compression of superior hemorrhoidal veins by pregnant uterus and the effect of progesterone on the smooth muscle in the wall of veins.

10. **What are the anatomical types of hemorrhoids?**
    The anatomical types of hemorrhoids are:
    - Internal hemorrhoids
    - External hemorrhoids
    - Interno-external hemorrhoids.

11. **What are internal hemorrhoids?**
    These are the dilated veins of the superior hemorrhoidal plexus above the mucocutaneous junction which are covered by mucosa. They represent the vascular cushions in the loose areolar submucosal tissues of the lower rectum.

12. **What are external hemorrhoids?**
    The external hemorrhoids occur below the dentate line beneath the anoderm and perianal skin.

13. **What are the complications of hemorrhoids?**
    The complications of hemorrhoids are:
    - Profuse hemorrhage, anemia
    - Strangulation
    - Thrombosis
    - Ulceration
    - Gangrene
    - Fibrosis, fibrous polyp
    - Suppuration, perianal or submucous abscess
    - Portal pyemia.

14. **What is an acute attack of piles?**
    When the complication of strangulation occurs, it is accompanied by considerable pain, hence complained as acute attack of piles.

15. How does a fibrous polyp form?

After thrombosis, an internal hemorrhoid gets fibrosed that is at first sessile, but by repeated traction during defecation it becomes pedunculated into a fibrous polyp.

16. How do you differentiate a fibrous polyp from an adenoma?

A fibrous polyp is white and firm while an adenoma is bright red and soft.

17. What is an arterial pile?

Entering the pedicle of each internal hemorrhoid is a terminal branch of superior rectal artery; sometimes this artery becomes hemangiomatous. Hence, this hemorrhoid is called as arterial pile.

18. How do you confirm the diagnosis?

The diagnosis is clinical and can be confirmed by anoproctoscopy.

19. How do you do anoproctoscopy?

A well lubricated anoproctoscope is passed into the anorectum and the obturator is removed. The instrument is then slowly withdrawn. Just below the anorectal ring the internal hemorrhoids, if present, bulge into the lumen of anoproctoscope.

20. How do you treat this disease?

The essentials of treatment are:
- No symptoms: No treatment. Avoid constipation and straining at defecation
- Small, nonprolapsing, symptomatic hemorrhoids: Bulking agents, injection sclerotherapy
- Prolapsing hemorrhoids arising above dentate line: Barron's band ligature
- Prolapsing piles straddling the dentate line, large to band or having a large symptomatic external component: Hemorrhoidectomy.

21. What do you do in injection treatment?

In this method, 5 percent phenol in almond oil or arachis oil is injected into the submucosal space above the main mass of each hemorrhoid. About 3 to 5 mL is injected into each hemorrhoid.

22. How does this treatment benefit in this disease?

The injection causes local inflammation and fibrosis thus obliterating the hemorrhoid.

23. How do you inject the hemorrhoids?

The injection is performed with a long hemorrhoidal needle (e.g., Gabriel) or a spinal needle through an injecting proctoscope (Fig. 5).

24. Does this procedure cause pain?

There is minimal pain if the injection is in the correct location.

25. How do you know that you are injecting in the correct plane?

If the tip of the needle is correctly placed a bleb appears having semitransparent mucosa containing visible blood vessels (striation sign) as the injection proceeds.

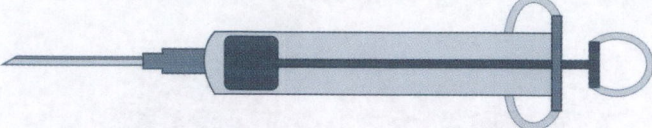

Fig. 5: Disposable type of Gabriel syringe for sclerotherapy of hemorrhoids

26. What are signs of injection into the mucosa?

If the injection is made into the mucosa more pressure is required on the plunger and a white featureless area appears on the mucosa.

27. What is done in cryosurgery?

The hemorrhoids are destroyed by freezing (-196^0C) with a cryo-probe using liquid CO_2 or N_2.

28. What are the disadvantages of this method?

The main disadvantage is uncontrolled sloughing of mucosa and associated foul smelling discharge from the anus for quite some time. The healing of the wound is delayed. Hence, this method is not popular.

29. How does the Barron's band ligation help in this disease?

The Barron's band ligation causes ischemic necrosis of hemorrhoids which slough off within a few days.

30. What is the technique of Barron's band ligation?

With the aid of proctoscope the redundant mucosa above the hemorrhoid is grasped with forceps advanced through the barrel of a special ligator, the rubber band is then placed snugly around the base of the pile mass.

31. How many pile masses can be treated in one sitting?

Ideally, one hemorrhoidal mass or at the most two should be treated at a time.

32. How much time should elapse between two ligations?

2 to 4 weeks.

33. What are the complications of this technique?

The complications are:
- Pain severe enough to require removal of band
- Infection
- Secondary hemorrhage.

34. What are the indications of hemorrhoidectomy?

The indications for hemorrhoidectomy are:
- Third and fourth degree hemorrhoids
- Interno-external piles
- Failure of nonoperative treatment in early hemorrhoids

35. What do you do in hemorrhoidectomy?

In this operation, the hemorrhoids are excised after defining and ligating their pedicles (Fig. 6).

36. What are the complications of hemorrhoidectomy?

The complications are:
- Acute retention of urine
- Hemorrhage
- Wound infection, submucous abscess

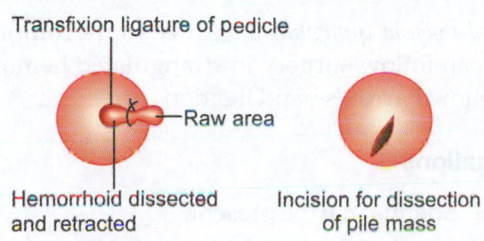

Transfixion ligature of pedicle

Raw area

Hemorrhoid dissected and retracted

Incision for dissection of pile mass

Other hemorrhoids are excised in the same manner

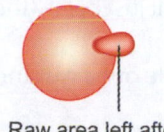 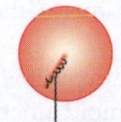

Raw area left after excision of pile mass at 3 o'clock position

Sutured wound after excision

Open method　　　　**Closed method**

Fig 6: Methods of hemorrhoidectomy

- Anal stenosis.
- Anal fissure
- Whitehead's anus.

37. **How do you treat strangulated hemorrhoids?**
   - The patient is put to bed rest and given analgesics and antibacterial drugs. Locally glycerine and tannic acid or lotio plumbi is applied. The piles gradually reduce over the ensuing few days. Subsequently an elective hemorrhoidectomy is done to cure the condition.
   - If the patient is not relieved an emergency hemorrhoidectomy may be required.

DISCUSSION

Hemorrhoids are symptomatic displaced anal cushions that are normal structures of the anal canal having a rich arterial supply leading directly into distensible venous spaces. Normally, anal cushions help in sealing the anal canal and contribute to continence. The hemorrhoids may be external, internal or internoexternal. The external hemorrhoids are external to the anal orifice and covered by skin. The internal hemorrhoids are internal to the orifice and covered by mucosa. The internoexternal hemorrhoids result from the progression of the internal hemorrhoids to involve the external hemorrhoidal plexus.

Etiology

Symptomatic hemorrhoids: These hemorrhoids are a symptom of some other disease, such as:
- Anorectal carcinoma because of compression or thrombosis of superior rectal vein

- Anorectal deformity, hypertonic anal sphincter
- *Ascitis:* Due to persistently raised intra-abdominal pressure
- Pelvic problems, e.g. pregnancy, uterine tumors, ovarian tumors, carcinoma of urinary bladder
- Neurological disorders, e.g. paraplegia, multiple sclerosis.

Primary Hemorrhoids

The exact cause is not known. Hence, many possible etiological factors were considered and discarded, such as portal hypertension, infection, diet and stool consistency, anal hypertonia and ageing. The current view is:
- Caudal displacement of anal cushions and mucosal trauma due to shearing forces.
- Loss of elasticity of the cushions that they do not retract following defecation due to fragmentation of supporting structures.

Pathology

The primary hemorrhoidal masses are situated at 3, 7 and 11 o'clock positions (Fig. 1) in accordance with the terminal divisions of superior rectal artery as there are two subdivisions on right side while the left branch remains single. There may be secondary hemorrhoids in between the primary hemorrhoids.

The pedicle of primary hemorrhoid is situated above the anorectal ring, covered by pale pink mucosa through which large tributaries of superior rectal vein are visible. Sometimes, a pulsating artery may be palpable here. Below the pedicle there is main pile mass covered by bright red or purple mucosa.

Clinical Features

1. *Bleeding:* Painless bleeding per rectum is the main and earliest symptom. Usually it is bright red and occurs during defecation. The blood drips or splashes in the pan. It may continue for months or years and may cause anemia.
2. *Prolapse:* As the disease advances the pile masses tend to prolapse out. Initially, the protrusion is small and occurs only during defecation and reduces spontaneously. As the disease advances they may not reduce by themselves and have to be reduced by a finger.
3. *Discharge:* The prolapsed hemorrhoids may be responsible for a mucoid discharge. The patient may have pruritus ani due to this discharge.

Anorectal Examination

In early cases anus is normal. In an advanced case redundant folds or tags of skin may be present at the sites of primary hemorrhoids. On making the patient strain down, the hemorrhoids may be visible transiently or may come out and remain prolapsed.

The digital palpation of anorectum is useless as they are not palpable till they are thrombosed.

Degree of Hemorrhoids

First degree: Bleeding without prolapse
Second degree: Prolapsing hemorrhoids reducing spontaneously
Third degree: Prolapsing hemorrhoids requiring manual reduction
Fourth degree: Permanently prolapsed hemorrhoids (Fig. 4).

Complications

If the hemorrhoids are not treated they may have the following complications:

1. *Hemorrhage:* It is a symptom of this disease but sometimes the bleeding is profuse. It is usually external, but it may be internal if the bleeding pile mass has gone in.
2. *Strangulation:* A prolapsed hemorrhoid may be gripped by external sphincter and may be strangulated. This complication commonly occurs in second degree hemorrhoids. Because of severe pain, the patients often call it "acute attack of piles."
3. *Thrombosis:* If the strangulated hemorrhoids are not reduced within 1 to 2 hours they get thrombosed. They become dark purple or black and feel solid. The anal margin is swollen due to edema. The pain disappears but the tenderness persists.
4. *Ulceration:* Strangulation and thrombosis are followed by ulceration of exposed mucous membrane.
5. *Gangrene:* If the grip of external sphincter is tight that arterial supply is also cut off, the pile mass becomes gangrenous resulting in localized superficial ulceration. The whole hemorrhoid may become gangrenous and slough out leaving an ulcer that heals gradually (auto-hemorrhoidectomy). Very rarely gangrene may extend into anorectum.
6. *Fibrosis:* Following thrombosis, a hemorrhoid may be fibrosed that is initially sessile, but repeated traction at defecation may make it pedunculated (fibrous polyp).
7. *Suppuration:* It is an uncommon complication. A thrombosed pile may be infected resulting in a perianal or submucous abscess.
8. *Portal pyemia (pylephlebitis):* It is a rare complication and can follow surgery in strangulated hemorrhoid, or follow Barron's band ligation.

Investigations

1. *Blood:* Anemia may be present.
2. *Anoproctoscopy:* An anoproctoscope is passed to its full extent and the obturator is removed. It is then slowly withdrawn. The bluish-pink pile masses will bulge into the lumen of the instrument just below the anorectal ring.
3. *Sigmoidoscopy:* It is done to rule out a carcinoma at the rectosigmoid junction.

Treatment

General measures: Early hemorrhoids are treated by addition of dietary fibre, stool softeners and avoidance of straining or prolonged sitting for stool. Early hemorrhoids may respond to this treatment and the bleeding stops.

Surgical treatment: Surgery is rarely needed for first degree disease. It is indicated when the medical measures fail in second degree, and all the cases of third degree.

1. *Band ligation:* In this method the pile masses are ligated 1 to 2 cm above the dentate line with rubber bands. It is indicated in second and third degree hemorrhoids. It is good for bulky piles. It is very effective for control of bleeding and prolapse. The pile mass is grapsed, pulled into the cylinder of a rubber band applier (Barron) and the rubber band is slipped at the base of the pile mass. The hemorrhoidal tissue sloughs out leaving a scar at the site of the pedicle. The rubber band should not be placed on the transitional zone or anoderm, and deep internal sphincter, otherwise the patient may have retention of urine.

In office practice one quadrant is ligated every 2 weeks. If symptoms are severe or there are significant external hemorrhoids three quadrants may be banded in the operating room under local anesthesia. The rubber bands usually fall off with the necrotic pile after 7 to 10 days. The complications of this procedure are retention of urine, severe sepsis and bleeding. The incidence of urinary retention after single ligation is less than 1 percent, and after multiple ligation 10 to 20 percent. Severe sepsis occurs in immune compromised patients and those with pelvic floor abnormalities where full thickness of distal prolapsing rectum has been ligated. This is a dangerous complication and requires intravenous antibiotic coverage for gram negative and anerobic bacteria, removal of rubber bands and hospitalization.

Bleeding may occur but it is usually minimal. Sometimes, it is significant requiring cautery or suture ligation of the bleeder. Nonsteroidal anti-inflammatory drugs or aspirin taken during 7 to 10 days after banding may increase the chances of hemorrhage when the band falls off.

2. *Injection sclerotherapy:* A mixture of 5 percent phenol in arachis or almond oil is injected submucosally to raise a bleb of mucosa at the base of each hemorrhoid with a spinal needle. It stops bleeding from first and second degree hemorrhoids, and obliterates the hemorrhoids by fibrosis. Further it hitches up the anorectal mucosa. About 5 mL of sclerosant is injected into the apex of the pile mass using a disposable (Gabriel) syringe. It is a painless procedure. The pain indicates that the needle is in the wrong place. The complications of a deep injection are pelvic sepsis, prostatitis, impotence and rectovaginal fistula. Too superficial injection is also avoided as it results in blebing of the mucosa followed by ulceration. The patient is examined after 8 weeks, if necessary repeat injections are given.

3. *Cryotherapy* (Lloyd Williams) and *infrared photocoagulation* (Leicester) are no more popular.

4. *Hemorrhoidectomy:* It is ideally done for large third and fourth degree hemorrhoids that cannot be treated on outpatient basis. Other indications are:
   - Internoexternal hemorrhoids where the external component is well defined
   - Second degree hemorrhoids not controlled by conservative methods
   - Acutely thrombosed incarcerated hemorrhoids with severe pain and impending gangrene
   - Patients on anticoagulant drugs.

Hemorrhoidectomy should not be done in elderly women with weak sphincters as it may result in frank incontinence. There are many methods of excising hemorrhoids. All of them can be done in lithotomy or prone, flexed position.

a. **Open method (Milligan Morgan):** Each hemorrhoid is caught by two artery forceps one at the lower angle and another at the apex and held by an assistant as to form a triangle. A V-shaped cut is made in the skin and the pile mass is dissected to expose the lower border of internal sphincter. Cuts are made on either side of the pile converging towards the apex and the pile mass is separated up to its pedicle that is ligated by a transfixation ligature of strong vicryl and the pile mass is removed. In this manner all the pile masses are excised. After hemostasis the wound is dressed with petroleum jelly gauze (Fig. 6).

b. **Closed method:** The pile mass is excised by an enclosing incision. After hemostasis, the wound is closed by a continous suture with the same suture that was used to ligate the pedicle (Fig. 6).

c. **Circumferential excision ("circumcision" of anus):** Sometimes there is a circumferential prolapse of primary and secondary hemorrhoids. This is best treated by circumferential excision of prolapsing piles. The results are good. The procedure can be done by a stapling gun (PPH, Ethicon). It is quick to perform and said to be less painful. The long-term results are not known.

The complications of these operations are retention of urine, bleeding, infection, fecal impaction and sphincteric damage. Urinary retention is the commonest complication. Many of these complications are preventable by proper use of analgesia in the immediate postoperative period. Bleeding is managed by cautery or suture ligation of the bleeding point. Anal stenosis is a delayed complication following circumferential excision of anoderm. It may respond to anal dilatation otherwise anoplasty is required.

Whitehead deformity: In this complication, there is eversion of rectal mucosa to form ectropion and stenosis of anal canal following excision of dentate line and anoderm. It requires an island advancement flap procedure which inserts normal skin into the anal canal to relieve the ectropion and stenosis.

Prevention

1. *Occurrence:* Majority of hemorrhoids are related to poor bowel habits. The patient should take fibre-rich diet and avoid straining at stool and sitting at the toilet for long periods of time.

2. *Recurrence:* Following successful treatment the hemorrhoids can recur if the same factors that caused the initial hemorrhoids are continued.

External Hemorrhoids

There are many conditions that are included under this term: perianal hematoma, interno-external hemorrhoids, dilatation of veins of anal verge, a sentinel pile of chronic anal fissure and genital warts (condylomata).

Perianal Hematoma
(Thrombosed External Hemorrhoids)

There is a small blood clot in peranal subcutaneous tissue usually superficial to corrugator cutis ani muscle caused by back pressure in an anal venule following straining at stool, coughing, or lifting a heavy weight. The patient presents with acute anal pain of sudden onset associated with a tense, tender swelling resembling a semiripe black currant. It is usually situated at the anal verge on the sides.

If not treated it may burst with extrusion of clot, resolve, suppurate, fibrose or end in a cutaneous tag. In majority of patients resolution or fibrosis occurs, hence called 'a 5-day painful, self-curing lesion.'

Treatment: Under local anesthesia the hemorrhoid is bisected and the two halves are removed together with 1.25 cm of skin in the vicinity. The wound is left/open to heal by granulations. If the hematoma is situated anteriorly or posteriorly it should be treated conservatively as the wound of operation is likely to result in a fissure.

Dilatation of Veins at Anal Verge

It occurs in persons leading a sedentary life. When the patient strains a bluish cushion-like ring appears at the anal verge. The patient is asked to modify the style of living.

CASE 2: BLEEDING FROM THE NIPPLE: DUCT PAPILLOMA

CLINICAL DIAGNOSIS

- The patient is usually a middle-aged female who presents with blood-stained discharge from the nipple (Fig. 7).
- The discharge is unilateral and comes from a single duct. It is a painless discharge
- The patient may come with the complaint of blood-staining of the undergarments
- On milking of a segment of the breast the discharge may appear from the mouth of the duct draining that segment
- Otherwise the breast is normal with axilla free. There is no lump.

VIVA VOCE

1. **What are the causes of discharge from the nipple?**
   The common causes of discharge from the nipple are:
   - Mammary duct ectasia
   - Fibrocystic disease
   - Duct papilloma
   - Galactorrhea.

2. **What is duct papilloma?**
   It is a benign tumor of lactiferous duct epithelium of unknown etiology characterized by painless serous or blood-stained discharge from the nipple.

3. **How do you differentiate it from duct carcinoma?**
   Clinically, it is not possible to differentiate. In a woman over 50 years of age, duct carcinoma is more likely. It may be possible to differentiate by cytology of discharge. Excision biopsy is the final court of appeal.

4. **What are the investigations?**
   The possible investigations are:
   - Cytology of the discharge or ductal washings
   - Mammography
   - Ductoscopy and ductography.

5. **What is the aim of cytology?**
   It is done to see for the presence of cancer cells, as a duct papilloma closely mimics a duct carcinoma.

6. **What are the results of cytology?**
   In duct papilloma it is negative for cancer cells, but a negative cytology does not rule out duct carcinoma. A positive cytology is indicative of carcinoma.

7. **What is the role of mammography?**
   It is done to detect impalpable mass lesions.

8. **What are the usual findings?**
   Usually there are no findings.

9. **What is the role of ductoscopy and ductography?**
   They are the newer methods of investigation but the results have been disappointing.

10. **Can we do endoscopic biopsy?**
    The problems in doing endoscopic biopsy are:
    - The affected duct may not be visualized by the microendoscope
    - The technology has not that developed so far.

11. **How do you treat a duct papilloma?**
    It is treated by microdochectomy which is the excision of the duct containing papilloma.

12. **What is the technique of microdochectomy?**
    Sometime before operation the duct is not pressed as an empty duct may be difficult to identify. Under general anesthesia a fine lacrimal duct probe or a stiff nylon suture is passed in the bleeding duct and a racquet incision enclosing the duct or periareolar incision is made. The duct is dissected out in its whole length by a very fine dissection. The distended duct is excised and the wound is closed.

13. **How do you treat a duct carcinoma?**
    It is treated like a T1 carcinoma of breast.

14. **Can Paget's disease of breast present with nipple discharge?**
    In Paget's disease of breast the discharge is from the nipple and, or the areola, and not from the lactiferous ductal orifice. In duct papilloma the nipple and areola are otherwise normal, but in Paget's disease there are eczematous changes in these structures.

DISCUSSION

The duct papilloma is a benign tumor of unknown etiology of duct epithelium of the breast. It is an uncommon lesion but a common cause of blood-stained discharge from the nipple (Fig. 7).

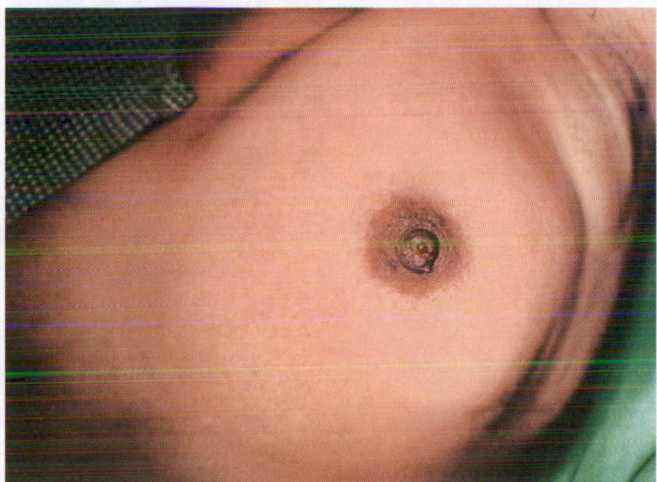

Fig. 7: Bleeding from left nipple due to a duct papilloma that was excised

Clinical Features

There is serous or blood-stained discharge from one of the openings of lactiferous ducts of the nipple. It may stain the undergarment of the breast. The bleeding is painless and occurs spontaneously from one of the ducts of the nipple. The discharge may appear on milking a segment of the breast from the mouth of the duct draining that segment. Usually there is no palpable lump.

Pathology

The duct papilloma is usually solitary and is situated in one of the larger lactiferous ducts. It may be associated with a cystic swelling under the aerola within 4 to 5 cm of its orifice on the nipple.

Investigations

*   Cytology of the discharge or the ductal washings is done for the presence of cancer cells, as it closely mimics a duct carcinoma. A negative cytology does not rule out malignancy which is more likely in women over 50 years of age.
*   Mammography is usually normal.
*   Ductography and ductoscopy may be tried, but so far the results have been equivocal.

Treatment

The excision of the involved duct system (microdochectomy) is the treatment. Sometime before the operation, the duct must not be squeezed or pressed as an empty duct may be difficult to identify. A fine lacrimal duct probe or a stiff nylon suture is passed into the affected duct to make it palpable during dissection. A racquet incision enclosing the duct or a periareolar incision is made and the duct is dissected out with a very fine dissection. The lesion is excised and the wound closed. The results of this surgery are very good.

CASE 3: JUVENILE RECTAL POLYP

CLINICAL DIAGNOSIS

1. The patient is a child between one to six years of age who presents with passage of bright red blood or blood-stained mucus per rectum.
2. The polyp may prolapse out during defecation causing pain and tenesmus.
3. On rectal examination, there is a small pedunculated swelling in the rectum that can be hooked out by a finger (Figs 8 and 9).
4. It is spherical, slightly lobulated and soft or firm in consistency.

VIVA VOCE

1. **What do you mean by a polyp?**
   Polyp is a mass of tissue projecting into the lumen of a hollow cavity or organ. It comprises a heterogeneous group of sessile or pedunculated, benign or malignant, mucosal, submucosal or muscular lesions. Polyp is a morphologic term and no histologic diagnosis is implied.

2. **What are the types of colorectal polyps?**
   They are enlisted below:
   - Neoplastic
     i. Adenoma
        1. Tubular adenoma (adenomatous polyp)
        2. Tubulovillous adenoma (villoglandular adenoma).
        3. Villous adenoma (villous papilloma).
     ii. Carcinoma.
     iii. Miscellaneous: Lipoma, leiomyoma, carcinoid.
   - Hamartomas
     i. Juvenile polyp.
     ii. Peutz-Jeghers polyp.
   - Inflammatory polyps or pseudopolyps
   - Metaplastic or hyperplastic polyps.

3. **What is the incidence of colorectal polyps?**
   In general population the incidence ranges from 9 to 60 percent. They are detected on barium enema in about 5 percent of patients.

4. **What is the site of occurrence?**
   They can occur anywhere in the rectum or colon. About 50 percent of polyps occur in sigmoid or rectum.

5. **How often are they multiple?**
   About 50 percent of patients with adenomas have more than one lesion, and 15 percent have more than two lesions.

6. **What is the potential of malignancy in a colorectal polyp?**
   - Adenoma is a premalignant lesion.
   - Cancer developing in association with hamartomas is rare.
   - Inflammatory polyps have no malignant potential.
   - Hyperplastic polyps do not become malignant.

7. **What are the factors on which the malignant potential of an adenoma depends?**
   The malignant potential of an adenoma depends upon:
   - Size
   - Growth pattern
   - Degree of epithelial atypia
   - Presence of a stalk.

8. **How does the size determine the malignant potential?**
   Cancer is found in 1 percent of adenomas under 1 cm in diameter, 10 percent of adenomas 1 to 2 cm in size, and 45 percent of adenomas larger than 2 cm.

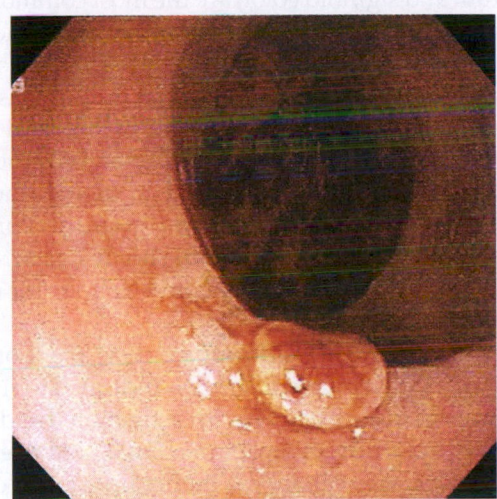

Fig. 8: Rectal polyp (*Courtesy:* Dr. Ajay Chaudhary)

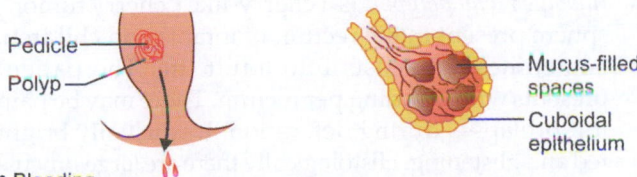

Pedicle
Polyp
Mucus-filled spaces
Cuboidal epithelium

- Bleeding
- Polyp coming out during defecation

Micropathology

Fig. 9: Juvenile rectal polyp

9. **How does the growth pattern modify the malignant potential?**
   About 5 percent of tubular, 22 percent of tubulovillous and 40 percent of villous adenomas become malignant.

10. **How does the epithelial atypia affect the malignant potential?**
    The potential for cancerous transformation goes on rising with increasing degrees of epithelial dysplasia.

11. **How does the presence of stalk affect malignant potential?**
    The sessile lesions are more often to be malignant than the pedunculated ones.

12. **How much time an adenoma takes to become malignant?**
    It probably takes at least 5 or more often 10 to 15 years for an adenoma to become malignant.

13. **What is the evidence that an adenoma is a premalignant lesion?**
    The evidence for the malignant potential of an adenoma is as follows:
    - Adenomas and cancers increase in incidence with each decade after 30 years of age.
    - Distribution of adenomas and carcinomas is similar.
    - About one third resected specimens of carcinoma also harbor adenomas.
    - All gradations of malignancy with remnants of adenoma may be seen in resected specimens.
    - The patients with familial adenomatous polyposis die of cancer at a young age unless the bowel is resected.
    - Chemical carcinogens produce adenomas and carcinomas indiscriminately in the colon of experimental animals.
    - Routine removal of rectal adenomas reduces the incidence of subsequent rectal carcinoma.

14. **How do you differentiate a juvenile rectal polyp from a polyp of familial colonic polyposis?**
    The differences are given in the following table:

Features	Juvenile polyp	Familial polyposis
Age	Infants and children	Puberty
Number	Single	Multiple
Pedicle	Present	Absent
Malignant potential	None	Present

15. **What are the complications of a rectal polyp?**
    The complications are:
    - Torsion
    - Intussusception.

16. **Do you know any other name of juvenile rectal polyp?**
    Cherry tumor.

17. **Does the juvenile rectal polyp ever become malignant?**
    No.

18. **What is the histologic appearance of a juvenile rectal polyp?**
    There is unique histological structure of large mucus-filled spaces covered by smooth surface of thin rectal cuboidal epithelium (Fig. 9).

19. **How do you treat a juvenile rectal polyp?**
    It is treated by transanal excision that can be done easily with forceps or a snare.

20. **What are the complications of excision?**
    The complications are:
    - Hemorrhage
    - Rectal injury.

21. **What is juvenile polyposis?**
    It is a rare autosomal dominantly inherited syndrome that has an increased risk of malignancy. It has a positive family history.

DISCUSSION

The rectum and sigmoid colon are the most common sites of polyps and carcinoma in the gastrointestinal tract. The neoplastic polyps of these structures may become malignant. This tendency is more: (i) if the polyp is more than 1 cm in diameter, (ii) increasing in size, and (iii) is sessile. Because of these reasons all polyps should be excised completely and subjected to histopathologic examination. It will detect carcinoma in situ and prevent local recurrence. Hence these lesions should not be treated by electrofulguration, which can only be done for a very small polyp.

Endoscopy: Initially sigmoidoscopy is done. If one or more polyps are detected, a colonoscopy is indicated to rule out further polyps higher up. This investigation decides the treatment because no tumor of the rectum should be excised till the existence of a carcinoma higher up is ruled out, as there is a risk of local implantation of cancer cells in the rectal wound.

As in colon, polyps can occur in the rectum. They are of many types:

1. *Juvenile rectal polyp:* It is a cherry-like ('cherry tumor') sphere present in the rectum of infants and children. Sometimes it persists into adult life. The patient presents with bleeding per rectum. There may be pain if it prolapses during defecation. It is usually bright red and glistening. Histologically there are large mucus-filled spaces covered by a smooth surface of thin rectal cuboidal epithelium (Figs 8 and 9). It is excised with forceps or a snare. It does not recur and does not become malignant.

2. *Hyperplastic polyps:* The patient has multiple, small, pinkish and sessile polyps of 2 to 4 mm diameter. These lesions are harmless.

3. *Pseudopolyps:* These polyps are edematous mucosa present in patients of ulcerative proctocolitis and other inflammatory bowel diseases. They can be recognized by signs of inflammation during endoscopy but may cause diagnostic difficulty during radiography.

4. *Villous adenoma:* It is a tumor having a characteristic frond-like appearance. It is often very large and may fill the whole rectum. These patients may have profuse mucus discharge per rectum resulting in fluid and potassium deficiency.

   This tumor can convert into cancer; this is more likely to occur when it is very large. It tends to become hard in consistency. Diagnosis can be made by biopsy. If it is not malignant, it is excised by submucosal resection endoscopically, surgically per anum or by sleeve resection transabdominally. Rarely rectal excision may be indicated. Transanal endoscopic microsurgery (TEM, Buess): Through a large operating sigmoidoscope the rectum is inflated by CO_2, the operating area is magnified by a camera inserted inside, and the images are seen on a monitor. Then the lesion is removed. It is a highly specialized technique. If malignant change has occurred, it is treated like carcinoma of rectum.

5. *Familial adenomatous polyposis (familial polyposis coli):* The patient is of puberty age and presents with bleeding per rectum. The diagnosis can be confirmed by colonoscopy that shows multiple adenomatous polyps in the rectum and colon.

   It is an autosomal dominantly inherited disease, where the adenomatous polyposis coli (APC) gene has been found on chromosome 5 (Bodmer). As this disease is precancerous, resection of the affected part has to be done. In colonic disease, colectomy is done; preserving the rectum, but regular endoscopic follow-up is required.

   If rectum is involved a restorative proctocolectomy is required where the rectum is replaced by a 'pouch' of folded ileum. A pan-proctocolectomy with permanent ileostomy is an alternative procedure.

Miscellaneous Cases

CASE 1: CARBUNCLE

CLINICAL DIAGNOSIS

1. The patient is usually a middle-aged person commonly a diabetic who presents with a varying combination of fever, toxemia and a pus discharging swelling.
2. The swelling can be present anywhere in the skin except palm and sole, but is commonly present on the nape of neck, dorsum of hand or fingers, trunk and gluteal region.
3. It discharges pus from multiple openings from the surface giving a sieve-like appearance (Figs 1 and 2).
4. It may be bluish-red in color or may appear red like fire.
5. It is tender and has diffuse induration.

VIVA VOCE

1. **What is a carbuncle?**
   It is a type of infective gangrene or extensive infection of skin and subcutaneous tissue starting from hair follicles caused by *Staphylococcus aureus*.

   It consists of several furuncles developing in adjoining hair follicles and coalescing to form a

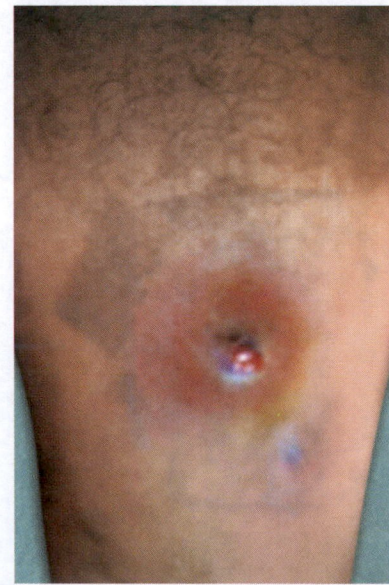

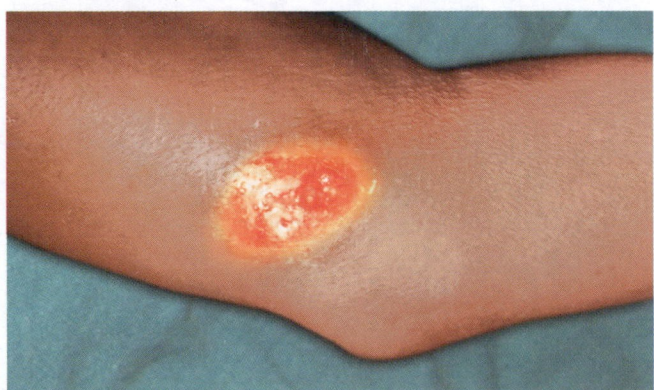

Fig. 1: Carbuncle of upper arm—many openings are seen

Fig. 2: Non-diabetic carbuncle of back of thigh in a young man. Three openings are visible

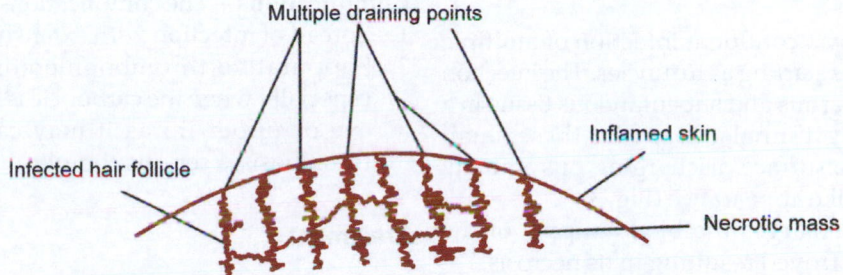

Fig. 3: Pathology of a carbuncle

conglomerate, deeply located mass with multiple discharging points (Fig. 3).

2. **How does this infection occur?**
   The infection occurs by local spread. In a carbuncle of nape of neck a stiff dirty collar may have some role. The carbuncles of dorsum of hand or fingers usually occur following wiping of nose with the dorsum of hand or fingers.

3. **Do you know of any predisposing factor?**
   Yes, carbuncles usually occur in diabetics. Other predisposing factors are malnutrition, cardiac failure, prolonged corticosteroid therapy, HIV disease, injection drug use and generalized dermatoses.

4. **Can a carbuncle occur in a non-diabetic?**
   Yes, but only occasionally.

5. **What is the pathology of this lesion?**
   It starts as a furuncle and then the infection dissects through the dermis and subcutaneous tissue in a myriad of connecting tunnels open on the surface with many pustular openings giving a sieve-like appearance (Fig. 3).
   Usually, there is one large central slough surrounded by a rosette of smaller areas of necrosis.

6. **Why does this lesion occur on the nape of neck commonly?**
   It may be due to repeated rubbing of the local skin with a dirty stiff collar.

7. **What is the mechanism of infection in a carbuncle of hand or fingers?**
   The infection occurs by wiping the nose with the dorsum of hand or fingers.

8. **What are the complications?**
   The complications are:
   - Local extension of infection
   - Extensive tissue necrosis
   - Thrombophlebitis, especially in a carbuncle of upper lip and adjoining areas (cavernous sinus thrombophlebitis)

9. **How do you treat a carbuncle?**
   The essentials of the treatment are:
   - Antibiotic therapy depending on culture and sensitivity—usually sodium dicloxacillin or cephalexin 1 g daily in divided doses orally for 10 days.
   - Control of diabetes mellitus
   - Excision of slough especially if extensive or invasive.
   Many carbuncles are aborted if antibiotics are given adequately in early stage of disease. Local treatment by osmotic pastes is often supplemented by infra-red, or short wave diathermy.

10. **If the culture report reveals infection by methicillin resistant *Staphylococcus aureus* (MRSA) what will you do?**
    The patient should be given doxycycline 100 mg twice daily, trimethoprim-sulfamethoxazole 320/1600 twice daily, and clindamycin 150-300 mg twice daily.

11. **How do you control diabetes?**
    The diabetes is controlled by diet control and insulin.

12. **Why don't you drain a carbuncle like an abscess?**
    Incision alone is inadequate as there is a lot of slough which does not drain following incision only.

13. **What is the technique of excision?**
    Excision includes all the sinus tracts and necrotic tissue. Usually it goes far beyond the cutaneous evidence of suppuration. It may leave behind a large open wound to granulate.

14. **Why don't you skin graft the raw area?**
    It is not required as the wound contracts and heals to a small scar. The carbuncles tend to occur in loose skin on the back of neck and on the buttocks where contraction is the predominant form of healing.

DISCUSSION

Carbuncle is a type of infective gangrene of the subcutaneous tissue commonly caused by *Staphylococcus aureus*.

Pathology

The lesion is formed by a confluent infection of multiple contiguous hair follicles starting as furuncles. The infection dissects through the dermis and subcutaneous tissue in a myriad of connecting tunnels. Many of these small extensions open to the surface discharging pus at many points giving a sieve-like appearance (Fig. 3).

As the carbuncle enlarges the blood supply of the overlying skin it is destroyed resulting in its necrosis.

Clinical Features

The patient is usually a middle-aged diabetic who presents with a painful swelling which discharges pus from more than one opening giving a sieve-like appearance to the swelling (Figs 1 and 2). It is commonly present on the nape of neck, dorsum of hand or fingers and buttocks. The patient may be febrile and toxic.

Complications—The complications include:
1. Spread of infection with extensive tissue necrosis.
2. Suppurative thrombophlebitis when near a vein especially when the carbuncle is located near the nose, eye or upper lip as it may cause central venous thrombosis, a serious complication.

Treatment

Carbuncle is often more extensive than the external appearance indicates. Incision alone is almost always inadequate and excision with electrocautery is required. Excision is continued until all the sinus tracts are removed. It is usually far beyond the cutaneous evidence of suppuration. It is sometimes necessary to produce a large open wound. This may appear to be drastic but it works.

CASE 2: TUBERCULOUS CERVICAL LYMPHADENITIS

CLINICAL DIAGNOSIS

1. The patient is usually a child or young adult who presents with cervical lymph node enlargement of insidious onset.
2. One or many nodes are enlarged.
3. They are mild to moderate in size, firm, nontender and matted.
4. The patient may present with a cold abscess, collar-stud abscess, sinus or ulcer in the neck (Figs 4 and 5).
5. The patient may have general symptoms of tuberculosis i.e. low-grade fever, loss of weight, appetite and night sweats.

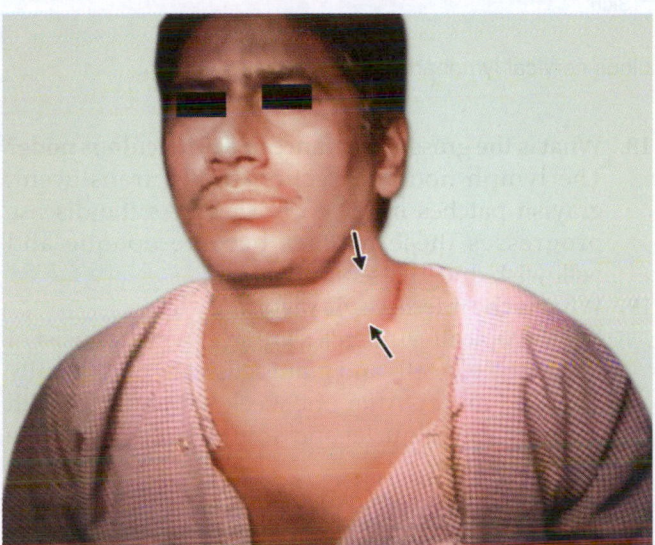

Fig. 4: Tuberculous cervical lymphadenitis of left lower neck with cold abscess formation

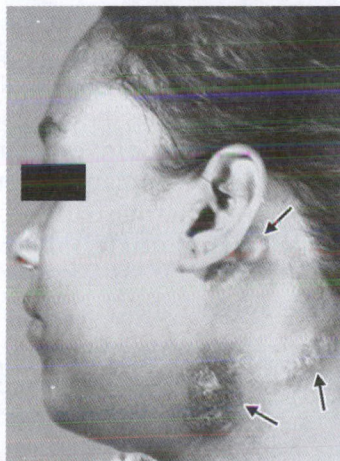

Fig. 5: Tuberculous lymph nodes of neck with skin involvement (scrofuloderma)

VIVA VOCE

1. **Do you know the total number of lymph nodes in the body?**
   Yes, there are about 800 lymph nodes in the body.
2. **How many lymph nodes are present in the neck?**
   About 300 lymph nodes are present in the neck.
3. **Which group of cervical nodes is usually involved in tuberculosis?**
   Upper jugular group
4. **What is King's evil?**
   Tuberculous cervical lymphadenitis with sinuses was known as King's evil, as for 600 years King's touch was believed to cure this disease (Fig. 5).
5. **What are the stages of this disease?**
   The stages of this disease are:
   1. Tuberculous adenitis
   2. Periadenitis
   3. Cold abscess
   4. Collar-stud abscess
   5. Sinus or ulcer.
6. **What are the clinical signs of tuberculous adenitis?**
   - The lymph node/nodes are enlarged, mild, nontender, firm but elastic and not matted.
   - In this stage the tuberculous disease cannot be differentiated from chronic nonspecific lymphadenitis.
7. **What are the signs of periadenitis?**
   The lymph nodes are enlarged, firm and matted. Matting is a specific feature of tuberculous infection (Fig. 6).
8. **What is the cause of matting?**
   It is because the infection enters by lymphatics into the subcapsular space resulting in the involvement of periphery of the lymph node (periadenitis).
9. **Why matting does not occur in tuberculous adenitis?**
   In this type which is relatively rare the infection enters by blood stream into the centre of lymph node resulting in adenitis.
10. **What are the signs of a tuberculous sinus?**
    The signs of a tuberculous sinus are –
    1. There is a single or multiple sinuses in the neck, axilla or groin, of insidious onset.
    2. The edge is pigmented and undermined.
    3. It discharges thin syrup-like pus which may have curdy flakes.
11. **Which mycobacterium tuberculosis is responsible for this infection?**
    In 70% of cases it is caused by human type, and in 30% bovine bacillus is responsible.

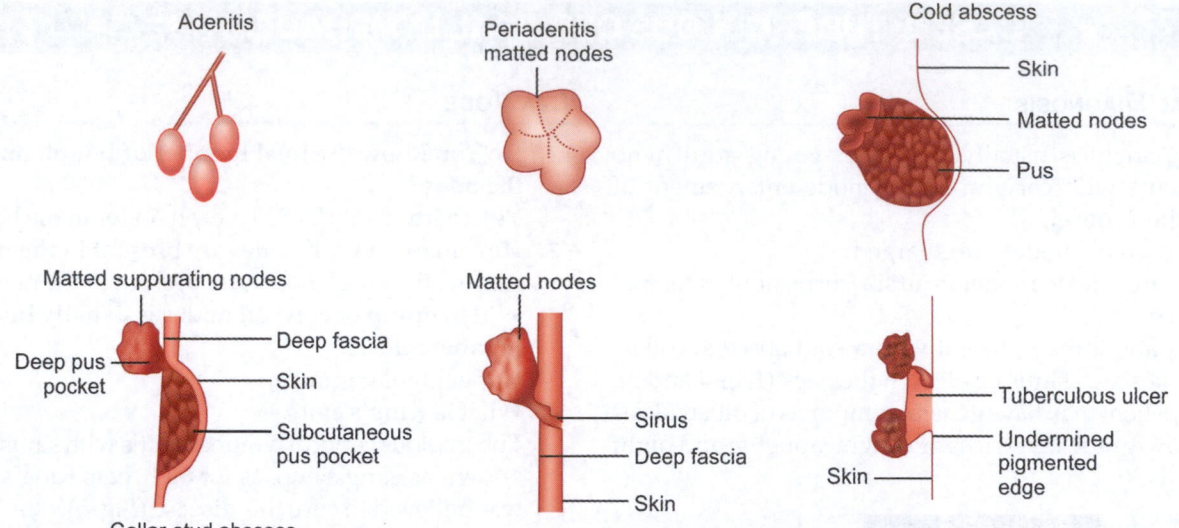

Fig. 6: Stages or types of tuberculous cervical lymphadenitis

12. **What is the source of infection?**

The common sources of infection are:
- Pharynx, including tonsils and adenoids
- Apex of lung

13. **How does the infection reach cervical nodes?**
- The infection is carried to lymph nodes by the lymphatics.
- It can rarely come by hematogenous route from a distant focus of infection.

14. **How does a cold abscess develop?**

The infected lymph node undergoes caseous necrosis, which liquefies and breaks through the capsule to cause a cold abscess.

15. **What is collar-stud abscess?**

This abscess has two compartments of pus joined together by a narrow track (Fig. 6).

16. **How do you diagnose a collar-stud abscess clinically?**

There are two fluctuant swellings in the neck in close proximity, one smaller, deeper at a higher level, and another larger, superficial and a little lower down. The compression of the upper swelling may make the lower swelling more prominent.

17. **What is the mechanism of formation of a collar-stud abscess?**

After the formation of a cold abscess the pus is initially confined by the deep cervical fascia. In a few weeks the deep fascia is eroded at one point and the pus flows through the small opening into the more commodious space in the superficial fascia. Thus, there are two pus containing cavities joined together by a narrow track in the neck.

18. **What is the gross appearance of a tuberculous node?**

The lymph node on section shows translucent, grayish patches in the early stage. As the disease progresses these patches become opaque and yellowish due to caseous necrosis.

19. **What is the microscopic picture?**

Microscopically, tubercles are seen which consist of the epitheloid cells and giant cells with peripherally arranged nuclei. After one week lymphocytes with darkly staining nuclei and scanty cytoplasm make their appearance.

By the end of second week caseation appears in the centre of the tubercle surrounded by giant cells and epitheloid cells around which remains a zone of chronic inflammatory cells (lymphocytes and plasma cells), surrounded by fibroblasts (Fig. 7).

20. **What is the role of tuberculin skin test?**

Tuberculin skin test has a limited diagnostic value, as a positive result is not necessarily diagnostic nor does a negative one excludes the presence of disease.

21. **What is the most diagnostic investigation?**

Recovery of the causative organism from the lesions or discharge, if any, is the most diagnostic.

22. **How will you differentiate tuberculous from metastatic nodes?**

The differences are given below:

Features	Tuberculous nodes	Metastatic nodes
Age	Young	Usually elderly
Consistency	Firm but elastic	Hard
Matting	Usually present	Usually absent
Cold abscess	Usually forms	Does not occur
Primary	Not present	Present

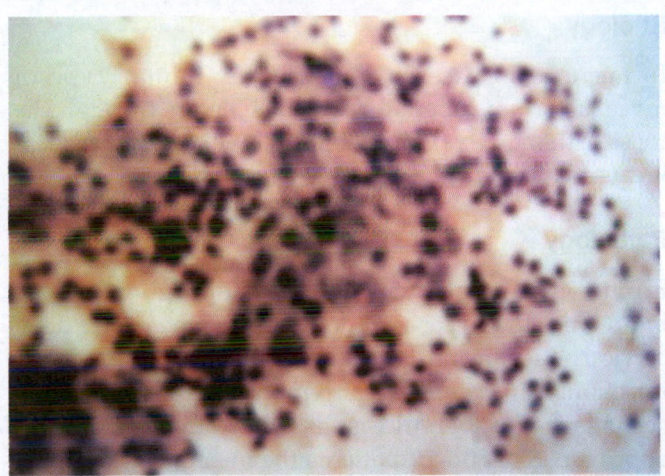

Fig. 7: Tuberculous lymphadenitis. FNAC smear shows collection of epitheloid cells, lymphocytes and Langhan's type of giant cells (*Courtesy:* Professor PK Agarwal)

23. What is drug treatment of this disease?

The treatment is started with isoniazid, rifampicin and pyrazinamide which is continued for 2-3 months. Then, pyrazinamide is withdrawn, and isoniazid and rifampicin are continued for 6-7 months (total drug treatment is for 9 months).

Antituberculous drugs:

Agent	Dose	Side effects	Remarks
Isoniazid	5 mg/kg daily or 300 mg daily	Peripheral neuropathy, hepatitis, rash, mild CNS effects	• AST and ALT are done • Bactericidal to both extracellular and intracellular mycobacteria • Pyridoxine 10 mg daily as prophylaxis, 50-100 mg daily for therapy of neuritis
Rifampicin	10 mg/kg daily or 600 mg daily	Hepatitis, fever, rash, flu-like sickness, GI upset, bleeding problems, renal failure	• Platelets, AST and ALT are done • Bactericidal • Colors urine orange
Pyrazinamide	15-30 mg/kg or 2 g daily	Hyperuricemia, hepatotoxicity, rash, GI upset, arthralgia	• Uric acid, AST, ALT • Bactericidal to intracellular bacteria
Ethambutol	20-25 mg/kg or 2.5 g daily	Optic neuritis (reversible)	• Eyes to be examined • Bacteriostatic • Use with care in renal disease
Streptomycin	15 mg/kg or 1 g daily	Auditory nerve damage, nephrotoxicity	• Vestibular function, BUN and creatinine • Bactericidal to extracellular bacteria • Use with caution in elderly

24. How do you manage drug resistance?

Primary resistance to these drugs is unusual. But if it is encountered the other drugs must be substituted depending upon sensitivity.

25. What are the indications for excisional surgery?

The indications for surgery are:
- Persistent lymph node enlargement.
- Cold abscess formation.
- Persistent sinus with tuberculous nodes.

26. What are the risks during operation?

The risks during operation are:
- Injury to large veins of the neck.
- Injury to the nerves of the neck, i.e. spinal accessory, cervical branch of facial and hypoglossal nerves.

27. How do you prevent injury to the veins of the neck?
- No tissue should be divided when stretched taut. If the nodes are closely related to internal jugular vein this vein should be identified first and then the nodes can be dissected away from it.
- If the internal jugular vein is involved to such an extent that freeing it is difficult or impossible, it can be ligated and a portion of it can be excised.

28. Is the ligation or excision of internal jugular vein harmful?

No, ligation of one internal jugular vein does not have any untoward effect.

29. How do you treat a cold abscess?
- Apart from antituberculous drugs, the abscess should be aspirated with a thick needle through healthy skin before it ruptures to form a sinus.
- If the aspiration does not help the abscess should be evacuated.

30. What are the dangers or disadvantages of aspiration?

The dangers or disadvantages of aspiration are:
- Formation of sinus.
- Failure to evacuate completely, especially the solid necrotic tissue.

31. What are the causes of sinus formation?

The causes of sinus formation are:
- Rupture of a cold abscess.
- Aspiration of the abscess through the most prominent part of involved skin.
- Drainage of cold abscess.
- Residual necrotic tissue.

32. How do you treat a collar-stud abscess?

Apart from antituberculous drugs, it is treated by evacuation of both the cavities.

33. How do you evacuate a collar-stud abscess?

After incision in a skin crease, the pus in the superficial compartment is mopped away and the opening in the deep fascia is enlarged to admit a small curette for scraping out the deeper cavity completely. The cavity is packed with a gauze piece which is brought out through a corner of the wound which is closed by primary suturing.

34. **What is the method of making a bacteriological diagnosis?**

Any fluid (aspirate) or tissue (biopsy material) can be used for detection and isolation of bacteria. The bacteria can be detected in a smear or culture.

35. **Will you like to send a swab for microbial study?**

No, it is useless to send a swab as these bacteria cannot be detected by this method.

36. **What are the stains used for mycobacterial detection?**

The stains used for mycobacterial detection are:
- Ziehl-Neelsen using light microscopy
- Auramine using fluorescence microscopy

37. **Which method of staining is more sensitive?**

The auramine using fluorescence microscopy is a more sensitive method.

38. **What are the limitations or disadvantages of smear method?**

Very small number of bacilli which is usual in this disease, may escape detection. Thus a negative smear does not exclude the diagnosis.

39. **What are the disadvantages of culture method?**

The disadvantages are:
- It requires special media.
- The growth of bacteria is very slow and takes 3 to 4 weeks.

40. **What determines the speed of growth?**

It is determined by many factors, especially by the number of organisms in the culture material. Specimens containing large number of mycobacteria will sometimes grow in 7-10 days whereas those with few organisms may take several weeks.

41. **What is the advantage of culture method?**

Once mycobacterium is grown, definitive identification and sensitivity testing can be done.

42. **Will you wait for starting the treatment till bacteriological diagnosis is made?**

As this diagnosis takes a lot of time, treatment is started on the basis of clinical diagnosis and results of other investigations.

43. **What are the results of treatment?**

The overall results after adequate treatment are very good.

Discussion

Tuberculous cervical lymphadenitis is a very common chronic infection of cervical lymph nodes caused by mycobacterium tuberculosis.

Etiology

In majority of cases it is caused by human type of mycobacterium tuberculosis, which enters through the tonsil of the corresponding side. In some cases, the disease is caused by bovine type of mycobacteria.

Pathology

From tonsil or pharynx, the infection goes via the lymphatics to the cervical nodes, hence the upper deep cervical nodes are most often affected. There is no systemic infection. Thus the cervical lymph node disease is not secondary to tuberculosis elsewhere in the body. In approximately 80% of patients the infection is virtually limited to clinically affected lymph glands.

Following infection, there is caseous necrosis of lymphatic tissue which may liquefy resulting in cold abscess, collar-stud abscess or sinus formation.

Gross pathology—The cut section of enlarged node shows translucent, grayish patches in early disease. Later, they become opaque and yellowish due to caseous necrosis.

Micropathology—It shows multiple tubercles consisting of epitheloid cells and giant cells with peripherally arranged nuclei in the early stage. After one week lymphoctyes appear in the lesion. They have darkly-stained nuclei and scanty cytoplasm.

At the end of second week the center of tubercle shows caseation surrounded by giant cells and epitheloid cells with a zone of chronic inflammatory cells and fibroblasts around.

Clinical Features

Age—This disease usually occurs in children and young adults.

Sex—The females are more commonly affected.

Symptoms—The main symptom is single or multiple swellings of insidious onset in the neck. Usually there is no pain.

Systemic symptoms are unusual in the young. In elderly patients, anorexia and some loss of weight may be present.

Signs—They depend upon the clinical stage of the disease, described below:
- *Adenitis*—The lymph node or nodes are mildly enlarged, nontender and firm but elastic, and not matted.
- *Periadenitis*—The lymph nodes are mild-to-moderate in size, firm and nontender, and matted.

- Cold abscess
  - There is a hemispherical, smooth, opaque and soft swelling related to enlarged nodes.
  - It does not have any signs of acute inflammation (redness, heat and tenderness).
- Collar-stud abscess
  - There is a hemispherical or hemioval, smooth and soft swelling a little below the enlarged node.
  - A track of communication between the soft swelling (abscess) and enlarged node may be felt as a firm, cord-like structure.
- Tuberculous sinus/ulcer
  - The sinus/ulcer is chronic and nonhealing.
  - It discharges thin syrup-like pus, may be with curdy flakes.
  - The edge is pigmented and undermined.
  - It is related to enlarged nodes in the neck.

Investigations

- Apart from routine the main investigation is FNAC (Fig. 7) or biopsy of the enlarged nodes which confirms the diagnosis.
- Aspirate from the lymph node or discharge from the sinus can be sent for mycobacterium tuberculosis culture, or nucleic acid (DNA and RNA) amplification test for mycobacterium tuberculosis which gives results within a few hours.

Treatment

1. Antituberculous drugs start with a combination of rifampicin, isoniazid and pyrazinamide for two months followed by rifampicin and isoniazid for seven months. It is ideal if they are given depending on culture and sensitivity report.
2. General measures such as good diet with vitamins and minerals, fresh air and sunlight help these patients recover early.
3. Surgical treatment is indicated in the following situations:
   - If the lymph nodes do not respond to drugs or show initial response but remain static after that.
   - If cold abscess has formed.

The nature of operation is given below:

1. *Lymph node excision* – The incision is made along the Langer's lines over the swelling. With careful dissection the surrounding adhesions are released and lymph nodes are excised.
2. *Cold abscess*—It may be aspirated by a thick cannula through the healthy skin in the upper part.
   Evacuation—Aspiration cannot remove the solid necrotic material, hence evacuation is recommended, especially for a large abscess. In this procedure, the abscess is opened and all the pus and necrotic material is removed. The cavity is cleaned and the wound is closed by suturing.

CASE 3: TUBERCULOUS EPIDIDYMITIS

CLINICAL DIAGNOSIS

1. The patient is an adult who presents with discomfort and swelling in the scrotum and low grade pyrexia of insidious onset.
2. The epididymis is enlarged and nontender (may be tender sometimes).
3. There are single or multiple nodules in the epididymis which are hard and irregular ('craggy' epididymis).
4. The vas is thickened and beaded ('craggy') (Fig. 8.1).
5. The scrotal rugae are usually smoothed out. In 30% cases there is a lax hydrocele of mild-to-moderate size.
6. The up and down mobility of the testes is restricted.
7. Later on, the epididymis may be fixed to the overlying skin resulting in formation of a sinus or ulcer posterolaterally discharging thin pus (Fig. 8A to D).
8. The testis is usually normal.
9. The prostate and seminal vesicles may feel hard and nodular (craggy).
10. There may be evidence of tuberculosis elsewhere, e.g. renal tuberculosis.

VIVA VOCE

1. **What is epididymitis?**
   It is inflammation of epididymis due to a variety of causes including tuberculosis.
2. **What is the incidence of tuberculous epididymitis?**
   It is the commonest cause of chronic epididymitis, and nearly 90% of cases of chronic epididymitis are tuberculous.

3. **What are the important clinical signs of this disease?**
   Induration, thickening and nodularity (craggy) of epididymis, and beading of vas deferens ('craggy' vas).
4. **What is the cause of 'craggy' vas?**
   It is due to subepithelial nodules (Figs 8A to D).
5. **Can a patient of tuberculous epididymitis have hydrocele?**
   Yes
6. **What is the incidence of hydrocele?**
   It is present in about 30% of patients.
7. **What is the nature of hydrocele?**
   It is a lax hydrocele (secondary hydrocele).
8. **How many patients present with a scrotal cold abscess or sinus?**
   It is present in 20% of cases.
9. **What happens to the body of testis?**
   It is not affected for a long period, often years.
10. **What is the cause of smoothing out of scrotal rugae?**
    It is due to wasting of subcutaneous cellular tissue including dartos.
11. **Can the patient have signs of disease anteriorly?**
    Yes, when the testis is anteverted, these changes are found in front of testis.
12. **What is the cause of this disease?**
    It is caused by mycobacterium tuberculosis human type.
13. **How does the infection reach there?**
    The infection reaches by two routes—retrograde along the vas deferens from an infected seminal vesicle and by hematogenous route (very rare).

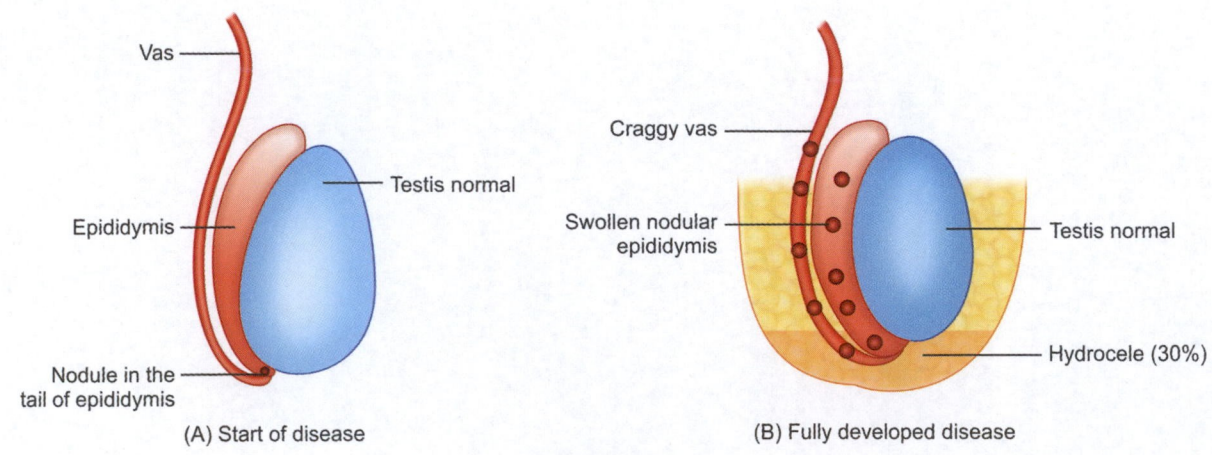

(A) Start of disease   (B) Fully developed disease

Figs 8A and B

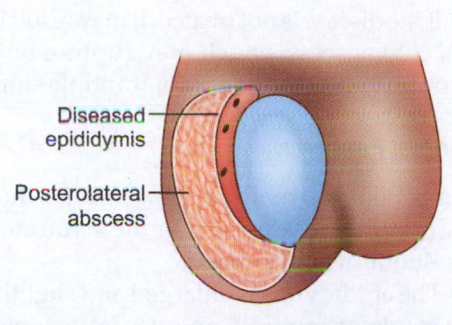

Posterolateral sinus of chronic
tuberculous epididymitis

Diseased
epididymis

Posterolateral
abscess

(C) Cold abscess formation

(D) Sinus formation

Figs 8A and D: Tuberculous epididymitis

14. **What is the site of commencement of this lesion?**
When the infection reaches through the vas, the globus minor is the first site of involvement.

15. **How does a sinus develop?**
Following caseation of tuberculous nodule, there occurs an abscess which involves the overlying skin of scrotum which reddens and breaks down, resulting in a sinus formation (Fig. 8A to D).

16. **What are the other tuberculous lesions associated with this disease?**
The other lesions are tuberculous seminal vesiculitis, tuberculous prostatitis, tuberculosis of kidney and tuberculous cystitis.

17. **What are the signs of tuberculous prostatitis?**
The prostate is enlarged and firm, and in advanced cases contains one or more discrete nodules.

18. **What are the investigations?**
The investigations are:
1. Blood - hemoglobin, blood counts and ESR
2. Urine examination including culture for mycobacteria
3. Culture of semen for mycobacteria
4. Ultrasound of scrotum to see the epididymis
5. FNAC may be done under US guidance
6. X-ray chest.

19. **What is the result of urinary culture for mycobacteria?**
Mycobacteria can be cultured in urine of about half the patients.

20. **What are the findings in chest X-ray?**
A chest X-ray frequently shows evidence of apical lung disease.

21. **How many patients have associated pulmonary tuberculosis?**
It is present in 76% of patients.

22. **Why do you want to do intravenous urography?**
To see the involvement of urinary tract in tuberculosis

23. **What are the urographic signs of urinary tuberculosis?**
The signs are –
1. Moth-eaten caseous cavities or bizarre irregular calices (kidney)
2. Strictures in straight rigid moderately dilated ureters
3. Contracted urinary bladder with vesicoureteral reflux

24. **What is the role of culture of semen?**
It is a useful means of confirming the tuberculous nature of epididymitis.

25. **What is the quick bacteriological method of confirming the diagnosis?**
DNA and RNA amplification for tuberculosis in urine and semen which gives results within a few hours.

26. **How do you treat this disease?**
• This disease resolves with antituberculous drug therapy in some patients.
• Others require epididymectomy, especially if there is formation of a sinus.

27. **What is the nature of antituberculous drugs?**
Usually the treatment is started with four drugs (rifampicin, INH, pyrazinamide and ethambutol). They are continued for two months, and then pyrazinamide and ethambutol are withdrawn, and rifampicin and INH are continued for 7-10 months.

28. **What is the result of antituberculous drug treatment?**
    The treatment with antituberculous drugs is less effective in genital tuberculosis than in urinary tuberculosis.

29. **What are the indications of surgery?**
    The indications of surgery are -
    1. When there is no sign of resolution within two months of drug treatment.
    2. When a cold abscess or sinus is present.

30. **What is the surgical treatment?**
    Epididymectomy.

31. **What is the incision employed for epididymectomy?**
    It is performed through a midraphe incision.

32. **What are the steps of operation?**
    The tunica vaginalis is opened and the vas is isolated and followed to the inferior pole of epididymis. As the upper pole of epididymis is reached, it is necessary to identify the main branches of testicular artery and the bifurcation, where the branch to the epididymis is found and separately ligated. The upper pole of epididymis can then be excised using sharp dissection.
    Occasionally sutures may have to be inserted into the upper pole of testis for satisfactory hemostasis.

33. **What are the complications of epididymectomy?**
    The complications are -
    1. Hemorrhage, scrotal hematoma
    2. Wound infection
    3. Sterility
    4. Testicular atrophy

DISCUSSION

It is a chronic granulomatous inflammation of epididymis caused by mycobacterium tuberculosis. The spread of infection is usually retrograde from a focus of infection in the seminal vesicle as indicated by the involvement of the tail of epididymis first.

Pathology

There is a firm discrete swelling of the lower pole of epididymis. Subsequently the whole of the epididymis may be thickend and nodular. Microscopically it has tuberculous inflammation with tubercle formation and caseous necrosis.

The vas is also involved. It has many subepithelial tubercles.

If the disease is not treated, it may result in the formation of a cold abscess, which may rupture on the skin of the scrotum to produce single or multiple sinuses.

Clinical Features

The patient is usually a young adult who presents with discomfort and a nodule in the scrotum. There may be low-grade evening pyrexia.

The epididymis is enlarged and slightly tender. There are single or multiple nodules in the epididymis which are firm, irregular ('craggy' epididymis), discrete and situated behind the testis.

The scrotal rugae are usually smoothed out, the up and down mobility of testis is reduced and in 30% of patients there is a lax secondary hydrocele.

Later a small soft cystic swelling appears in the epididymis which ruptures on skin to produce a single or multiple sinuses which discharge thin watery pus. The testis is normal.

The vas is thickened and beaded ('craggy' vas). The prostate and seminal vesicles may feel hard and nodular (tuberculous involvement). In two-thirds of patients there may be signs of renal tuberculosis.

Investigations

Urine and semen are examined repeatedly for tubercle bacilli. DNA and RNA amplification for tuberculosis may be done for rapid diagnosis.

Ultrasonography reveals the nodule in the epididymis with a normal testis. FNAC may be done at the same time.

Chest radiography and intravenous urography are done to rule out pulmonary and renal tuberculosis, respectively.

Treatment

Antituberculous treatment (four drugs) is given. The lesion may disappear though this treatment is less effective.

Epididymectomy – If the lesion does not disappear within 2 months of antituberculous drugs, epididymectomy is done, alongwith the sinus/sinuses if present.

The antituberculous drugs should continue till a full course is completed.

CASE 4: PHIMOSIS

CLINICAL DIAGNOSIS

1. The patient presents with difficulty or inability to retract the prepuce behind the corona.
2. The prepucial orifice is narrowed.
3. The prepuce may or may not be retractable.
   - It may be freely retractable on flaccid penis but not on erection.
   - It may be retractable with difficulty on flaccid penis, or
   - It cannot be retracted at all (Fig. 9).
4. If the prepuce can be retracted:
   - Discomfort is produced.
   - A constriction ring is visible.
   - Whitish or pale white flakes of smegma may be present in the coronal sulcus (Fig. 10).
5. The micturitioin is normal in most of the cases.
6. If the prepucial orifice is very narrow like a pinhole, the prepuce may distend with urine (secondary bladder) during micturition.

VIVA VOCE

1. **What is phimosis?**
   It is the difficulty or inability to retract the prepuce due to narrowing of prepucial orifice.
2. **What are the causes of difficulty or inability to retract the prepuce?**

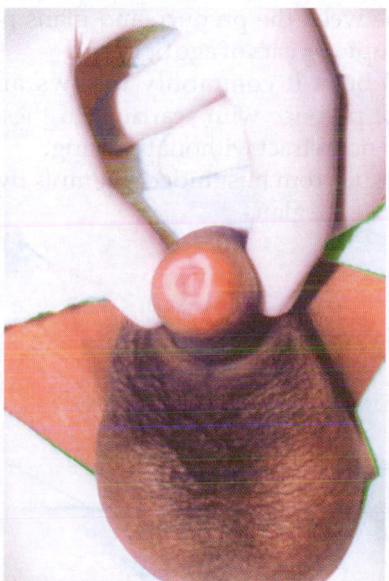

Fig. 9: Phimosis (*Courtesy:* Professor Ashish Wakhlu)

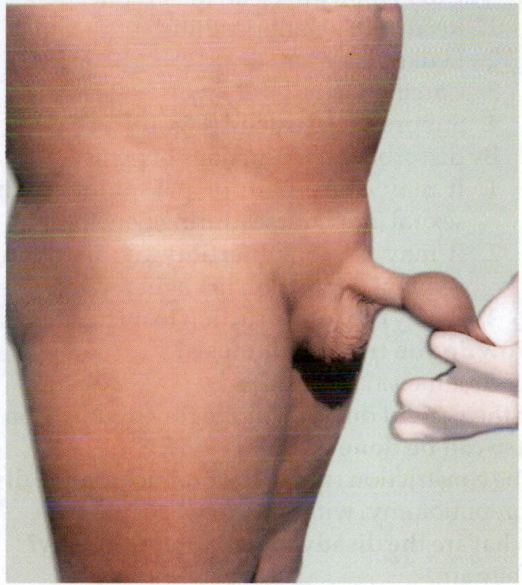

Fig. 10: Phimosis with club-like swelling of distal penis due to retained smegma

The causes of difficulty or inability to retract the prepuce are:
1. Phimosis
2. Subprepucial adhesions
3. Diabetic posthitis
4. Elephantiasis of prepuce
5. Prepucial carcinoma

3. **What are the causes of phimosis?**
   The causes of phimosis are:
   1. Recurrent or chronic infection of prepuce (posthitis) due to poor local hygiene
   2. Ammoniacal dermatitis of prepuce
   3. Congenital (rare)
   4. Diabetic posthitis
   5. Elephantiasis of penis
   6. Balanitis xerotica obliterans.

4. **What are the grades of phimosis?**
   The grades of phimosis are –
   Grade I (mild)—It is the inability to retract the prepuce on erect penis but not in flaccid state.
   Grade II (moderate)—The prepuce is retracted with difficulty but with a constriction ring on a flaccid penis.
   Grade III (severe)—The prepuce cannot be retracted at all even on a flaccid penis.

5. **What is 'secondary bladder'?**
   In extreme cases of phimosis the prepuce balloons out during micturition and drains gradually out with a weak stream. This ballooning of prepuce is called as secondary bladder.

6. **How can this problem harm the patient?**
It may harm the patient in many ways -
a. Due to inability to clean the prepucial sac –
   1. Recurrent balanoposthitis
   2. Leukoplakia
   3. Carcinoma
   4. Subprepucial calculi (Fig. 10)
b. By disturbing the functions of penis –
   1. It may cause pain or paraphimosis during sexual intercourse (during penetration).
   2. It may cause subfertility by disturbing the seminal deposition in vagina.
   3. It may cause obstruction to micturition.

7. **How do you treat of phimosis?**
By circumcision (Fig. 11)

8. **If the patient does not agree for circumcision what else can be done?**
The constriction ring of the prepuce may be divided (preputiotomy) without removal of prepuce.

9. **What are the disadvantages preputiotomy?**
They are –
1. Recurrence can occur
2. The prepucial skin which may not be healthy is retained.

10. **What are the complications of circumcision?**
The complications are - bleeding, wound infection, priapism, injury to glans penis, meatal ulcer.

11. **How do you treat phimosis in a child?**
- If it is not causing any obstruction during micturition and the child is less than 3 years of age, it does not need any treatment as it may correct itself with time.
- If the child is more than 3 years of age and/or there is obstruction to flow of urine, it should be treated by circumcision.

12. **If a middle-aged obese person comes to you with phimosis of recent onset, what will you do?**
The patient should be investigated for diabetes mellitus.

13. **How will you treat diabetic phimosis?**
The diabetes should be corrected by diet control and drugs. The defect usually corrects itself and circumcision is rarely required.

14. **What are the indications for circumcision?**
The indications of circumcision are –
1. Social or religious reasons
2. Phimosis due to any cause
3. Recurrent attacks of balanoposthitis

15. **What is the technique of doing circumcision using a plastibel?**
Plastibel (Hollister) is a circular bell-like device which has a groove at its edge. The prepuce is freed from glans penis and post-coronal sulcus. The device is fitted on glans within the prepuce and then the prepuce is ligated over the bell and the redundant prepuce is excised.
The ring separates between 5 and 8 days postoperatively.

16. **What is your opinion regarding cutting away the prepuce by applying a clamp or bone forceps across the prepuce?**
This must not be practiced as it is a blind method which may injure the glans penis.

DISCUSSION

Phimosis is the inability to retract the prepuce due to narrowing of prepucial orifice.

Etiology

Congenital phimosis is very rare. The inability to retract prepuce in infants is usually due to physiological adhesions between the prepuce and glans penis which may persist upto 6 years of age or more.

In small boys it commonly follows ammoniacal dermatitis of prepuce with scarring. In these cases the prepuce will not retract without fissuring.

It may result from misguided attempts by parents to forcibly expose the glans.

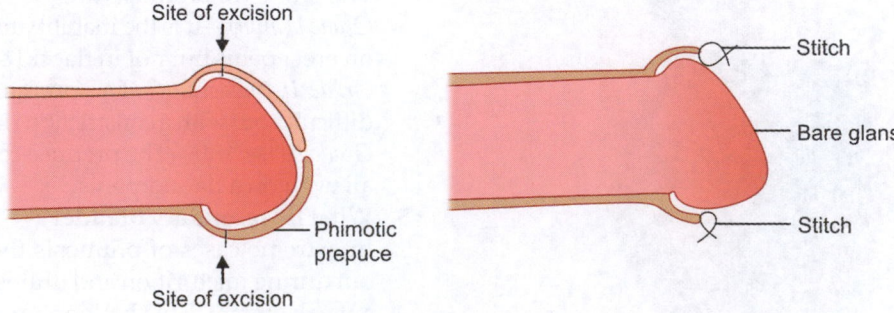

Fig. 11: Circumcision for phimosis

In a middle-aged person it may be due to diabetic balanoposthitis. It is a common finding in filarial elephantiasis of penis and scrotum.

It can occur as a result of balanitis xerotica obliterans.

Pathology

The prepuce is scarred and may be thickened. In these patients it is difficult to maintain penile hygiene. Hence the patient may have balanoposthitis, leukoplakia or carcinoma.

If the prepucial orifice is very narrow it may lead to distension of prepuce during micturition (secondary bladder). If the patient presents with obstructive uropathy with back pressure effects on ureters and kidneys, it is more commonly due to meatal atresia or stenosis masked by phimosis.

Treatment

It is treated by circumcision (Fig. 11). If the patient wants to retain the prepuce then division of constriction ring or dorsal slitting of narrowed prepuce (preputiotomy) is indicated.

The common complications of these procedures are – hemorrhage, wound infection and priapism.

CASE 5: PARAPHIMOSIS

CLINICAL DIAGNOSIS

- Acute paraphimosis
  1. The patient presents with pain and swelling of penis associated with dysuria or retention of urine.
  2. The glans is exposed, congested and edematous (Figs 12 and 13).
  3. The inner layer of prepuce is markedly edematous and everted, especially in the lower part.
  4. The constriction ring can be seen by retracting the penile skin.
  5. There may be ischemic changes in the distal penis.
- Chronic paraphimosis
  1. The patient presents with swelling, may be ulceration of penis and dysuria of insidious onset.
  2. The glans is exposed and may be slightly swollen (edematous).

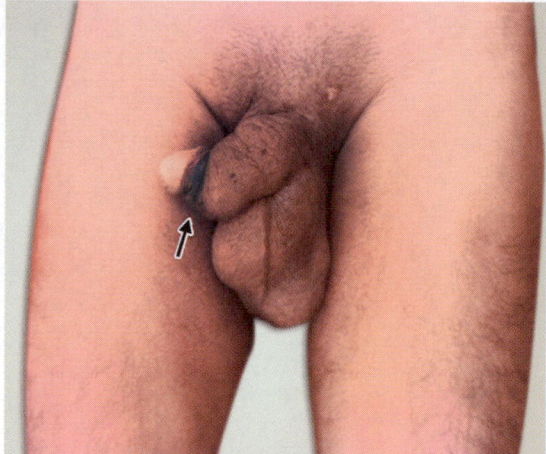

Fig. 12: Paraphimosis

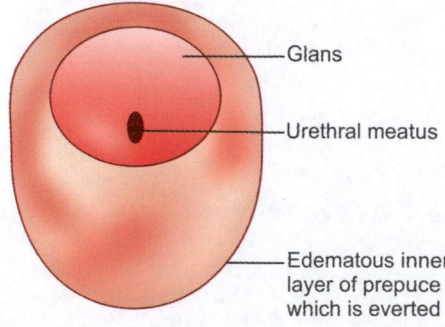

Glans

Urethral meatus

Edematous inner layer of prepuce which is everted

Fig. 13: End on view of penis in paraphimosis with "bearded glans" appearance

3. It is surrounded in the lower part by edematous and everted inner layer of prepuce giving a 'bearded glans' appearance (Fig. 13).
4. The penis may be angulated at the site of constriction ring with the glans pointing upwards.
5. The constriction ring is not visible as such but can be seen by retracting the penile skin backwards. It feels like a tight string.
6. The patient may present with ulceration of glans.

VIVA VOCE

1. **What is paraphimosis?**
   It is a complication of phimosis where the phimotic constriction ring gets engaged in the coronal sulcus and the prepuce fails to return to original position.
2. **What are the causes of this condition?**
   It is a complication of phimosis and occurs -
   1. If the prepuce is retracted forcibly.
   2. During penetration for sexual intercourse.
   3. Playing with phimotic penis.
   4. Retraction of prepuce for urethral catheterization or instrumentation and then forgetting to bring it back to original position (iatrogenic paraphimosis).
3. **Why the retracted prepuce fails to reduce?**
   If fails to reduce as the constriction ring gets engaged proximal to, or in the coronal sulcus. With prolonged retraction, edema of glans and inner layer of prepuce aggravates the condition.
4. **What are the effects or complications of this problem?**
   The effects or complications are –
   1. Edema of penis distal to constriction ring.
   2. Ischemia of distal penis. It may result in ischemic ulceration and rarely gangrene of penis.
   3. Difficulty in micturition or retention of urine.
5. **What are the causes of exposed glans?**
   The causes of exposed glans are –
   1. Following circumcision, preputiotomy
   2. Paraphimosis
   3. Hypospadias
6. **What is 'bearded glans' appearance?**
   It is because of edema of the inner layer of prepuce by the side of frenum of prepuce. The edematous prepuce bulges out and hangs down the exposed glans giving the 'bearded glans' appearance (Fig. 13).
7. **How do you treat this condition?**
   It is treated by reduction. If it fails then by preputiotomy or circumcision.

8. What is the technique of reduction?

The swollen penis is held in a warm sponge (not hot otherwise the penis will be burnt) for 2-5 minutes and sustained but gentle pressure is applied to reduce edema. Now the penis is held in three fingers each of both hands and the glans is manipulated back with both the thumbs, while the prepuce is brought forwards with fingers.

9. Do you know of any other method to reduce the edema?

Yes, by local hyaluronidase injection

10. What is preputiotomy?

In this operation a dorsal midline incision is given in the prepuce to divide the constriction ring so that the prepuce can be reduced.

11. What is the definitive treatment?

Circumcision

Discussion

Paraphimosis is a complication of phimosis which is characterized by inability to reduce a previously retracted foreskin. The constriction ring of prepuce becomes fixed in the retracted position usually proximal to the corona.

Pathology

With prolonged retraction there occurs edema of the inner layer of prepuce which everts and bulges, and thus increases the circumferential pressure on the shaft proximal to the glans. If the condition is not relieved ischemic ulceration of distal penis can occur. The pressure on urethra can cause dysuria and retention of urine.

Clincial Features

Clinically it is of two types - acute and chronic. The patient presents with pain and swelling of the penis associated

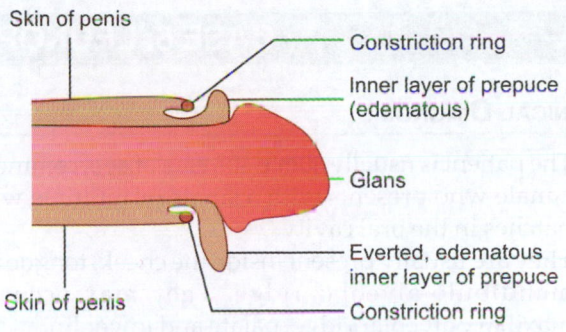

Fig. 14: Paraphimosis

with dysuria and pain. The glans is exposed, congested and edematous. The inner layer of the prepuce is markedly edematous and everted, especially in the lower part. The constriction ring can be seen by retracting the penile skin proximally. There may be ischemic changes in the distal penis, including ulceration. The penis may be angulated at the site of constriction ring with the glans pointing upwards (Fig. 12).

Treatment

- The swollen penis is held on a warm sponge (not hot) and gently pressed for sometime to reduce the edema.
- Initially manual reduction is attempted in which the index fingers of both hands pull the prepuce distally while both the thumbs push the glans backwards into the prepuce.
- If this measure fails the constriction ring is divided (dorsal slit, preputiotomy) and the prepuce is reduced with ease.
- Later on, circumcision may be done as an elective operation when the edema subsides.

CASE 6: LEUKOPLAKIA OF ORAL CAVITY

CLINICAL DIAGNOSIS

1. The patient is usually above 40 years of age, commonly a male who presents with a single or multiple white patches in the oral cavity.
2. They are usually present inside the cheek, tongue and mandibulo-alveolar ridge. They may occur on maxillary alveolar ridge, palate and lower lip.
3. The whiteness varies from faintly translucent to grayish, yellowish or brownish gray (Fig. 15).
4. The patches may be thick and fissured or cracked (cracked white paint appearance).
5. They may be macular or plaque-like.
6. They may feel rough or leathery, and cannot be wiped off.

VIVA VOCE

1. **What do you mean by leukoplakia?**
   It is a white patch which is slightly elevated from the surface and remains despite attempts to rub it off.
2. **What is its cause?**
   It is of multifactorial etiology. The important causative factors are—drying and chemical effects of tobacco smoking, ill-fitting oral prosthesis, chewing tobacco and snuff and cheek biting. The susceptibility to leukoplakia may be augmented by syphilis and alcoholism.

3. **What are the sites of its occurrence?**
   It can occur in the oral cavity, larynx, prepucial sac, vulva and perianal region.
4. **Which is the commonest site?**
   Oral cavity is the commonest site.
5. **Which is the commonest site in the oral cavity?**
   Cheek
6. **Which is second commonest site in the oral cavity?**
   Mandibulo-alveolar ridge
7. **What is the other name of leukoplakia of tongue?**
   Chronic superficial glossitis
8. **What is the macropathology of this lesion?**
   There are two outstanding features –
   1. Cracked white paint appearance due to areas of grayish white plaques of abnormal keratinizing epithelium.
   2. Raw beef appearance at the areas where the plaques are shed.
9. **What is the microscopic appearance?**
   The epidermis is greatly thickened and shows hyperplasia and all degress of cellular atypia ranging from mild dysplasia to carcinoma *in situ*.
10. **What is the mechanism of development of cracks and fissures?**
    They are due to contraction of the underlying scar tissue caused by chronic inflammation.
11. **What are the complications of this lesion?**
    It may undergo malignant transformation (Fig. 16).

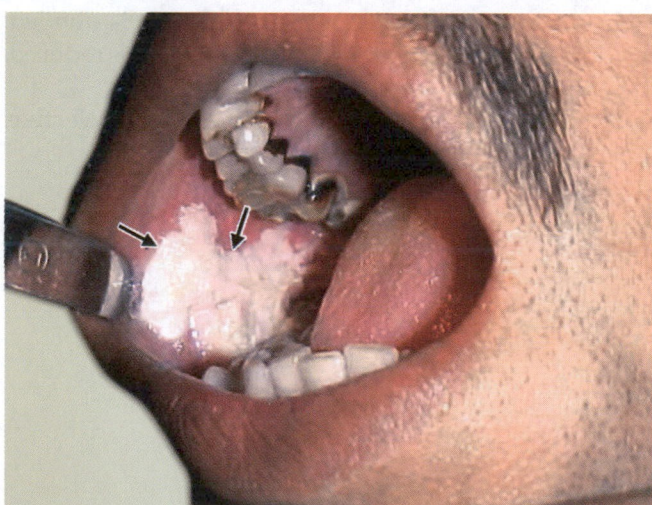

Fig. 15: Severe leukoplakia of right cheek (*Courtesy:* Professor Sandeep Kumar)

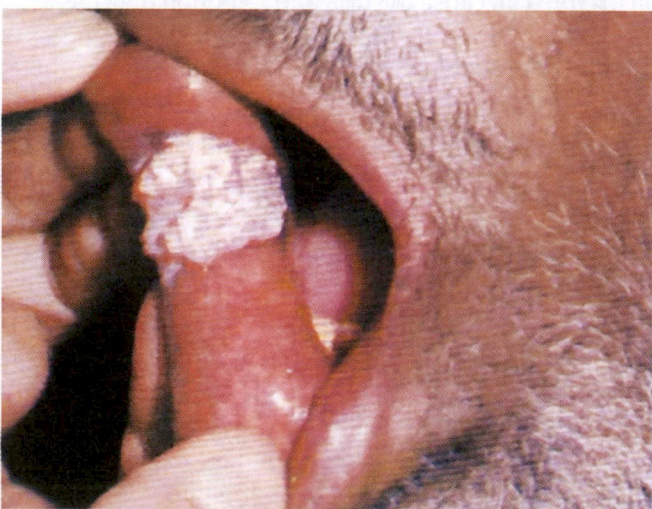

Fig. 16: Leukoplakic carcinoma at the commissure of lips. The carcinomatous change can be seen at the anterior edge. (*Courtesy:* Professor RK Agrawal and Professor AK Khare, Udaipur)

12. **What is the nature of malignancy?**
It is a squamous cell carcinoma.

13. **What are the stages of leukoplakia?**
It has four clinical stages -
- *Stage I*—Appearance of a thin gray transparent milky patch.
- *Stage II*—It becomes opaque and white. In the beginning it is soft but soon cracks and fissures appear.
- *Stage III*—Appearance of small nodules and warty outgrowths. Some areas appear smooth, red and shiny due to desquamation.
- *Stage IV*—Appearance of carcinoma as local thickening in the fissures.

14. **What are the investigations?**
The investigations are:
- Biopsy
- Serological tests for syphilis

15. **How do you treat this lesion?**
The essentials of the treatment are:
1. Removal of the causative factor
   - Stop smoking and tobacco chewing
   - No alcohol
   - Correct ill-fitting dental appliances
   - Avoid habitual lip or cheek biting
2. Beta carotene may cause partial regression.
3. If dysplasia is present the lesion should be excised.
4. Some small lesions may respond to cryosurgery or electrofulguration.

16. **What is the role of radiotherapy?**
Radiotherapy may improve the condition initially but increases the chances of malignant transformation.

17. **How do you differentiate it from candidiasis?**
- The leukoplakic patch cannot be wiped away while that of candidiasis can.
- The leukoplakia occurs in middle-aged people while candidiasis commonly occurs in young children.

DISCUSSION

It is a persistent white patch on the oral mucosa with no histological correlation which remains in position despite the attempts are made to rub it off (Fig. 15).

Etiology

It is due to chronic or persistent irritation of the oral mucosa in a susceptible person. The causes of irritation are drying and chemical effect of tobacco smoking, ill-fitting oral prosthesis, chewing tobacco and snuff and cheek-biting. The susceptibility to leukoplakia may be augmented by syphilis and alcoholism.

Pathology

- Apart from oral cavity it may occur in the larynx, prepucial sac, vulva and perianal region.
- In the oral cavity it may occur anywhere with the largest number of lesions occurring on mandibulo-alveolar ridge, gingivae and bucco-gingival fold with lesions of the buccal mucosa, palate, maxillary ridge, floor of mouth, lower lip and tongue in that order of frequency.
- There are two outstanding features: (1) Cracked white paint appearance—there are areas of grayish white plaques of abnormal keratinizing epithelium, and (2) Raw beef appearance—it represents the areas of shed plaques.
- Micropathology: The mucosa is greatly thickened and shows hyperplasia and hyperkeratinization. Microscopically it is of two types—without cellular atypia and with cellular atypia. The first type shows varying combinations of hyperkeratosis, parakeratosis and acanthosis (simple leukoplakia). The second type, apart from the features of leukoplakia shows varying degrees of dyskeratosis or atypia which may be minimal, moderate or severe. The severe atypia is difficult to distinguish from carcinoma in situ.

Staging—The leukoplakia is described to have 4 stages –
- I: Presence of thin, gray or milky transparent film which may be widespread.
- II: The film becomes opaque and white. Initially it is soft and then cracks and fissures appear.
- III: Appearance of small nodules and warts. Desquamation at places may result in smooth, red and shiny areas.
- IV: Appearance of carcinoma within the fissures as local thickening.

Speckled leukoplakia—It is a variation of leukoplakia occurring on an erythematous base. It has the highest rate of cancerous change.

Biopsy is the main investigation, which is very important to rule out malignant transformation.

Differential Diagnosis

- It has to be differentiated from the white oral lesions that can be wiped away, e.g. candidiasis, aspirin burns.
- It has to be differentiated from the white lesions that cannot be wiped away, e.g. traumatic and frictional keratosis,

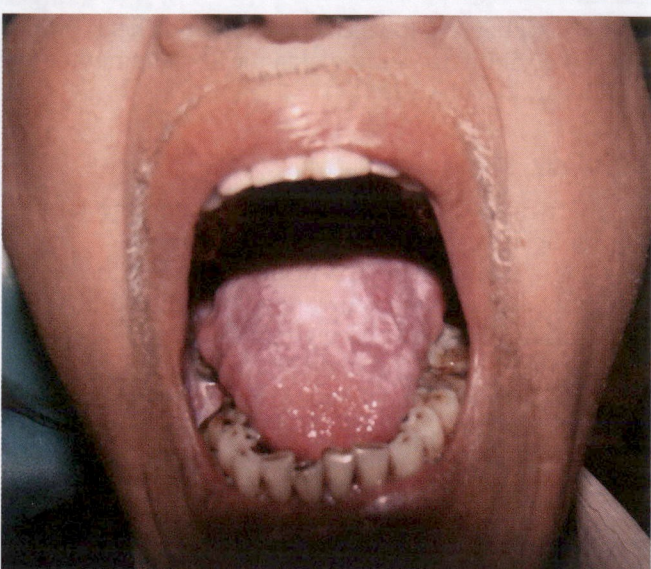

Fig. 17: Lichen planus of tongue (*Courtesy:* Professor Divya Mehrotra)

lichen planus (Fig. 17), veruccous carcinoma, lupus, oral hairy leukoplakia, leukokeratosis nicotina palati.

Treatment

- *Simple leukoplakia*—The cause is eliminated. If the lesion does not disappear within 3-4 weeks it is excised. Beta carotene may help.
- *Dyskeratotic leukoplakia*—Excision or ablation (electrofulguration or cryosurgery) is the treatment of choice. It may be removed by laser.

Prognosis

- The lesion is curable if treated properly early, but it can recur with 35% recurrence rate.
- Four percent of initially benign lesions subsequently turn malignant. It is more likely to become malignant if present on the floor of mouth and the ventral surface of tongue, especially in younger women even in the absence of associated risk factors.

CASE 7: SUBMUCOUS FIBROSIS OF ORAL CAVITY

CLINICAL DIAGNOSIS

1. The patient is usually a middle-aged person who presents with limited mouth opening (Fig. 18) and restricted movement of the tongue of insidious onset.
2. The patient is a habitual pan masala/areca nut chewer.
3. When the patient is asked to open the mouth, fibrous bands stand out beneath the buccal mucosa (Fig. 19).

VIVA VOCE

1. **What is submucous fibrosis of oral mucosa?**
   It is a disease of oral cavity of unknown etiology characterized by formation of fibrous bands beneath the oral mucosa.
2. **What is the cause of this condition?**
   The exact cause is not known but the studies done so far have shown that it is associated with the use of pan masala-areca nut. This disease affects only the Asian population.
   Alcohol and tobacco use may be contributing factors.
3. **What are the pathological changes?**
   There is subepithelial fibrosis with associated atrophy and hyperplasia of the overlying epithelium. There may be epithelial dysplasia.
4. **What are the risks associated with submucous fibrosis?**
   It is a medium-risk lesion associated with malignant transformation.

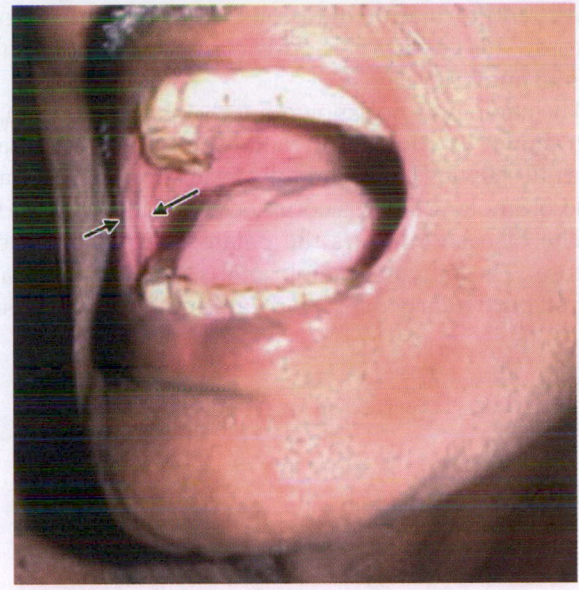

Fig. 19: Submucous fibrosis of right cheek. The mucosa is elevated at the site in the form of longitudinal bands. The opening of the mouth is restricted (*Courtesy:* Professor Sandeep Kumar)

5. **How do you treat this condition?**
   - To stop pan masala-areca nut chewing
   - Intralesional steroid injection may improve the mouth opening
   - Surgical excision and skin grafting is indicated in severe disease (Fig. 20).

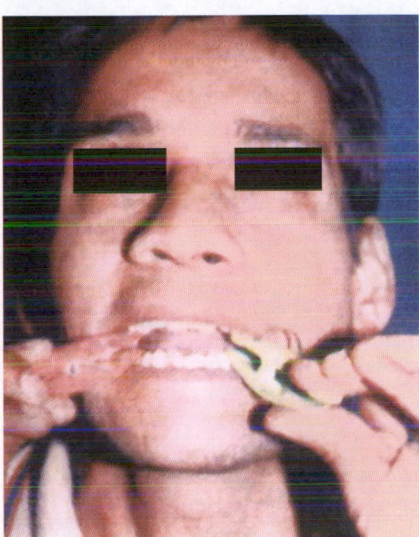

Fig. 18: Submucous fibrosis of cheek resulting in restriction of opening of the mouth (*Courtesy:* Professor RK Agrawal and Professor AK Khare, Udaipur)

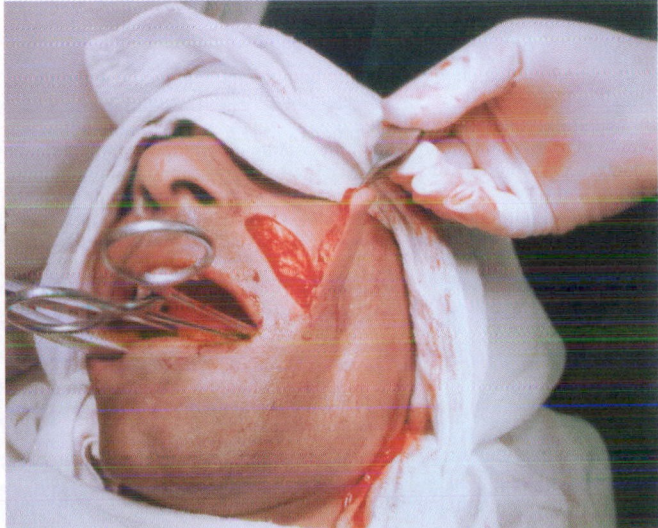

Fig. 20: Nasolabial flap being reflected to be rotated inside the cheek to repair submucous fibrosis (*Courtesy:* Professor Divya Mehrotra)

DISCUSSION

Oral submucous fibrosis is characterized by subepithelial fibrosis and formation of fibrous bands beneath the oral mucosa. This condition is quite common in our country (Figs 18 and 19).

The etiology is not known but the studies done so far have shown its etiological relationship with pan masala-areca nut chewing habit. It may be related to alcohol use and tobacco. Smoking alone is not associated with this disorder.

The disease involves the palate, tongue and cheek mucosa. The mucous membrane is pale, atrophic and scarred particularly over the palate and buccal mucosa.

The epithelium may have dysplasia, when this condition can lead to development of carcinoma.

The patient presents with limited mouth opening, restricted tongue mobility and pain during chewing.

Treatment

- Elimination of the etiological factor.
- Intralesional injection of corticosteroids may be helpful.
- In severe cases the fibrous tissue is excised followed by skin grafting.

CASE 8: INGROWING TOE NAIL (ONYCHOCRYPTOSIS)

CLINICAL DIAGNOSIS

1. The patient presents with pain and swelling by the side of the nail of great toe.
2. The lesion is more common in adolescent or young adult males.
3. The nail may be more convex from side to side than normal.
4. The side of the nail is lost into the nail fold and appears growing or digging into it (Fig. 21).
5. The nail fold may be swollen, red, hot and tender.
6. If the nail fold can be pulled away the digging nail jagged with spikes may become visible.

VIVA VOCE

1. **What is ingrowing toe nail?**
   In this condition the side of the nail curls inwards and grows to form a lateral spike which causes infection of over-hanging nail fold.
2. **What is the cause of this condition?**
   The predisposing factors are:
   - Nail abnormalities
     – A cut short and curved nail
     – Hypercurved nail—Congenital, peripheral arterial disease, pulmonary disease, aging
   - Soft tissue abnormalities—Soft and lax nail pulp due to debilitating diseases, hyperhidrosis
   - Crowded foot in an ill-fitting or pointed shoe

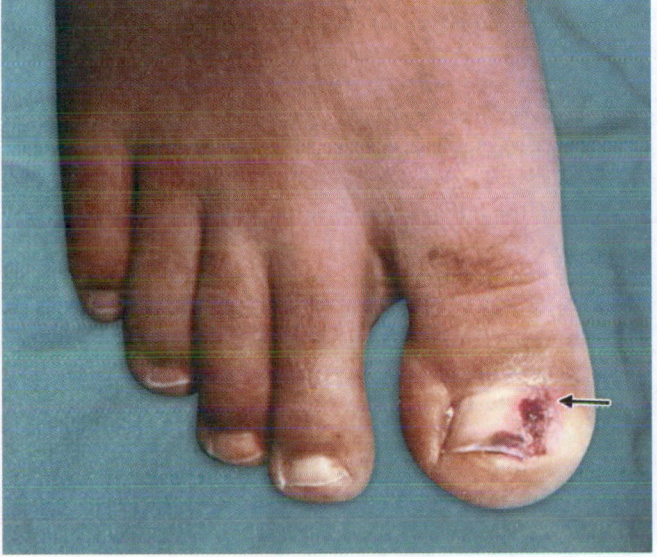

Fig. 21: Ingrowing toe nail

- Bone abnormalities such as subungual exostosis causing the nail plate to be domed.
3. **How does cutting the nail short and curved predispose to this lesion?**
   It allows the unsupported pulp of the toe to roll over the nail edge when upward pressure is exerted during walking.
4. **How can an ill-fitting shoe cause this condition?**
   In an ill-fitting or narrow pointed shoe the toes are crowded together which causes lateral pressure from both the sides resulting in pressure between the nail plate and nail fold.
5. **How does an ingrowing nail produce symptoms?**
   The lateral edge of toe nail cuts and grows into the adjacent soft tissue of nail fold. Infection (bacterial and fungal) also enters the tissues causing inflammation and exuberant granulation tissue formation.
6. **How do you treat this disease?**
   The early disease is treated by conservative measures while severe disease is treated by excision of nail partially or completely.
7. **What are the conservative measures?**
   The conservative measures include the following:
   1. Soaking, washing and carefully drying the feet everyday, and applying an emollient
   2. Wearing clean socks and wide fitting shoes.
   3. Trauma, especially pressure to be avoided.
   4. Nail should be cut properly (transversely).
   5. A cotton wool pledget may be placed under the corner of the nail to help it grow out from the nail fold.
      These measures are successful in a good number of patients of early disease.
8. **What are the indications for operation?**
   The indications for operation are:
   1. When the conservative measures fail
   2. In late or severe disease
9. **What is the nature of operation?**
   The nail is excised partially or completely.
10. **What is the result of this surgery?**
    Following these operations the nail regrows and if the measures described under conservative treatment are followed the new nail is expected to grow normally.
11. **Can this disease recur?**
    Yes
12. **How do you treat recurrent disease?**
    It is treated by wedge resection or Zadek's operation.

13. **What do you do in wedge resection?**

    It removes 25% of the width of the nail and the nail bed on the affected side. The nail bed is made smooth and plain and the hypertrophied nail fold should be debulked by raising a skin flap of nail fold (Fig. 22).

14. **What do you do in Zadek's operation?**

    The entire nail bed is excised so that there is no toe nail.

15. **What is the technique of Zadek's operation?**

    An incision is given on the three sides of the nail except the distal end. Two proximal extension are made from the edges of nail fold towards the distal interphalangeal joint so that a wide flap of skin can be raised to allow access to the root of nail and the matrix.

    The nail is excised, the limits of matrix are dissected out, and a block of tissue containing the matrix is excised to leave the bare phalynx. The flap is then replaced and sutured to the proximal end of the remaining nail bed.

16. **What is onychogryposis?**

    It is crooked overgrowth of a toe nail usually of the big toe occurring in elderly people, especially if bedridden. It may become so curled as to resemble a Ram's horn.

17. **How do you treat this condition?**

    It is treated by cutting through its base by a Gigli saw and the residual by filing. If necessary, nail bed may also be removed.

DISCUSSION

Ingrowing toe nail is a common problem in adolescents and young adults, and most commonly affects the hallux, other toe nails may be affected. One should be very careful in making this diagnosis in the elderly as in them, it is often a manifestation of peripheral vascular disease.

An ingrowing toe nail is caused by the lateral edge of the toe nail cutting and growing into the adjacent soft tissues of the nail fold. Superimposed infection (bacterial or fungal) causes inflammation of tissues and attempted tissue repair results in exuberant granulation tissue

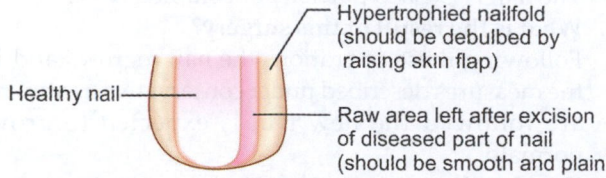

Fig. 22: Wedge resection of ingrowing toe nail

formation. A combination of the following factors is the cause of this condition:

1. Tight fitting shoes
2. Cutting (or picking) the nail down into the nail fold rather than transversely
3. Sweaty feet and poor foot hygiene.

Clinical Features

The patient may present with anything ranging from the nail fold riding up on to the nail, or a grossly infected, painful nail fold with cellulitis and weeping granulation tissue. It may be unilateral or bilateral disease.

Treatment

a. Early disease:
   1. Soaking and washing and carefully drying the feet everyday and applying an emollient to keep the nail healthy.
   2. Wearing clean socks and wide fitting shoes.
   3. Trauma, especially pressure must be avoided.
   4. The nail should be cut properly (transversely).
   5. A cotton wool pledget may be placed under the corner of the nail to help it grow out from the nail fold.

   These measures are successful in a good number of cases.

b. **Late or severe disease:** Operation is indicated and the aim of operation in the acute disease is to remove the ingrowing nail from the nail fold so that the wound can heal. It can be achieved by –
   1. Excision of the whole nail
   2. Excision of ingrowing portion of the nail. Following avulsion, the nail regrows and if the treatment described above is followed, the new nail is expected to grow normally.

c. **Recurrent disease:** More severe measures are indicated such as wedge resection or Zadek's operation.
   1. *Wedge resection*—It removes 25% of the width of nail and the nail bed on the affected side. The nail bed is made smooth and plain. The nail fold of the diseased side is frequently hypertrophied (enlarged). It is better if it is debulked by raising a small skin flap from the nail side. Thus the area is prepared to receive the about-to-grow nail in a correct manner (Fig. 22).
   2. *Zadek's operation*—The entire nail bed is excised so that there is no toe nail. The wound heals by fibrosis. This operation is reserved for severe disease.

CASE 9: POST-BURN CONTRACTURE

CLINICAL DIAGNOSIS

1. The patient presents with deformity, restriction of movement or loss of function of the affected part following healing of wounds of burns.
2. It commonly occurs across the areas of flexion such as neck, axilla and cubital fossa.
3. The structures on either side of the joint are brought together.
4. There is significant cosmetic problem (Figs 23 and 24).

VIVA VOCE

1. **What is a contracture?**
   A contracture is a pathologic end stage of healing of a wound related to the process of contracture of newly formed scar tissue.

2. **What is the cause?**
   Contractures usually develop when a wound heals with excessive scarring followed by contracture of scar tissue. The cause of excessive scarring is not known.

3. **What is the mechanism of contracture?**
   The mechanism of contraction of the wound is not understood, but it is considered to develop via smooth muscle contractile elements in myofibroblasts.

4. **What are the effects of contractures?**
   The effects are cosmetic and functional.

5. **What are the types of contractures?**
   The contractures are of two types:
   - Flexion contractures are common which can develop in any flexible tissue, e.g. eyelids, lips, and across areas of flexion such as neck, axilla and cubital fossa.
   - Extension contractures are rare except for extension contractures of the toes and the metacarpophalangeal joints of the digits (hyper-extension deformity).

6. **How do you treat contractures?**
   It is better and prudent, to prevent development of a contracture, by proper wound care. It is simpler than the treatment.

7. **What are the preventive measures?**
   - The wounds of the flexion areas are covered with flaps or grafted early with thick split-thickness grafts to reduce scarring and stop the process of contraction.
   - Following grafting the part is splinted in position of extension during the healing phase, and 2-3 weeks more after the healing is completed.

8. **How do you treat established contractures?**
   It depends upon the type of contracture –
   - Narrow bands of contracture are excised and the contracture is released with one or more Z-plasties.
   - Large contractures are incised (cut) from the medial to lateral axis across the flexion surface and opened up by full extension of the affected joint. The resulting defect is covered with a skin flap or skin graft.

9. **What is the role of passive stretching and physiotherapy?**
   In established contractures they have hardly any role.

10. **How do you treat recurrent contracture?**
    It is treated by release of contracture and covering it by a fasciocutaneous flap.

11. **What is the postoperative care?**
    - After the operation the affected part is splinted in extension which continues for about 2 weeks after the wound or graft has healed.
    - After healing of the wound physiotherapy is beneficial.

DISCUSSION

Contracture is a pathologic end-stage of healing of a wound related to the process of contraction (Figs 23 and 24) of scar tissue.

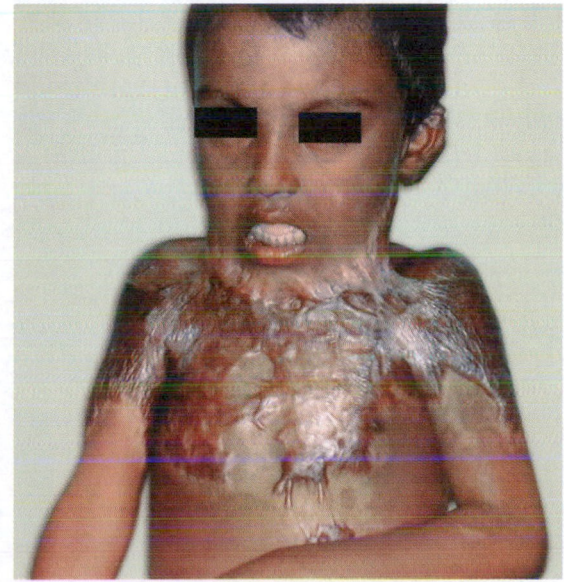

Fig. 23: Extensive post-burn contracture of neck, both shoulder regions and chest wall (*Courtesy:* Dr. Divya Narain)

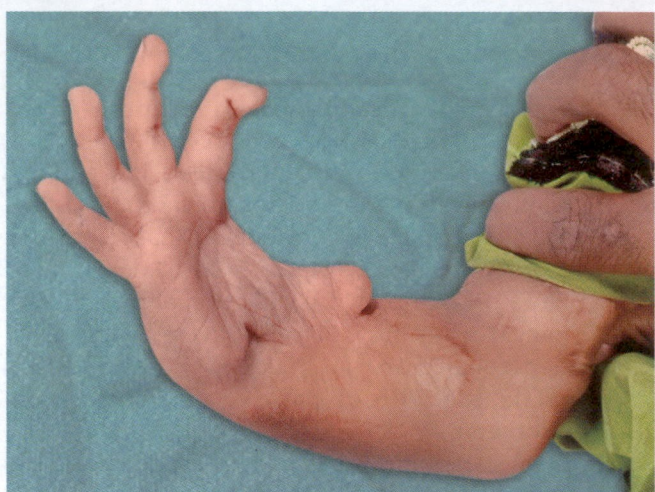

Fig. 24: Post-burn contracture of hand and forearm
(*Courtesy:* Professor Rajiv Agarwal)

Pathology

Contractures usually develop when a wound heals with excessive scarring followed by contraction of scar tissue which results in distortion of surrounding tissues. Contractures can develop in any flexible tissue, e.g. eyelids, lips, etc. but they commonly occur across areas of flexion such as neck, axilla and cubital fossa. The contracture or tight web brings together the structures on either side of the joint (hyperflexion deformity) restricting the range of movement, especially extension, both active and passive.

Extension contractures are rare except for extension contractures of the toes and the metacarpophalangeal joints of the digits (hyperextension deformity).

The mechanism of contraction is not understood. It is considered to develop via smooth muscle contractile elements in myofibroblasts.

Prophylaxis

It is better and prudent to prevent development of a contracture than to treat it, by proper wound care. The wounds in the flexion areas are covered with flaps or grafted early with thick split-thickness grafts to reduce scarring and stop the process of contraction. Following this, the part is splinted in a position of extension during the healing phase, and 2-3 weeks more after the healing is completed. Vigorous physical therapy is of benefit.

Treatment

- The passive stretching and physiotherapy do not help.
- Narrow bands of contracture are excised and released with one or more Z-plasties.
- Large contractures are incised from the medial to lateral axis across the flexion surface and opened up by full extension of the affected joint. The resulting defect is covered with a skin flap or skin graft.
- Recurrent contracture is treated by a fasciocutaneous flap. After the operation the affected part is splinted in extension which continues for about 2 weeks after the wound or graft has healed.

CASE 10: HALLUX VALGUS

CLINICAL DIAGNOSIS

1. The patient is usually a middle-aged or elderly person who comes with pain in the great toe, deformity of the forefoot and difficulty in wearing shoes (Figs 25 and 26).
2. The great toe is deviated laterally and the head of first metatarsal is protruded medially with a bony prominence.
3. An adventitious bursal swelling may be present on the bony prominence (Fig. 26).
4. The second toe may have hammer deformity (hammer toe)—the MP joint is hyperextended and PIP joint is flexed. A corn or bursa is often present on the dorsum of PIP joint.
5. The forefoot looks widened.
6. A bunionette may be present on the metatarsal head.

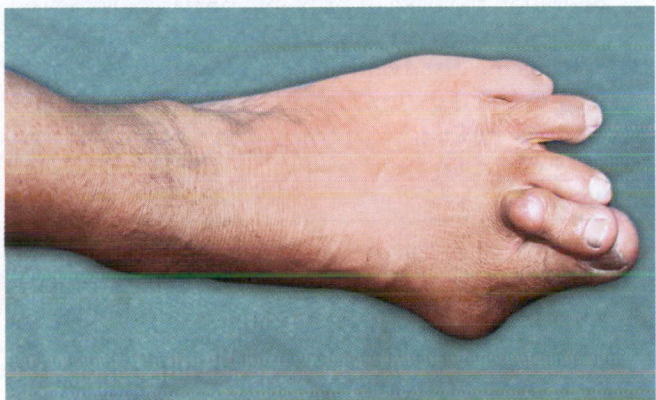

Fig. 25: Hallux valgus as seen from above. The great toe is deviated laterally with over-riding second toe. The metatarsophalangeal joint of great toe is very prominent medially

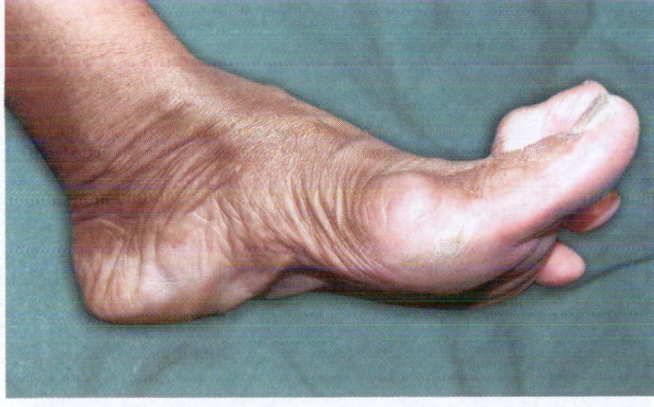

Fig. 26: Hallux valgus as seen from the medial side. The over-riding second toe can be seen

VIVA VOCE

1. **What is hallux valgus?**
   It is a deformity of great toe in which it is abducted at metacarpophalangeal joint (Fig. 25).
2. **What is the incidence?**
   It is probably the most common deformity of foot.
3. **What is the cause of this condition?**
   The factors which may be responsible for this condition are:
   1. Wearing narrow-pointed shoes
   2. Heredity
   3. Metatarsus primus varus
   4. Long first metatarsal
   5. Hypermobility of the first digital ray.
4. **What is metatarsus primus varus?**
   It is angulation of the first metatarsal bone toward the midline of the body, producing an angle sometimes of 20^0 or more between its base and that of the second metatarsal bone.
5. **What is digital ray?**
   A digit of the hand or foot (finger or toe) and the corresponding portion of the metacarpus or metatarsus is considered as a continuous structured unit and called a digital ray.
6. **What do you mean by an adventitious bursa?**
   It is an abnormal bursa-like structure due to chronic or repeated friction or some mechanical cause that contains fluid like synovial fluid.
7. **What is hammer toe?**
   It is a deformity in which the MP joint is hyperextended and the PIP is flexed causing a claw-like appearance.
8. **What is a corn?**
   It is a horny induration and thickening of the stratum corneum of the skin produced by recurrent friction and pressure. It forms a conical mass pointing down into the corium producing pain.
9. **What is a bunionette?**
   It is an abnormal prominence of the inner aspect of the first metatarsal head, accompanied by bursal formation seen in hallux valgus.
10. **What are the investigations?**
    Radiography of the foot is done to see the deformities, their extent, and osteoarthritic changes in the MP joint (Fig. 27).
11. **What is hallux valgus angle?**
    It is the angle between the longitudinal axis of first metatarsal bone and the proximal phalanx. Normally it is nearly a straight line.

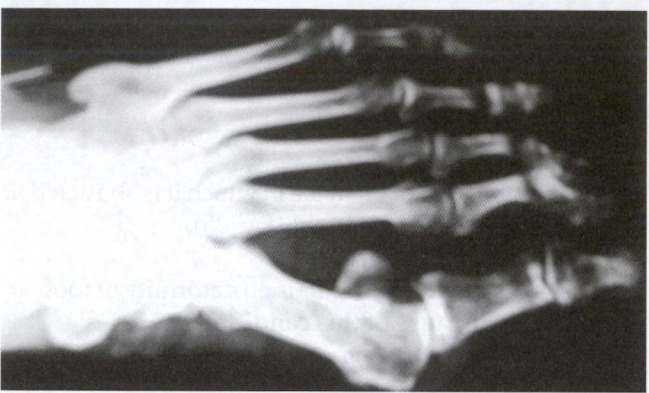

Fig. 27: X-ray of the foot, superoinferior view showing marked deviation of metatarsal bone medially and the phalanges laterally. The sesamoid bone of the head of metatarsal is visible laterally

12. **How do you treat hallux valgus?**
   - Asymptomatic hallux valgus may not be treated except the advice regarding the change to a wide toe comfortable shoes.
   - Symptomatic hallux valgus is treated by surgical correction of the deformity.
13. **How do you correct the deformity?**
   Three types of operations are in use for correcting the deformity—osteotomy, arthrodesis and arthroplasty.
14. **What do you do in an osteotomy?**
   It is the correction of the deformity by dividing the bone which is deviated. Two types of osteotomies are done for correcting hallux valgus—distal osteotomy and proximal osteotomy.
15. **What do you do in distal osteotomy?**
   Through a medial approach a proximally based V-shaped osteotomy is done. The distal fragment is displaced laterally by about one third of the diameter of metatarsal head and the medial prominence is excised. The osteotomy is held in position by internal fixation.
16. **When do you do distal osteotomy?**
   It is the operation of choice in younger patients less than 50 years of age, and when hallux valgus angle is less than 25^0.
17. **What do you do in proximal osteotomy?**
   Here the osteotomy is done near the base of metatarsal bone. It is combined with division of the tendon of contracted adductors of the first web space and tightening of the medial collateral ligament (Fig. 28A and B).
18. **When do you do proximal osteotomy?**
   It is done in patients less than 50 years of age and when hallux valgus angle is between 25-45^0.
19. **When do you do arthrodesis?**
   It is done in elderly men, especially when the MP joint is osteoarthritic.
20. **When do you do arthroplasty?**
   It is done in elderly women with arthritis and when the hallux valgus angle is more than 45^0. In this operation the base of proximal phalanx is excised (Keller's operation, excision arthroplasty).
21. **What is the disadvantage of arthroplasty?**
   It defunctions the toe. Hence, it is avoided in an active woman.

DISCUSSION

Hallux valgus is an osteoarticular deformity in which the great toe is abducted at metatarsophalangeal joint (MP joint). It is probably the most common problem affecting the forefoot (Figs 25 and 26).

Etiology

A number of factors may be responsible for this condition:
- Wearing narrow-pointed shoes
- Heredity

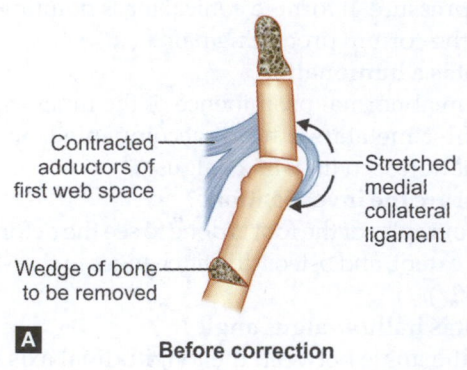

Contracted adductors of first web space — Stretched medial collateral ligament — Wedge of bone to be removed

A **Before correction**

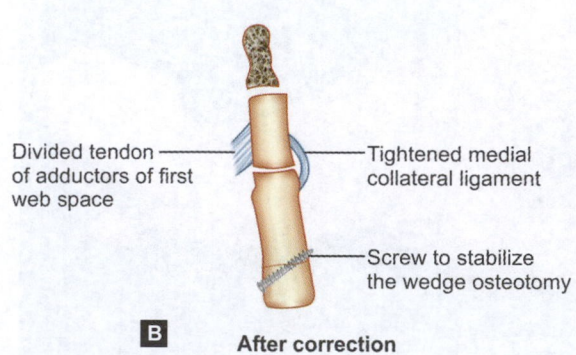

Divided tendon of adductors of first web space — Tightened medial collateral ligament — Screw to stabilize the wedge osteotomy

B **After correction**

Fig. 28: Correction of hallux valgus (left)

- Metatarsus primus varus, congenital or acquired
- Long first metatarsal
- Hypermobility of the first ray.

Pathology

Two structures prevent the great toe from going into valgus the medial collateral ligament and abductor muscle of great toe. As the toe starts to go into valgus the medial part of the capsule of MP joint stretches and the abductor shifts below the metatarsal head due to its attachment to medial sesamoid. As a result of this shift the first metatarsal deviates medially in relation to the great toe and its sesamoids. Because of the changed mechanics of MP joint of great toe it suffers with secondary osteoarthritis.

Clinical Features

The patient is usually a middle-aged or elderly person who presents with the deformity of the great toe and pain. It may be a bilateral disease. There is difficulty in wearing the shoes.

The diagnosis is clinical but radiography of the forefoot is done to exactly assess the deformity and to measure the hallux valgus angle and the angle between the first and second metatarsal (Fig. 27).

A clinical photograph of the patient should also be taken.

Complications

- Ulceration can occur at the pressure points.
- Secondary osteoarthritis of MP joint of great toe
- Infection of the adventitious bursa.

Treatment

- Ill-fitting or tight shoes are avoided.
- Surgical treatment is indicated for recurrent infection or ulceration and increasing deformity. Many types of operation are available, the choice of the procedure depends on the age, hallux valgus angle, the angle between the first and second metatarsal, the mobility of first tarsometatarsal joint and the osteoarthritic changes in the first MP joint. Three types of operations are in use.
- *Distal osteotomy*—It is the operation of choice in younger patients less than 50 years of age, and when hallux valgus angle is less than 25^0. In Chevron osteotomy, through medial approach, a proximally based V-shaped osteotomy is done. The distal fragment is displaced laterally by about one third of the diameter of metatarsal head and the medial prominence is excised. The osteotomy is held in position by internal fixation.
- *Proximal osteotomy*—It is the operation of choice for patients less than 50 years of age, and when hallux valgus angle is between 25-45^0. It is combined with procedures to balance the distal soft tissues by dividing the tendon of contracted adductors in the first web space and lightening the stretched medial collateral ligament. It is a difficult procedure but gives good results.
- Arthrodesis is best for elderly men especially when the MP joint is osteoarthritic.
- Excision arthroplasty (Keller) is done in elderly women with arthritis and when the hallux valgus angle is more than 45^0. The base of the proximal phalynx is excised. It defunctions the toe, so it is avoided in an active woman.

CASE 11: SUBMANDIBULAR SALIVARY CALCULUS

CLINICAL DIAGNOSIS

1. The patient (unusual in children) presents with pain and swelling in the submandibular region which appears or worsens just before or during meals.
2. There may be a swelling in the submandibular region especially after meals which is mild to moderate in size, smooth or lobulated, firm, well-defined and tender.
3. The opening of the Wharton's duct is inflamed, edematous and pouting. It may exude turbid fluid or purulent saliva which increases on pressing the submandibular swelling.
4. The stone is usually palpable in the floor of mouth as an indurated nodule along the course of Wharton's duct.
5. Sometimes the stone is visible as it is projecting from the mouth of the duct. It is gray-yellow in color.

VIVA VOCE

1. **What happens in this disease?**
   In this disease, a stone forms in the Wharton's duct or submandibular salivary gland.
2. **What is the cause of this condition?**
   - The cause is not known. It is nothing to do with serum calcium, and the diseases of teeth, gum and oral cavity.
   - The submandibular saliva contains higher concentrations of calcium and phosphate and it is highly viscous. Further, the Wharton's duct is longer and runs an upward course (against gravity) in the terminal course.
3. **What is the site of occurrence?**
   Usually the stone is situated in the main duct, often at the junction of the duct with the gland or near its orifice. Sometimes it may be present in the gland itself.
4. **What is a secondary salivary calculus?**
   Stones may develop in the stagnant duct system proximal to the primary stone; they are known as secondary salivary calculi.
5. **What are the complications of this disease?**
   The complications include:
   - Chronic submandibular sialadenitis.
   - Secondary salivary calculi.
   - Submandibular abscess.
   - Salivary fistula.
6. **What are the investigations?**
   X-ray of the floor of the mouth is required to see the stone. A CT scan may be done.

7. **What are the X-ray signs?**
   It usually shows an ovoid or rounded shadow in the floor of mouth by the side of midline (Fig. 29).
8. **How do you take the radiograph?**
   The patient holds a dental X-ray plate in between the teeth, and the rays are directed upwards from under the chin.
9. **How do you treat this disease?**
   - A stone in the Wharton's duct is removed by cutting the duct at the stone.
   - If the stone is present in the proximal part of the duct or hilum of the gland, submandibular sialadenectomy is the treatment.
10. **What is the anesthesia used?**
    The stone can be removed both in general or local anesthesia.
11. **What is the anesthesia of choice?**
    General anesthesia.
12. **What is the disadvantage of local anesthesia?**
    It may cause local edema and swelling making the stone impalpable, hence difficult to remove.
13. **What are the precautions during operation?**
    A stitch is passed around the duct proximal to the stone to prevent it from slipping back into the gland.
14. **What are the complications of submandibular gland excision?**
    The complications are:
    - Injury to the cervical branch of facial nerve.
    - Hemorrhage (injury to facial artery).

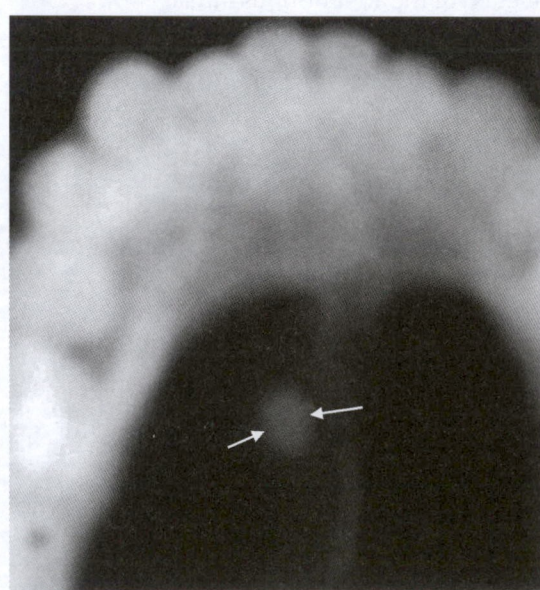

Fig. 29: Radiograph of floor of mouth showing a stone in the submandibular duct

- Injury to the hypoglossal nerve.
- Opening of the oral mucosa.

DISCUSSION

Calculus disease is more common in the submandibular than in the parotid salivary system. 80 percent of salivary stones occur in the submandibular salivary system.

Etiology

It is unknown, apart from the fact that in chemical composition, a salivary calculus resembles the dental tartar:

Phosphates of Ca and Mg	—	79%
Salivary mucus	—	12.5%
Ptyalin	—	1%
Animal matter	—	7.5%

The occurrence of this stone is not related to any disease of teeth, gums or jaws, or to any systemic factor such as plasma calcium.

Pathology

The primary stone usually lies in the main duct, often at the junction of the duct with the gland. It varies in size from millet seed to pigeon's egg; but usually it is small and ovoid in shape. It is yellowish in color (Fig. 30).

In the stagnant duct system proximal to the primary stone, secondary calculi which are spherical, may form.

The gland may suffer due to obstruction and superadded infection.

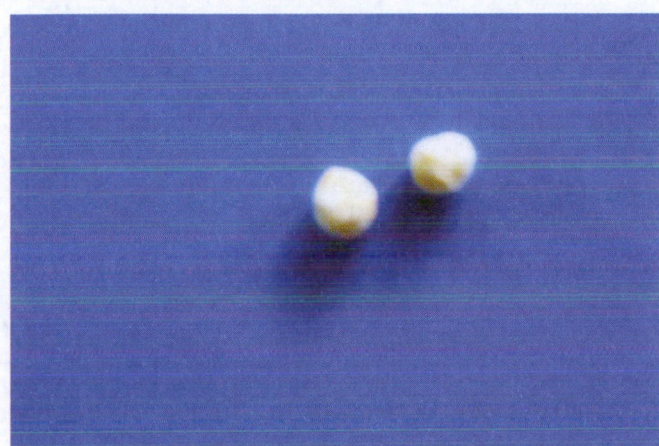

Fig. 30: Salivary calculi removed from submandibular duct

Clinical Features

This disease can occur at any age, although relatively unusual in children. It is symptomless till it produces obstruction. The gland then swells and may be painful.

The symptoms nearly always start during a meal and the duration is usually brief lasting minutes rather than hours or days. The attack subsides suddenly with a gush of salty saliva from the affected duct into the mouth.

If the patient is given a little lemon juice to taste, the attack is precipitated. The saliva pours out from the normal side while nothing comes from the affected side where the gland swells and may be painful.

Between attacks there may be no signs. The calculus may be visible as an elevation in the floor or sometimes visible in the opening of the duct. It is palpable within the duct in the floor of mouth or at the hilum of the gland by bimanual palpation with a finger in the floor of mouth and the other hand below the lower jaw.

The submandibular gland may be enlarged, firm and slightly tender. Sometimes on pressing it, pus comes out from the orifice of Wharton's duct.

Radiography

The plain X-ray of floor of mouth usually reveals the stone. The patient holds a dental X-ray plate in the mouth between the teeth and the rays are directed upwards from under the chin.

Eighty percent of submandibular stones are radiopaque. A CT scan will show the better details of the disease.

Treatment

1. A stone in the Wharton's duct can be removed under general or local anesthesia (the edema of local anesthesia may make the stone impalpable). The tongue is drawn to the opposite side with a stitch or towel clip, and a stitch is passed around the duct proximal to the stone and pulled so that the stone does not slip into the gland. The duct is opened with a knife upto the stone which is removed. No sutures are required as suturing usually leads to stricture formation.
2. If the stone is present in the proximal part of the duct or the hilum of the gland, and if there is chronic sialadenitis, the gland is excised by a skin crease incision 5 cm below the lower border of mandible. One should not try to remove a hilar stone by intraoral approach as there is real risk of injury to the lingual nerve.

CASE 12: CLEFT LIP AND CLEFT PALATE

CLINICAL DIAGNOSIS

1. The patient is a neonate who is having a cleft in the upper lip, alveolus and, or palate since birth (Figs 31 to 33).
2. It is unilateral or bilateral and situated by the side of midline.

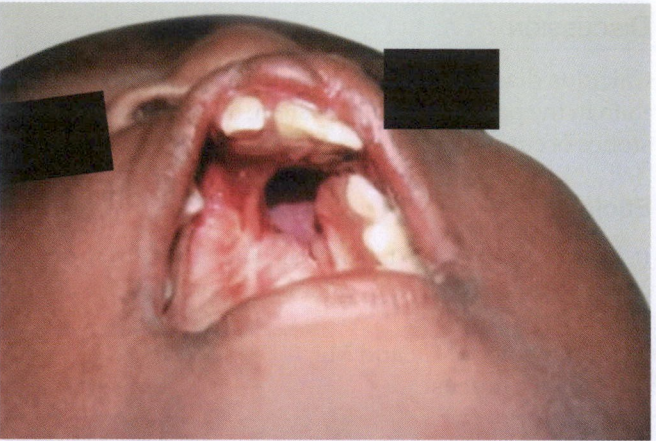

Fig. 33: Cleft palate. The labial defect can also be seen (*Courtesy:* Professor Divya Mehrotra)

3. The nose on the side of the defect is flattened with a wider nostril.
4. There may be a cleft in the soft palate with or without involvement of hard palate and alveolus.
5. The cleft of the lip and the cleft of the palate may occur together or may occur as an isolated defect.
6. The cleft may be associated with feeding and breathing problems.

VIVA VOCE

1. **What is the incidence of cleft lip and cleft palate?**
   - The cleft lip and cleft palate are the most common congenital anomalies of oro-facial region (Figs 31 to 33).
   - The cleft lip and cleft palate occurs once in 600 live births, and the cleft palate alone once in 1000 live births.
   - The relative incidence of cleft lip is 15 percent, cleft palate 40 percent and cleft lip and palate 45 percent.
   - These anomalies are more common in males but an isolated cleft palate occurs more commonly in female newborns.

2. **What do you know about the etiology of these defects?**
   The etiology is both genetic and environmental. The genetic factor is more significant in cleft lip and palate than in isolated cleft palate where the environmental factors include maternal epilepsy and some drugs, e.g. steroids, diazepam and phenytoin.

3. **What is the development of face?**
   At about 6th week of intrauterine life, a depression appears in front of the head called stomodeum or

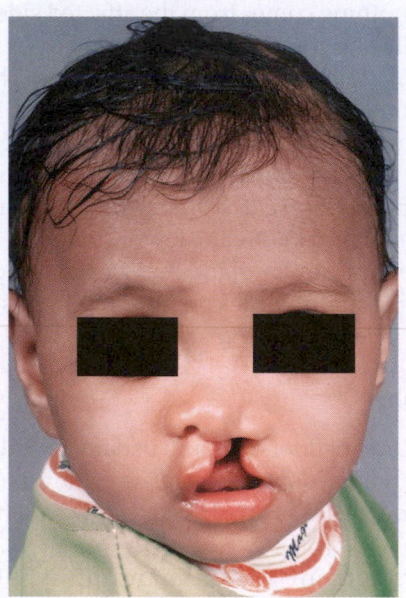

Fig. 31: Unilateral (left) complete cleft lip and palate (*Courtesy:* Professor Rajiv Agarwal)

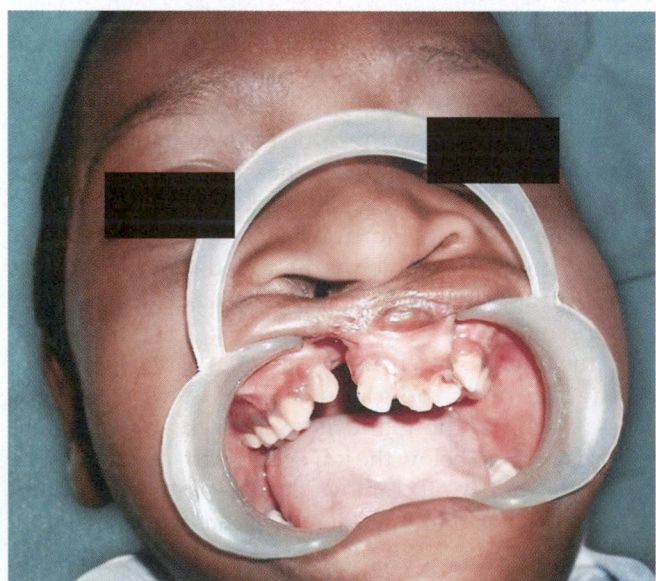

Fig. 32: Right-sided cleft alveolus (*Courtesy:* Professor Divya Mehrotra)

primitive mouth. Around it appears five processes – a frontonasal process at the head end and a maxillary and a mandibular process on each side. Fusion of all these processes results in the formation of face which is completed in a period of 3 weeks (Fig. 34).

4. **What is the mechanism of cleft lip formation?**
   The cleft lip is considered to be caused by failure of fusion of maxillary and medial nasal processes. Another theory says that it may be due to incomplete mesodermal ingrowth into these processes with subsequent breakdown of epithelium.

5. **What is the mechanism of cleft palate formation?**
   The cleft palate is due to failure of fusion of palatal shelves of the maxillary processes which are initially separated by tongue, which descends down by the 8th week of pregnancy allowing the shelves to fuse. The fusion starts anteriorly and is followed by the development of centers of ossification which form the hard palate.

6. **What are the structural and functional problems caused by a cleft lip?**
   The cleft lip can cause the following problems:
   - Cosmetic defect because of the cleft lip and the deformity of the nose.
   - Defective dentition: The teeth may come out through the gap.
   - Defective speech, especially the labials, e.g. M, P.

7. **How do you classify the clefts?**
   The clefts are classified according to LAHSHAL system where the complete clefts of lip, alveolus, hard palate and soft palate are labeled by capital LAHS, respectively, and the incomplete clefts are indicated by small letters.
   LAHSHAL stands for complete bilateral cleft lip and palate while the paraphrase lahSh indicates an incomplete right unilateral cleft lip and alveolus and complete cleft of the soft palate going partly into the hard palate (Fig 35).

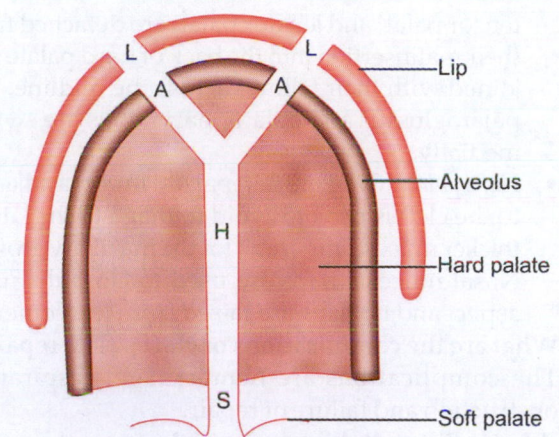

Fig. 35: LAHSHAL classification of cleft lip and palate

8. **When do you repair a cleft lip?**
   The cleft lip is usually repaired at 3 to 6 months of age.

9. **What is the "rule of ten"?**
   The "rule of ten" was used for deciding the optimal time for repair by the following factors:
   - Body weight 10 lb or more
   - Hemoglobin 10 gram% or more
   - At least 10 weeks of age.

10. **Can the lip repair be made easier by narrowing the cleft preoperatively?**
    Yes. It may be achieved by an orthodontist fitting a series of presurgical splints which draw the two halves of the maxilla together.

11. **What is the technique of cleft lip repair?**
    The skin incisions are given to restore displaced tissues: Skin, mucosa, muscles and cartilage to their normal position. For good approximation without tension subperiosteal undermining of the anterior maxilla is done. The nasolabial muscles are sutured to the premaxilla, the oblique fibers of the orbicularis oris are anchored to the base of the anterior nasal spine and nasal septum, and then the horizontal fibers are sutured to restore the ring of oral sphincter. There should be accurate alignment of mucocutaneous junction, construction of Cupid's bow, correction of shape of nostril and repair of nasal floor.

12. **When do you repair a cleft palate?**
    The cleft palate is repaired at 6 to 18 months of life.

13. **How do you repair a cleft palate?**
    The aim of repair is to bring together mucosa and muscles with minimal scarring. The palate can be repaired in one or two stages. The two stages repair results in narrowing of hard palate which reduces the dissection during the second stage.
    - *Soft palate:* The abnormally situated muscles in the soft palate are identified and repositioned. The

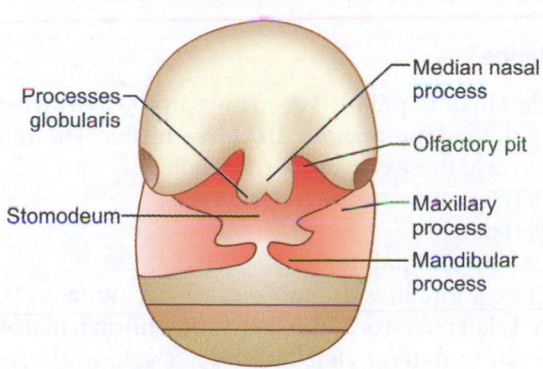

Fig. 34: Development of face

tensor palati and levator palati are detached from their malinsertion into the back of hard palate and joined with their fellows across the midline. The palatoglossus and palatopharyngeus are swung medially.

- *Hard palate:* Only the thin palatal mucosa adjacent to the cleft is used to avoid damage to the lateral thicker mucosa important for the maxillary growth. Nasal mucosal flaps are used to close the nasal aspect and no flaps are raised from the vomer.

14. **What are the complications of cleft palate repair?**
The complications are hemorrhage, respiratory obstruction and failure of repair.

15. **What is Pierre-Robin syndrome?**
It is characterized by a palatal defect associated with a receding lower jaw and posterior dislocation of tongue obstructing the oropharyngeal airway.

16. **What is the significance of this syndrome?**
It may cause sudden infant death due to respiratory obstruction.

17. **Do these patients need any further treatment?**
After the repair of clefts, the patient needs further treatment as described below:
- Most of the patients require orthodontic treatment throughout the growth period with greater stress in the early phase of permanent dentition. Around the age of 10 to 11, bone grafting in the alveolar defect should be done to allow the teeth to migrate into the normal position in the line of defect (Figs 36 and 37).
- Rhinoplasty and submucous resection: When the growth is complete at around 18 years, these procedures may be necessary to correct the deformity of nasal bone.

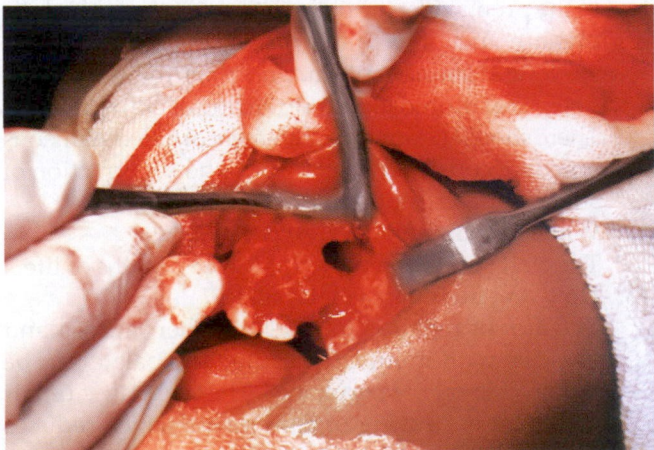

Fig. 36: Alveolar cleft of maxilla (*Courtesy:* Professor Divya Mehrotra)

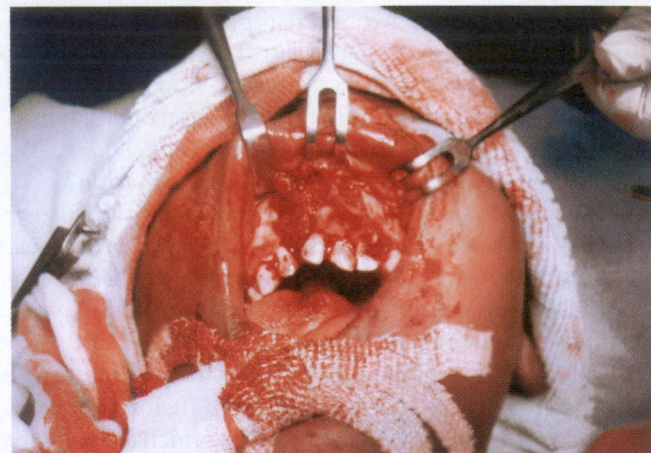

Fig. 37: Bone grafting has been done in the alveolar cleft (*Courtesy:* Professor Divya Mehrotra)

- Speech therapy is required to correct cleft palate speech due to nasal escape of air.
- Later in life, further help may be required depending upon the problems, e.g. cleft lip revision, transplantation of teeth, etc.

DISCUSSION

The cleft lip and palate are the most common congenital anomalies of orofacial region. They usually occur as isolated abnormalities but may be associated with other developmental defects.

Development of Face

At about 6th week of intrauterine life, a depression appears in front of head called stomodeum or primitive mouth. Around it appears five processes—a frontonasal process at the head end and a maxillary and a mandibular process on each side. Fusion of all these processes results in formation of face which is completed in a period of 3 weeks.

Incidence

The cleft lip and palate is seen once in 600 live births and cleft palate alone once in 1000 live births. The relative incidence of these defects is given below:

Cleft lip	: 15%
Cleft palate	: 40%
Cleft lip and palate	: 45%

These anomalies are more common in males, but an isolated cleft palate occurs more commonly in females than males. In unilateral cleft lip, the left side is affected in 60 percent of patients.

Etiology

It is both genetic and environmental. The genetic factor is more significant in cleft lip/palate than isolated cleft palate where the environmental factors play a larger role. The environmental factors include maternal epilepsy and some drugs, e.g. steroids, diazepam and phenytoin. More than 150 syndromes are associated with cleft lip and palate.

Pathological Anatomy

- *Unilateral cleft lip:* The nasolabial and bilabial muscle rings are disrupted on one side leading to an asymmetrical deformity involving the nasal cartilages, nasal septum and anterior maxilla (premaxilla). These defects involve the mucocutaneous tissues also.
- *Bilateral cleft lip (Fig. 38):* The defect is more pronounced but symmetrical. Both the superior muscular rings are disrupted on both sides causing flaring of nose, a protruding premaxilla and prolabium in front of premaxilla which is devoid of muscle.
- *Cleft palate:* The primary palate consists of the structures in front of the incisive foramen, i.e. the alveolus and upper lip.
  The secondary plate consists of the rest of the palate posterior to incisive foramen, i.e. hard palate and soft palate. The cleft palate occurs due to failure of fusion of two palatine shelves. When the cleft of hard palate remains attached to the nasal septum and vomer, the cleft is incomplete. When the nasal septum and vomer are completely separated from the palatine process the cleft is complete.

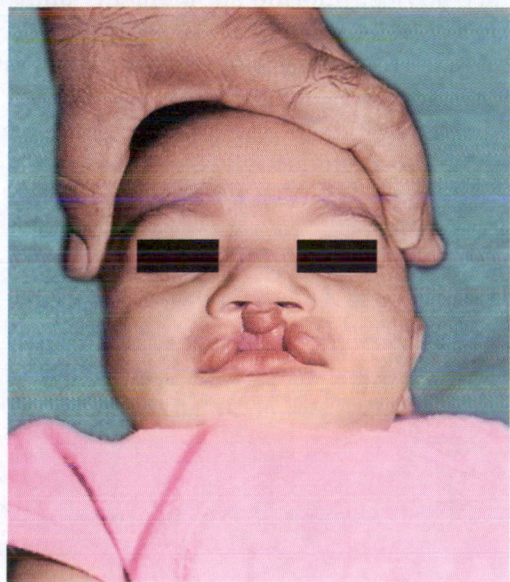

Fig. 38: Bilateral cleft lip (*Courtesy:* Dr. Sanjeev Bhatia)

- *Soft palate:* The closure of the velopharynx is achieved by five muscles working in a coordinated manner. The muscle fibers in the soft palate are transversely oriented with hardly any attachment to the hard palate. In a soft palatal cleft the muscle fibers are oriented antero-posteriorly inserting into the posterior edge of the hard palate.
- *Hard palate:* It is covered by a layer of fibromucosa, which is divided into three zones:
  1. Palatal fibromucosa is the central mucosa that lies below the nasal floor. It is a very thin layer of tissue.
  2. Maxillary fibromucosa lies lateral to palatal fibromucosa. It is a thick layer that contains the greater palatine vessels and nerves.
  3. Gingival fibromucosa lies more laterally near the teeth.

Clinical Features

- *Worried parents:* The cleft lip can be seen by ultrasonography after 18 weeks of gestation. Hence the worried parents may come for advice. As this defect can be corrected by appropriate surgery, they are advised to continue the pregnancy. The cleft palate cannot be seen by ultrasonography.
- *Feeding difficulties:* A cleft baby finds it difficult to suckle the nipple due to interruption of oral sphincter in cleft lip, and because of the difficulty in creating negative pressure in the oral cavity due to palatal leak. Further, the palatal cleft interferes with swallowing with escape of milk into the nose.
- *Breathing difficulties:* Usually there is no breathing problem except in babies with Pierre Robin syndrome where hypoxic episodes during sleep and feeding may occur.
- *Cosmetic problem:* It may be difficult for the parents to accept the defective baby.
  A cleft lip, apart from the lip abnormality, produces deformity of alar cartilage and deviation of nasal skeleton. The nose is flat and wide on the side of the cleft. A cleft of the alveolus is associated with dental deformities and abnormalities.
- Speech defects are not seen these are minor if the baby is treated and the defects are corrected according to the time table. In untreated babies, the cleft lip is associated with difficulty in speaking labials, e.g. papa, mama; and cleft palate with linguo-palatals, e.g. kho-kho with a nasal twang to the sound.
- *Hearing abnormalities:* A cleft palate may be associated with shorter Eustachian tubes with straight. Eustachian canals allowing entry of milk into the middle ear producing chronic middle ear infection and later impaired hearing.

Types of Clefts (Fig. 39)

The clefts are classified according to LAHSHAL system where the complete clefts of lip, alveolus, hard palate and soft palate are labeled by capital LAHS, respectively, and incomplete clefts are indicated by small letters.

LAHSHAL stands for complete bilateral cleft lip and palate, while the paraphrase 'lahSh' indicates an incomplete right unilateral cleft lip and alveolus with complete cleft of soft palate going partly into the hard palate (Fig 35).

Treatment

- Feeding difficulties: The feeding difficulty is studied and appropriate advice is given accordingly. Good feeding may be achieved with soft bottles and modified teats.
- Breathing difficulties may be overcome by nursing the baby prone. More severe problems may need labioglossopexy.

Repair of the Cleft

- *Timing:* The cleft lip is usually repaired at 3 to 6 months of age while the cleft palate is repaired at 6 to 18 months of life. The aim of surgery is restoration of normal or near normal anatomy. Emphasis is put on the muscular reconstruction of the lip, nose, face and soft palate.
- *Cleft lip:* The skin incisions are given to restore displaced tissues – skin, muscles and cartilage to their normal position. For good approximation without tension subperiosteal undermining on the anterior maxilla is done. The nasolabial muscles are sutured to the premaxilla, the oblique fibers of orbicularis oris are anchored to the base of anterior nasal spine and nasal septum, and then the horizontal fibers of both sides are sutured to restore the ring of oral sphincter.
- *Cleft palate:* The aim of cleft palate repair is to bring together mucosa and muscles with minimal scarring. The palate can be repaired in one or two stages. The two-stage repair results in narrowing of hard palate defect in first stage that reduces the dissection during the second stage.

Secondary Management

After the repair of cleft the child goes home. As he grows and develops, with the age many problems appear that require continued care and treatment:

- **Hearing:** All patients should be assessed before 12 months of age by auditory brainstem response (ABR) and tympanometry for sensineural and conductive hearing loss, respectively. The former is treated by a hearing aid. The latter is due to secretory otitis media which may require myringotomy.
- **Speech:** Regular speech assessment is done to detect speech problems, which may be velopharyngeal incompetence and articulation problems. The velopharyngeal incompetence produces a nasal or hypernasal speech that may be due to inadequate muscle repair. The articulation problems are due to compensatory mechanism to overcome velopharyngeal incompetence or due to jaw, dental or occlusal abnormalities. Video-fluoroscopy nasal airflow studies (aerophonoscopy) and nasoendoscopy are done to find the cause of speech defect.

  The speech problems are treated by speech and language therapy, secondary palatal surgery including intravelar veloplasty or pharyngoplasty and speech training devices.
- **Dental problems** are common. They are managed by dietary advice, fluoride supplements and fissure sealants. A well-maintained and disease-free dentition is the main requirement for orthodontic treatment which is done in two phases:
  1. Mixed dentition (8-10 years) to expand maxillary arches as a prelude to alveolar bone graft.

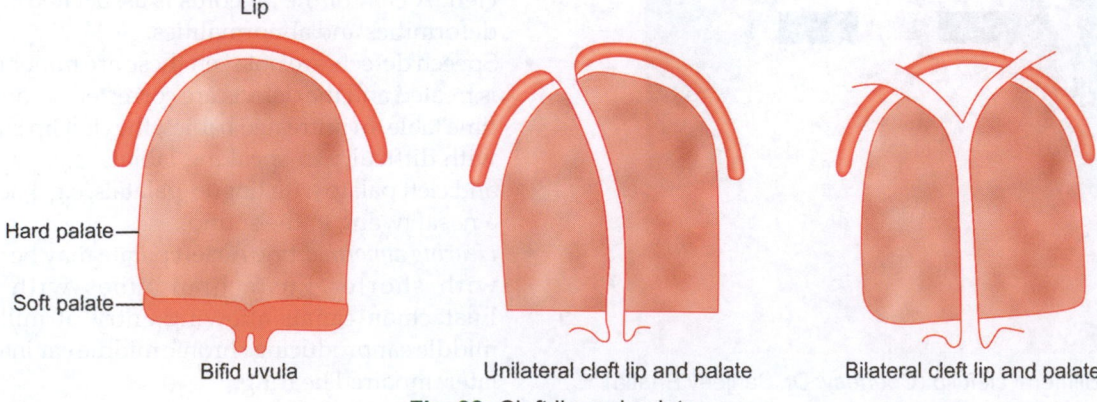

Fig. 39: Cleft lip and palate

2. Permanent dentition (14–18 years) to provide a normal functioning dental occlusion. It may require surgical correction of a malplaced/retrusive maxilla by osteotomy.

Secondary Surgery

Secondary surgery may be required to correct the deficiencies and defects of primary surgery. The following are the procedures that may be required:

1. Revision of cleft lip repair.
2. Alveolar bone grafting.
3. Repair of a palatal fistula.
4. Transplantation of teeth, insertion of osseo-integrated dental implants.
5. Orthognathic surgery.
6. Open septorhinoplasty.
   Overall it is a long-term treatment, but the results are good and rewarding.

CASE 13: INCOMPLETELY DESCENDED TESTIS

CLINICAL DIAGNOSIS

1. The patient is usually a male child who is brought with the complaint of empty scrotum which is underdeveloped (Fig. 40).
2. The testis may be palpable as a rounded or oval, firm or soft nodule along the course of its normal descent, i.e. in the inguinal canal or at the external ring (Fig. 41).
3. The testis may not be palpable (cryptochidism) (Fig. 40).
4. An ipsilateral inguinal hernia is usually present.
5. Other congenital anomalies may also be present, the commonest being a hypospadias.

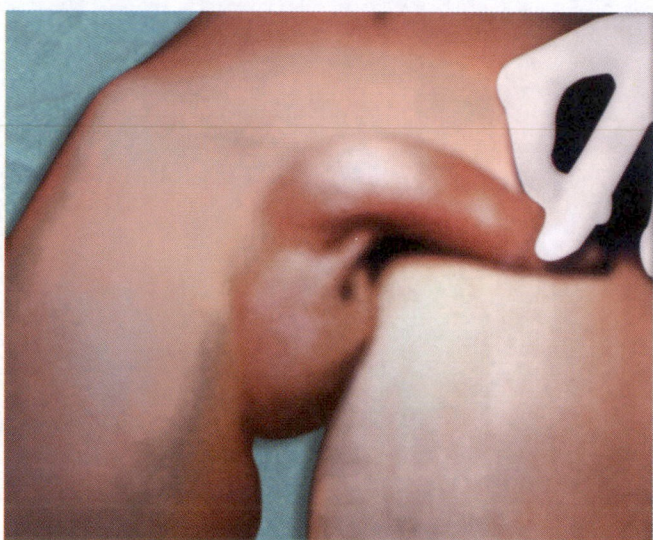

Fig. 40: Right undescended testis with empty underdeveloped right hemiscrotum (cryptorchidism)

VIVA VOCE

1. **What do you mean by imperfectly descended testis?**
   It includes all types of abnormalities of descent of testis - incompletely descended testis, ectopic testis and retractile testis.
2. **What is incompletely descended testis?**
   The testis may be arrested anywhere in the line of normal descent.
3. **What is ectopic testis?**
   The ectopic testis has come out of the abdomen and then it deviates from its normal route of descent and may lie at the root of the penis, in the femoral triangle or in the perineum (Fig. 42).
4. **What is retractile testis?**
   It is a normally descended testis that is intermittently pulled up by overactive cremaster reflex to lie in the superficial inguinal pouch.
5. **What is the harm in having an incompletely descended testis?**
   It is harmful in 2 ways:
   - If the testis is not brought down before 5 to 6 years of age it is likely to undergo gradual atrophy with loss of function.
   - It is likely to have some complications.
6. **What is the cause of atrophy of testis?**
   The main factor is temperature. The scrotal temperature is 2 to 5° C lower than the body temperature.
7. **What are the changes in the testis, if it is not brought down?**
   The undescended testis is normal at birth. If it is not brought down, it gradually degenerates till at puberty it is small, flabby and soft. Histologically, the

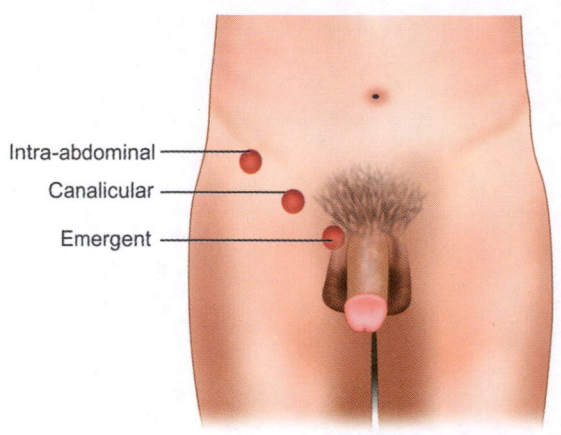

Fig. 41: Incompletely descended testis

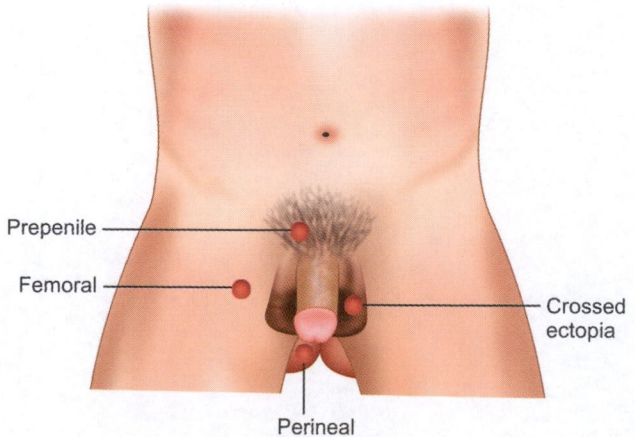

Fig. 42: Ectopic testis

functional parenchyma is immature or destroyed. Hence, there is no spermatogenesis and the production of androgens is halved.

8. **What are the complications of incompletely descended testis?**
   The complications are:
   - Infertility due to hypospermia or aspermia
   - More liable to torsion and trauma because of increased mobility
   - Complications of inguinal hernia that is invariably associated
   - More liable to malignant transformation

9. **If malignancy develops, what is the nature of the tumor?**
   It is usually a seminoma.

10. **What is cryptorchidism?**
    It is when the imperfectly descended testis is neither visible nor palpable.

11. **What are the causes of cryptorchidism?**
    The causes are:
    - Intra-abdominal testis
    - Absent testis (anorchia)
    - Testicular atrophy.

12. **How will you visualize the testis in cryptorchidism?**
    The testis may be visualized by ultrasound, CT scan, MRI or laparoscopy.

13. **What is 'vanishing testis'?**
    It is when during laparoscopy the blind ending vas and vessels are seen without any evident testis.

14. **How do you treat the incompletely descended testis?**
    It is treated surgically by bringing the testis down and fixing in the scrotum (orchiopexy).

15. **Is there any medical treatment?**
    Human chorionic gonadotropin has been tried, but it is useless as the incomplete descent is usually due to mechanical reasons.

16. **What are the essential steps of operation?**
    The essential steps of operation are:
    - Exposure of testis by a groin crease incision
    - Herniotomy of associated inguinal hernia
    - Lengthening of the cord by mobilization, division of adhesions and cremaster, including retroperitoneal mobilization
    - The testis is brought to the scrotum without torsion and fixed in an extradartos pouch.

17. **What is the role of microvascular surgery?**
    An intra-abdominal testis is treated by a single-stage microvascular transfer with the gonadal vessels being divided high near the renal vessels and anastomosed to the inferior epigastric vessels, thereby gaining the length of the cord to bring the testis down into the scrotum.

DISCUSSION

Imperfect descent of testis is one of the most common congenital abnormality (Fig. 40). It may be present in 5 percent of male infants born at full term falling to about 1 percent at one year of age.

Embryology

- **Development:** The development of gonads begins during the 4th week of intrauterine life. During the 6th week of the testis determining factor encoded by SRY (sex determining region of Y chromosome) is expressed and the developing gonad differentiates into testis.
- **Descent:** The testicular descent begins in the 7th week. It occurs in two stages: abdominal phase and inguino-scrotal phase.
  - *Abdominal phase:* The Sertoli cells release a Mullerian Inhibiting Substance (MIS) that causes regression of Mullerian structures and enlargement of gubernaculum. The fetal abdominal structures grow away from the testis that is anchored near the internal ring due to gubernaculum. This gives an appearance of abdominal descent.
  - *Inguinal phase:* It occurs during the 30 to 38 weeks of intrauterine life and is largely under control of testosterone which is thought to act on the nucleus of genitofemoral nerve in the spinal cord to cause the ipsilateral release of calcitonin gene-related peptide from the end of the nerve. It is postulated that this peptide induces swelling and cavitation of the gubernaculum into which the processus vaginalis protrudes. The testis passes into scrotum, possibly driven by intra-abdominal pressure.

Types

A fully descended testis resides in the scrotum with its lower pole touching the lower limit of scrotum.

- **Incompletely descended testis:** This testis is arrested somewhere in the line of normal descent. Depending upon its site it may be (1) intra-abdominal, (2) canalicular, and (3) emergent (Fig. 41).
- **Ectopic testis:** This testis has come out of abdomen and then deviates from the normal line of descent. Thus it can be (1) prepenile, (2) crossed to opposite scrotum, (3) femoral, and (4) perineal depending upon where it settles down (Fig. 43).
- **Retractile testis:** This testis has an overactive cremasteric reflex. The testis is in the scrotum when the child is warm and fully relaxed but retract into the superficial inguinal pouch on slightest provocation.

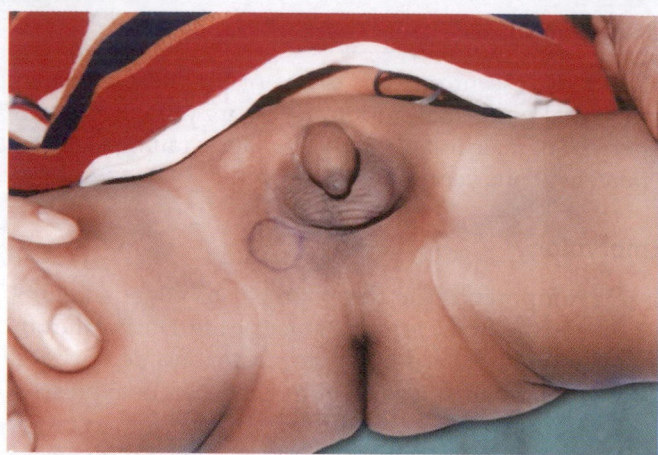

Fig. 43: Ectopic testis (right) (*Courtesy:* Professor Ashish Wakhlu)

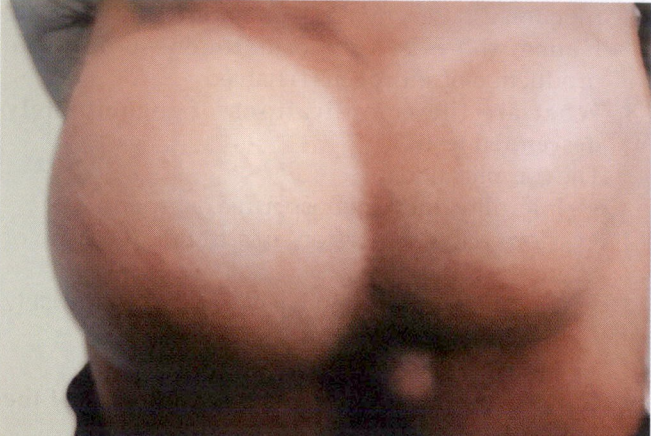

Fig. 44: Bilateral large inguinal hernias in a patient 52 years of age with bilateral undescended testis. Hernias are reducible. The penis is visible below the swellings. Ultrasound confirmed the diagnosis. The hernias look like buttocks

Clinical Features

The patient is brought or comes with empty hemiscrotum or scrotum at one year. The causes of this phenomenon are:
1. Incompletely descended testis.
2. Truly absent testis.
3. Retractile testis.
4. Ectopic testis.

A retractile testis can be coaxed into the scrotal sac while an ectopic and incompletely descended testis cannot be brought down.

Palpability: Depending upon the palpability the imperfectly descended testis is of two types: palpable and impalpable. All ectopic testes are usually palpable.

Complications

1. Infertility: It is inevitable in bilateral, common in unilateral, and frequent in those who have had undescent treated.
2. Torsion.
3. More likely to get traumatized than normal testis.
4. Inguinal hernia, a common association with undescent (Fig. 44).
5. Malignant transformation, usually seminoma. Orchiopexy does not reduce the risk but it may help in early detection.
6. Epididymo-orchitis in an incompletely descended testis on the right side resembles acute appendicitis.

Pathology

The testis in imperfectly descended testis is normal at birth and remains so for quite some time (5-6 years), then gradually degenerative changes start occurring in it and at puberty it is small, flabby or soft and poorly developed as compared to normally placed testis.

Histologically the epithelial cells are immature and by 16 years of age irreversible destruction occurs. It prevents spermatogenesis and halves the production of androgens.

If orchidopexy is done early in life the testis develops and functions satisfactorily.

Investigations

A palpable testis does not require any investigation. It is the impalpable testis which needs visualization, and it is done by ultrasonography, CT scan, MRI or laparoscopy. They give information whether it is absent or present, and if present where is it situated.

Treatment

Human chorionic gonadotropin has been used but it has not helped because imperfect descent is usually due to mechanical reasons. The treatment is surgical, which must be done as early as possible usually at the age of 1 year. However, if the child is brought late but before puberty with normal testis, orchidopexy should be done; and if brought with atrophic testis, orchidectomy is the usual practice. Orchidopexy has the following advantages:
1. The testis remains 2 to 5° C cooler than body temperature which is essential for spermatogenesis.
2. It enables early detection of malignant transformation.
3. It produces a good cosmetic result.

Palpable testis: It is treated by a single stage open orchidopexy under general anesthesia as a day case. The testis is exposed through a groin crease incision and mobilized by dividing gubernaculum. The associated patent processus vaginalis is dissected out and herniotomy is performed. The testis is delivered from within the tunica vaginalis and the hydatid of Morgagni is excised if present. The testis is placed in the scrotum in an extra-dartos pouch where it is secured by co-apting the dartos around the spermatic cord. The results of this procedure are good.

Impalpable testis: It is diagnosed and treated by laparoscopy. The vas and testicular vessels must be seen throughout their full extent. The possibilities are:

1. Blind-ending vas and vessels with no evident testis: the 'vanishing testis'.
2. Normal or attenuated vas and vessels entering the inguinal canal through the internal ring.
3. Good sized testis within the peritoneal cavity.

The first type does not need any further treatment.

The second type is treated by open inguinal canal exploration with orchidopexy of a normal testis or excision of a small testicular remnant that does not have any function but have enhanced malignant potential.

The third type is treated by a single-stage microvascular transfer with the gonadal vessels being divided high near the renal vessels and anastomosed onto the inferior epigastric vessels; or a two-stage Fowler-Stevens orchidopexy.

CASE 14: HYPOSPADIAS

CLINICAL DIAGNOSIS

1. The patient is usually a child or young adult who presents with some defects in the penis since birth (Fig. 45).
2. The floor of the urethra is absent partially or completely with external urinary meatus being situated on the undersurface of penis rather at the tip.
3. The meatus is smaller than normal.
4. There may be blind depression at the normal site of meatus on the glans penis.
5. The prepuce is hood-shaped and is absent on the ventral surface.
6. The glans is flattened on its ventral aspect (Fig. 45).
7. The penis may be ill-developed and may have a ventral curvature (chordee).
8. The patient may have dysuria. In a grown up person there may be sexual dysfunction.

VIVA VOCE

1. **What is hypospadias?**

   It is a congenital abnormality of urethra (and penis) where the external urinary meatus is situated on the ventral surface of penis proximal to the normal site.

2. **What are the types of hypospadias?**

   Hypospadias is of the following types (Figs 46 and 47):

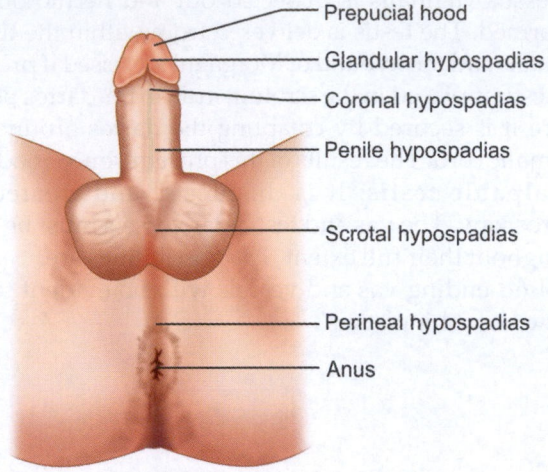

Fig. 46: Types of hypospadias

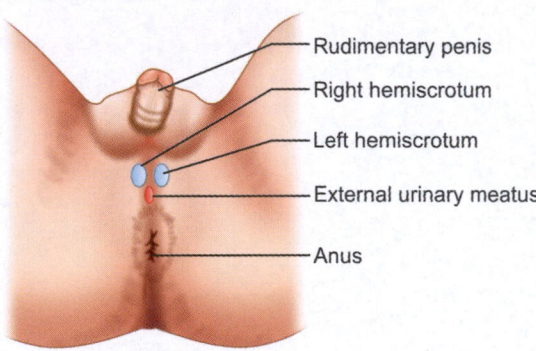

Fig. 47: Perineal hypospadias

- *Glandular type*—The external meatus is situated on the undersurface of glans penis. There is no chordee and the penis is straight.
- *Coronal type*—The meatus is situated at corona. In this type there is minimal chordee.
- *Penile or balanic*—The meatus is situated on the ventral surface of shaft of penis. The chordee is a prominent feature of this type.
- *Penoscrotal*—The meatus is situated at penoscrotal junction.
- *Scrotal*—The meatus opens up on the median raphe of scrotum. The scrotum is small and partially bifid.
- *Perineal*—The scrotum is completely bifid and the meatus opens either between the two halves or anywhere along the perineal raphe. The penis is very small with severe chordee.

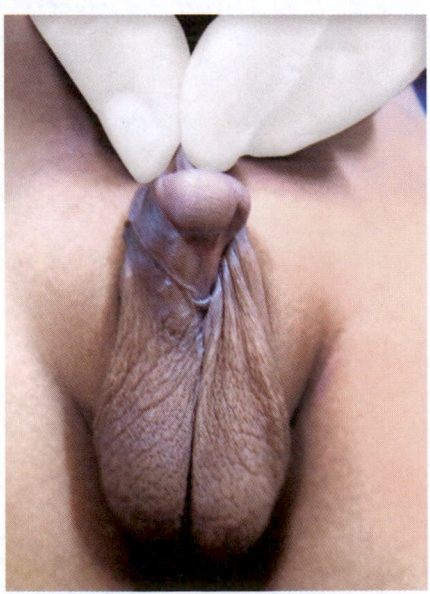

Fig. 45: Coronal hypospadias

3. **What is the cause of penile hypospadias?**
It is due to failure of fusion of anterior part of the medial labial folds.

4. **What is the cause of perineal hypospadias?**
It is due to complete failure of fusion of genital folds after the rupture of urogenital membrane.

5. **What is chordee?**
Chordee is a fibrous cord situated distal to ectopic meatus at the site of absent urethra and corpus spongiosum. Contracture of this fibrous cord results in a downward curvature of penis. The more proximal is the site of urinary meatus the more severe is the chordee (Fig. 48).

6. **Why is the prepuce hood-shaped?**
The prepuce is hood-shaped as it is deficient on ventral aspect due to failure of fusion of genital folds.

7. **Why are the glandular and coronal hypospadias more common than the posterior ones (scrotal, perineal)?**
It is because the fusion of medial labial folds begins posteriorly and then proceeds anteriorly, hence the deficiency of fusion is more common towards the tip of penis.

8. **What are the other common congenital abnormalities associated with a hypospadias?**
The other associated abnormalities are –
1. Imperfectly descended testes.
2. Bifid scrotum with female type of appearance of perineum.

9. **How does a hypospadias disturb penile function?**
The penile dysfunction depends upon the type of hypospadias, i.e. in glandular type there is hardly any penile dysfunction while in perineal type there is hardly any penile function.
   - Micturition:
     1. The urinary stream is deflected downwards resulting in soiling of garments. It is due to
ventral situation of meatus and curvature of penis (Fig. 49).
     2. Dysuria, if there is meatal stenosis.
   - Sexual function:
     1. Because of chordee the penetration may be difficult.
     2. During erection, the curvature may be exaggerated resulting in priapism.
     3. The semen may not be deposited at the proper place in the vagina. Hence, scrotal and perineal hypospadias are associated with infertility.
     4. The posterior type of hypospadias may be associated with bilateral undescended testes with very small penis. These patients may not have any sexual desire and function.

10. **How do you treat hypospadias?**
The essentials of treatment are:
a. Glandular hypospadias
   1. Usually no treatment is required.
   2. If meatal stenosis is there, meatotomy or meatoplasty is done.
b. Other types are treated by operative reconstruction which is usually done in two stages:
   Stage 1—Straightening of penis by excision of chordee.
   Stage 2—Reconstruction of urethra.

11. **What is the age of chordee correction?**
It is done preferably between one and a half to two years.

12. **What is age for urethral reconstruction?**
It is done preferably between 4 to 6 years.

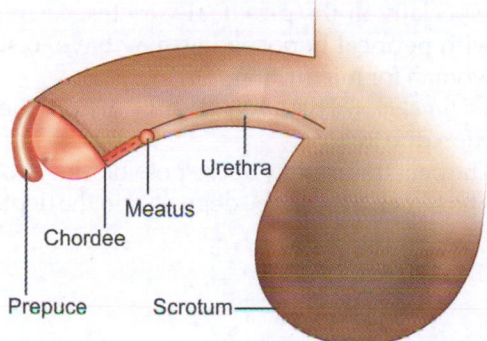

Fig. 48: Pathology of penile hypospadias showing bending of penis due to the presence of chordee

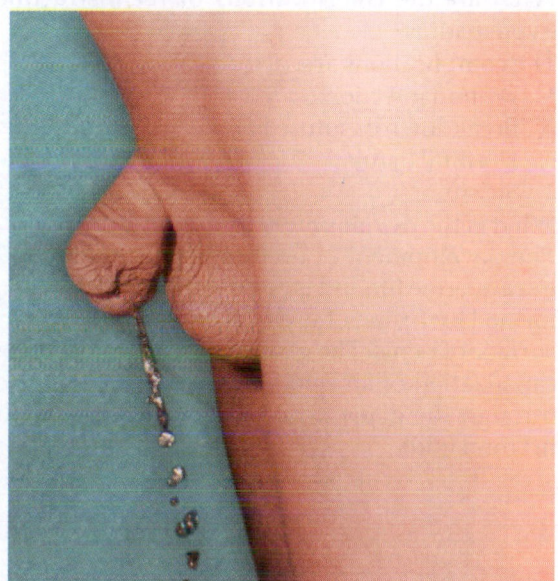

Fig. 49: A patient of coronal hypospadias passing urine. Note the vertical fall of stream (*Courtesy:* Professor Ashish Wakhlu)

13. **What happens to the urethral meatus after chordee correction?**

Following chordee correction the urethral meatus recedes proximally towards the perineum. Thus a coronal hypospadias becomes penile, and a distal penile becomes a proximal penile hypospadias.

14. **How do you reconstruct a new urethra?**

There are many methods of reconstruction of urethra but the following are the common methods:
1. From penile skin.
2. From prepucial skin.
3. From scrotal skin.

15. **How is the urethra reconstructed from penile skin?**

In this method (Denis Browne) the urethral tube is made by burying a strip of skin along the line of urethral meatus which grows out from the edge into a complete tube.

16. **A patient of hypospadias wants circumcision for religious purposes, will you do it?**

No, it should not be done.

17. **Why?**

Because the prepucial skin may be used for urethral reconstruction.

18. **What is the disadvantage of making urethra from scrotal skin?**

The hair will grow in the urethra and may cause dysuria or urethral obstruction.

19. **How does the patient pass urine till a new urethra is formed?**

The urine is diverted by any of the following methods-
1. Perineal urethrostomy (anterior types).
2. Suprapubic cystostomy (posterior types).

20. **What are the complications of reconstruction in hypospadias?**

The complications are:
1. Wound infection.
2. Breakdown of suture line.
3. Urethral fistula.
4. Stricture.

21. **What is the development of urethra?**

The development of urethra begins at 8th week of intra-uterine life and is completed by 15th week. It is formed by fusion of urethral folds along the ventral surface of penis. The glandular urethra develops by canalization of an ectodermal cord that has grown through the glans to communicate with the fused urethral folds.

22. **What is chordee without hypospadias?**

It is a rare anomaly which is caused by a short urethra, and fibrous tissues surrounding the corpus spongiosum or both. It is a ventral chordee.

DISCUSSION

Hypospadias is a congenital malformation of urethra in which the external meatus opens up more proximally on the undersurface of penis or perineum (Fig. 45).

Anatomical types—It is classified into 5 types according to the position of the meatus (Figs 46 and 47)-

1. *Glandular type*—The meatus is situated on the undersurface of glans penis. The normal site of urethral meatus is marked by a blind pit which may be sometimes connected by a channel to the ectopic meatus. It is the commonest hypospadias.
2. *Coronal type*—The meatus is situated at the junction of glans with the shaft (corona) on the undersurface of penis.
3. *Penile type*—The meatus is on the undersurface of shaft of penis. About 70 percent of hypospadias are distal penile or coronal.
4. *Perineal type*—It is the most severe type. The scrotum is bifid and meatus is sited in between its two halves. The testes may be maldescended and penis very small. Hence, it may be difficult to determine the sex of the child.

Chordee—The urethra and corpus spongiosum distal to the ectopic opening are absent, and represented by a fibrous cord which deforms the penis in a downward direction. This is chordee. The more severe is the hypospadias the more pronounced is the bowing (Fig. 48).

Pathophysiology

- *Micturition*—The micturition function may be disturbed due to:
  1. Meatal stenosis which is quite common.
  2. The projection of urinary stream may be lost, especially in the proximal varietes, e.g. a patient with perineal hypospadias may have to sit like a woman for micturition.
- *Sexual function*—This anomaly may disturb the sexual function due to:
  1. The penetration may not be possible due to chrodee.
  2. The semen may not be deposited in the depth of the vagina.

These alterations in the sexual function are proportionate to the severity of hypospadias.

The glans penis is splayed out and exposed. The prepuce is hood-shaped and not present on the inferior aspect of penis.

Investigations

- In distal type no investigations are usually required.
- In severe or proximal types an IVU may be done to detect additional congenital anomalies of kidneys and ureters.
- Urethroscopy and cystoscopy are done to find whether the internal male sexual organs are normal.
- Buccal smear and karyotyping may be done to establish the genetic sex.

Treatment

Glandular hypospadias—It does not require any treatment unless the urethral meatus is narrowed in which case a meatotomy is performed.

Other types—They all require some plastic reconstructive procedure to correct the chordee and reconstruct the urethra that is missing by making a skin tube from prepuce, penile skin or scrotum. Hence, no circumcision is done in these patients.

Currently repair is being done using island flap grafts taken from bladder or oral mucosa. The oral mucosa is being preferred more and more.

The chordee correction is confirmed by producing artificial erection by injecting saline into corpus cavernosum and placing a tourniquet at the root of penis.

The defect should be corrected usually in a single stage before the child goes to school.

CASE 15: EPISPADIAS

CLINICAL DIAGNOSIS

1. The patient is usually a child or young adult who presents with the external urinary meatus on the dorsum of penis (Figs 50 and 51).
2. The meatus may be situated on the dorsum of glans (glandular), shaft (penile) or at the root of penis (total epispadias).
3. The meatus may be narrow.
4. The penis is usually smaller than normal.
5. The patient may have dysuria or dribbling of urine.

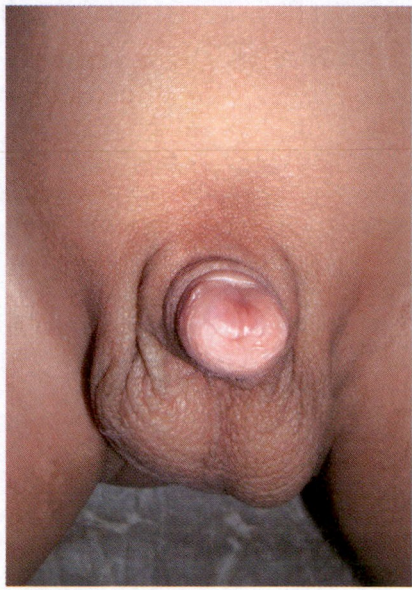

Fig. 50: Epispadias (*Courtesy:* Professor Rajiv Agarwal)

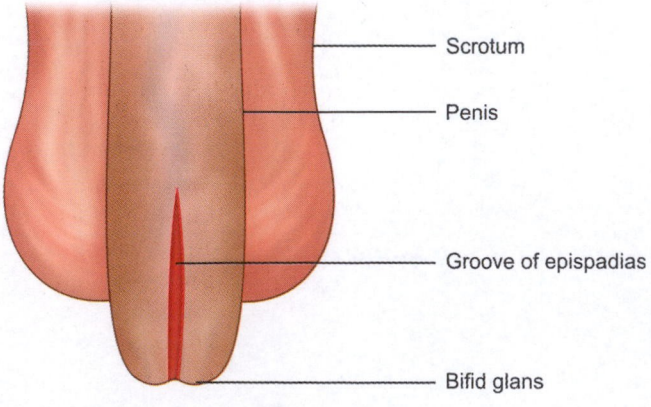

- Scrotum
- Penis
- Groove of epispadias
- Bifid glans

Fig. 51: Epispadias

VIVA VOCE

1. **What is epispadias?**
   It is a congenital anomaly in which the external urinary meatus is situated on the dorsal aspect of penis (Figs 50 and 51).
2. **What is its incidence?**
   It is a rare anomaly, occurring once in 30,000 births.
3. **What are the types of epispadias?**
   It is of three types—glandular, penile and total.
4. **What is glandular epispadias?**
   In this type, the external meatus is situated on the dorsum of glans penis.
5. **What is penile epispadias?**
   Here, the meatus is situated on the dorsum of shaft of penis.
6. **Is there a chordee present?**
   Yes, similar to hypospadias a chordee may be present.
7. **What is epispadias totalis?**
   In this type, the urethra is totally deficient. It is usually associated with ectopia vesicae.
8. **What is the most significant symptom of total epispadias?**
   Constant dribbling of urine.
9. **How do you treat this lesion?**
   - The glandular type may not require any treatment, or it may be treated like penile type.
   - The penile type is treated by Duplay's operation.
   - The penopubic type is treated by Cantwell-Ransley repair.
10. **What is Duplay's operation?**
    The edges of the open urethra are made raw, undermined and sutured over a catheter.
11. **What is Cantwell-Ransley repair?**
    It involves dissection of urethra from the corpora, urethral reconstruction and displacement of neourethral tube ventrally.

DISCUSSION

Epispadias is a congenital abnormality of urethra and penis in which the external urethral meatus is situated on the dorsum of penis. In contrast to hypospadias this anomaly is very rare. It is seen once in 30,000 live male births.

Types

It may occur in isolation, or more commonly in association with ectopia vesicae as a part of the exstrophy-epispadias complex. The most consistent finding with the latter type is some degree of separation of pubic symphysis. The isolated variety is of three types—penopubic, penile and glandular. The first type is associated with incontinence, which may or may not be present in the second type. There is no incontinence in glandular type.

Distal to the opening there is a mucosal groove alongwith a flattened glans. The penis is curved upwards and may be underdeveloped.

Isolated epispadias is seen less commonly in a female. It is associated with bifid clitoris.

Treatment

- The glandular variety does not need any treatment, or may be treated like penile type.
- The penile type is treated by Duplay's operation which is done at the age of 3 years. The edges of open urethra are made raw, undermined and sutured over a catheter, or reconstructed by island flap technique.
- The penopubic type is treated by Cantwell-Ranslay repair which involves the dissection of urethra from the corpora, urethral reconstruction and displacement of neourethral tube ventrally.
- The total type is treated by repair of ectopia, urethroplasty and reconstruction of a sphincter.

CASE 16: CONGENITAL TALIPES EQUINOVARUS (CLUB FOOT)

CLINICAL DIAGNOSIS

1. The patient is a newborn who is brought with unilateral or bilateral deformity of the foot.
2. The foot is plantar flexed, inverted and adducted and the sole faces inwards (Figs 52A and B).
3. The foot is smaller and cannot be fully dorsiflexed.

4. The outer border of the foot is convex (Fig. 53). In late disease there may be callosities on the lateral aspect of foot.

VIVA VOCE

1. **What is the incidence of congenital talipes equinovarus (CTEV)?**
   - It occurs once in 1000 live births.
   - It is more common in boys than girls.
   - It is bilateral in about half the cases.
2. **What is the cause of this condition?**
   - It is a congenital anomaly which may be due to many factors. There is 20 times increased risk if it occurs in a first-degree relative.
   - There is racial prevalence among Polynesians.
   - It may be syndromic or associated with arthrogryposis.
3. **What do you mean by equinus?**
   Equinus is derived from *equine* that means a horse who walks on toes. In this deformity the foot is fixed in plantar flexion.
4. **Which is the commonest deformity of foot?**
   Congenital talipes equinovarus is the commonest deformity of foot.
5. **Which is the next common deformity of foot?**
   The next common deformity is talipes calcaneovalgus which is just opposite to CTEV.
6. **What are the types of CTEV depending upon the severity?**

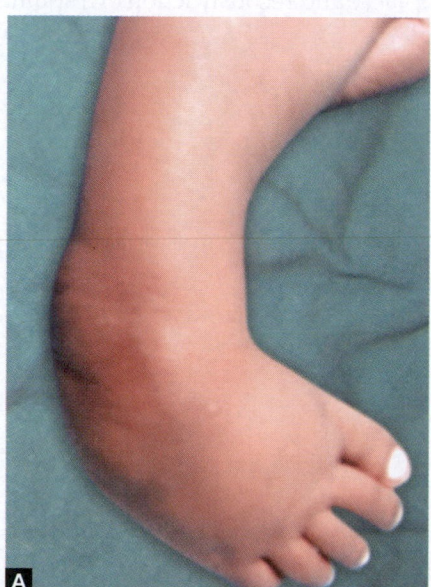

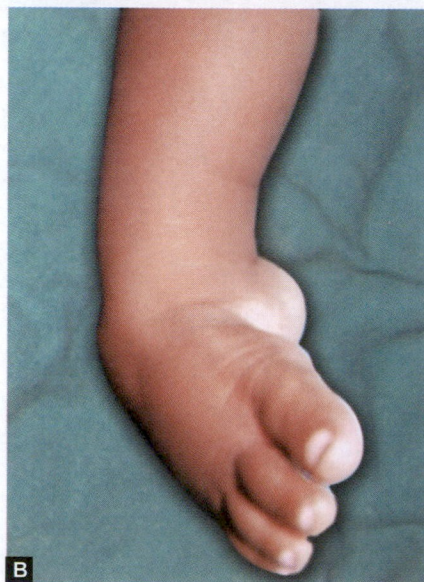

Figs 52A and B: Congenital talipes equinovarus
(*Courtesy:* Dr Uttam Garg)

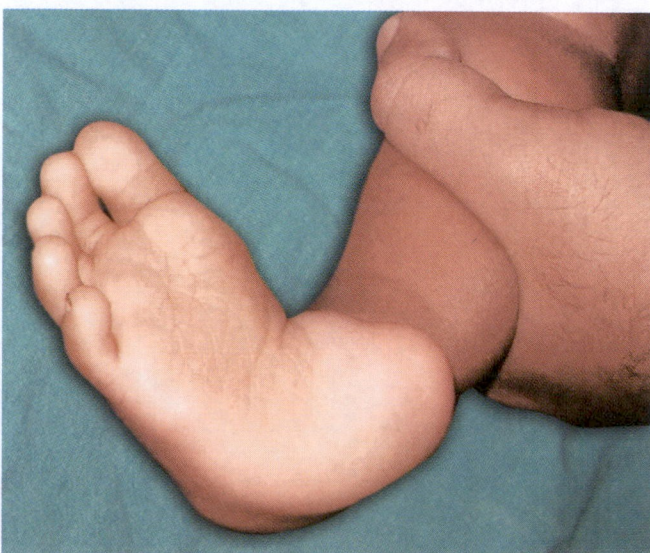

Fig. 53: Congenital talipes equinovarus—Plantar view
(*Courtesy:* Dr Uttam Garg)

It is of two types:
- Postural form: It is easily treatable by simple measures.
- Severe form: It is associated with arthrogryposis or tibial deficiency.

7. What are the changes in the bones of foot?

The bones are smaller than normal. The neck of the talus is angulated. Hence the head of talus faces downwards and medially. The calcaneum is also smaller and concave medially.

8. What are the changes in the joints of foot?

- The joints of the foot are malpositioned. The equinus occurs at ankle joint and the inversion occurs at subtalar joint.
- The inverted calcaneum takes the foot with it so that the sole faces medially.
- The adduction of forefoot occurs at midtarsal joints, mainly the talonavicular joint. There is excessive arching of the foot at the midtarsal joint.

9. Can a patient of this deformity walk?

If the deformity is not treated, the child walks on the lateral border of foot.

10. What are the effects of this walking?

As a result of walking on the deformed foot, the deformity is exaggerated and callosities and bursae develop on the bony prominences on the lateral border of the foot.

11. What is Kite's angle?

It is the angle between the long axes of talus and calcaneum (talocalcaneal angle).

12. What is its importance?

It is reduced in CTEV. Normally it is more than 35^0.

13. When will you treat this condition?

The treatment is started as early as possible.

14. How do you treat CTEV?

Mild disease is treated by nonoperative measures whereas severe disease requires surgical measures.

15. What is the criterion of successful treatment?

The criteria of successful treatment is given below:

- The foot, especially the heel should go flat on the ground (plantigrade foot)
- The patient must be able to wear normal shoes.
- The joint mobility is preserved as much as possible.

16. What is nonoperative treatment?

It consists of the following:

- Stretching or manipulation
- Strapping or serial plastering
- Splintage and special boots.

17. What is the technique of manipulation or stretching?

The mother manipulates the foot after every feed in an opposite direction to the deformity – the foot is dorsiflexed and everted. During stretching sufficient pressure is maintained for 5 seconds at a time.

18. What is the technique of keeping the foot in corrected position?

When the child is about one month old the foot is manipulated under sedation—the adduction is corrected first followed by inversion and then equinus deformity. Following reduction a below knee plaster cast is given which is changed every 2 weeks and continued till the deformities are corrected.

19. If this sequence in reduction is not followed what is the harm?

It may result in a rocker-bottom foot where the heel remains equinus and there is mid-foot breach.

20. What is the posttreatment care?

The feet are kept in corrected position by using a Denis-Brown splint. When the child starts walking CTEV shoes are used during the day and D-B splint at night (Fig. 54).

21. What is special about CTEV shoes?

They have a straight inner border to prevent forefoot adduction, outer shoe raise to prevent inversion and have no heel to prevent equinus.

22. What will you do if the nonoperative treatment fails?

In such cases surgical treatment is required. Most of the cases do well if the posterior, medial and plantar soft tissues are released and tendon lengthening is done.

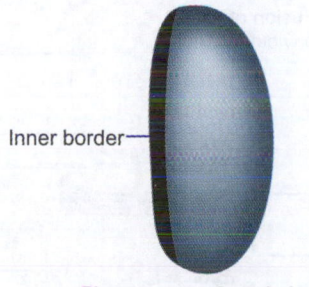
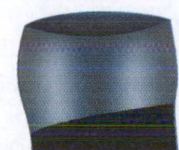
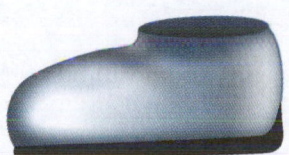

Inner border—

Shoe as seen from below showing straight inner border

Posterior view of the shoe showing outer raise of heel

Shoe without raised heel as seen from side

Fig. 54: CTEV shoes

23. **What is actually done in soft tissue release?**
    • Posteriorly the tendo-Achilles is lengthened (Fig. 55) and posterior capsules of ankle and subtalar joints and posterior tibiofibular and calcaneofibular ligaments are released.
    • Medially tibialis posterior, flexor digitorum longus and flexor hallucis longus tendons are lengthened and their contracted sheaths are excised. Further talo-navicular, superficial part of deltoid and spring ligaments are released. In severe disease interosseous talocalcaneal ligament, and capsules of naviculocuneiform and cuneiform-first metatarsal joints may have to be released.
    • Inferiorly release of plantar fascia, short flexors of toes and abductor hallucis from their origin on the calcaneum is required.

24. **What is the role of tendon transfer?**
    It may be required in children more than 5 years of age. To balance the weak peronei (evertors) the tibialis anterior is transferred to the outer side of the foot as there are two strong invertor tendons—tibialis anterior and tibialis posterior.

25. **What is Dwyer's osteotomy?**
    It is an open wedge osteotomy of calcaneum done in children more than 3 years of age to correct varus of the heel (Fig. 56).

26. **Why osteotomy is done in children more than 3 years of age?**
    Because before 3 years of age the calcaneum is cartilaginous.

27. **What is Dilwyn-Evan's operation?**
    In this operation the posteromedial soft tissue release is combined with calcaneocuboid fusion to reduce the growth of the lateral side of foot. It is done at 4 to 8 years of age.

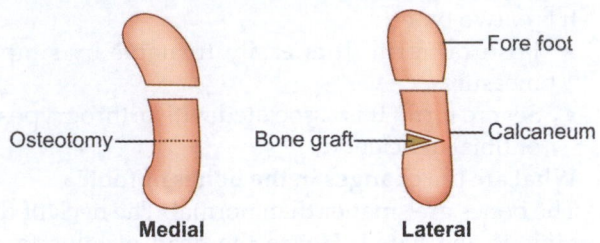

Fig. 56: Correction of varus by Dwyer's osteotomy

28. **What is the role of wedge tarsectomy?**
    It is indicated in neglected disease at 8 to 11 years of age. A wedge of bones from the mid-tarsal area with its base on the dorsolateral side is removed. It brings the foot in normal position.

29. **What is triple arthrodesis?**
    This operation is done after 12 years of age and consists of fusion of subtalar, calcaneocuboid and talonavicular joints after removing appropriate wedges to correct the deformity (Fig. 57).

30. **What is Ilizarov's technique?**
    Here, the different components of the deformity are corrected by gradual stretching using an external fixator followed by plastering.

31. **What are the indications of Ilizarov's technique?**
    It is indicated in neglected club foot and in recurrent deformity.

DISCUSSION

CTEV is a deformity of foot in three planes involving many joints and consists of a number of deformities of the shape of the foot, i.e.
• *Equinus (equinus means a horse):* The foot is fixed in plantar flexion.
• *Calcaneous:* The foot is fixed in dorsiflexion.
• *Varus:* The foot is inverted and adducted at the midtarsal joints so that the sole faces inwards.

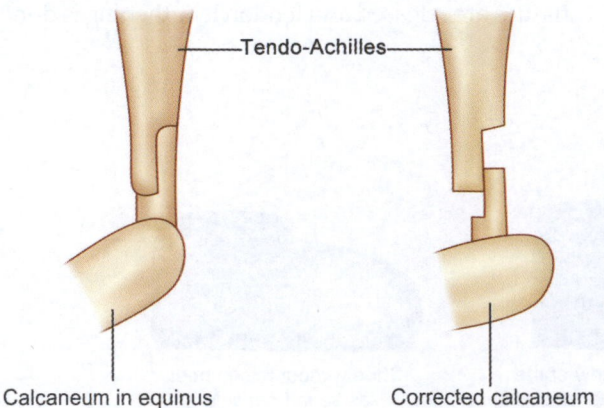

Fig. 55: Lengthening of tendo-Achilles by Z-plasty

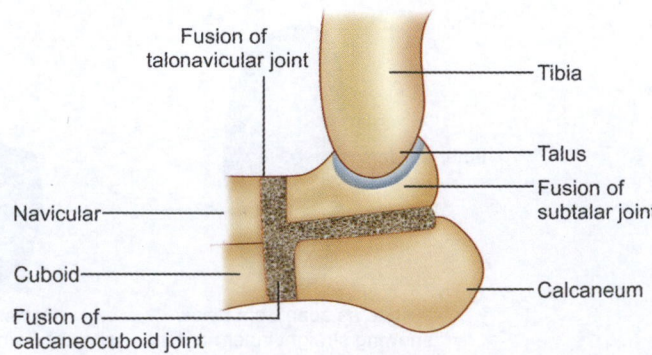

Fig. 57: Fusion of 3 joints of foot after correction of deformity

- Valgus: The foot is everted and abducted at the mid-tarsal joints. Hence, the sole faces outwards.

Usually a combination of deformities occur, the commonest being equinovarus and the next common is calcaneovalgus (Figs 52 and 53).

Incidence

- The deformity is usually obvious at birth. It occurs once in 1000 live births.
- It is more prevalent in boys than girls.
- Both the lower limbs are involved in up to 50% of patients.

Etiology

- *Idiopathic CTEV:* It is a congenital deformity which may be the result of multifactorial inheritance. There is 20 times increased risk if it occurs in a first degree relative. There is racial prevalence among Polynesians. Increased intra-uterine pressure may be etiologically related to this deformity. The most difficult cases are syndromic or are associated with arthrogryposis multiplex congenita.
- *Secondary:* CTEV type deformity may occur in some paralytic disorders leading to local muscle imbalance, e.g. poliomyelitis, spina bifida and myelodysplasia. If the invertors and plantar flexors are stronger than the evertors and dorsi-flexors, equinovarus will occur.

Pathology

All the tissues of the foot have developmental abnormality:
- *Bones:* The bones are smaller than normal. The neck of the talus is angulated so that the head of talus faces downwards and medially. The calcaneum is concave medially.
- *Joints:* The deformities are due to malpositioning of joints of the foot. The equinus occurs at the ankle joint and the inversion occurs at subtalar joint. The inverted calcaneum takes the whole foot with it so that the sole faces medially.

  The adduction of the forefoot occurs at midtarsal joints, mainly the talonavicular joints. There is excessive arching of the foot at the midtarsal joints.
- *Muscles:* The following muscles are contracted – tendo-Achilles, tibialis posterior, flexor digitorum longus and flexor hallucis longus.
- *Ligaments:* The ligaments of the postero-medial side of the foot are shortened.
- *Skin:* The skin of the medial side of the sole is shortened and have deep creases. If the deformity is not treated and the child walks on the deformed foot, the deformity is exaggerated and callosities and bursae develop on the bony prominences on the lateral border of foot.

Clinical Features

The problem may be detected at birth or the child may be brought for treatment during infancy or late childhood.
- The foot is smaller and is in equinus, varus and adduction. It cannot be fully dorsiflexed while normally the foot touches the anterior aspect of shin when dorsiflexed
- The heel is small and not in line with the leg. The calcaneum may be felt with difficulty
- The head of talus and the lateral malleolus are more prominent
- The outer border of the foot is convex. There may be cavus with a palpably tight band in the sole
- In late disease, there may be callosities on the lateral aspect of foot. The calf muscles are wasted.

Full physical examination of the patient is done to rule out other congenital abnormalities, especially of the hip and spine.

Investigations

- Radiography of the foot both anteroposterior and lateral is done with the foot in whatever corrected position possible. The talo-calcaneal angle (the angle between the long axes of talus and calcaneum—Kite's angle) is determined. It is reduced in CTEV, normal being more than 35°. For greater details of the pathologic anatomy CT scan may be done.
- Radiography, CT scan or MRI of the spine may be done if there is some associated spinal problem.

Treatment

- The parents must be told that the foot cannot be made normal. It is likely to be stiffer and smaller than normal. Also the calf will remain thin.
- The treatment is started as early as possible and consists of correction of deformity by nonoperative and operative methods, followed by maintenance of foot in corrected position. It is continued till one is sure that there will be no recurrence.
- Non-operative treatment:
  1. The mother is taught to manipulate the foot after every feed in an opposite direction to the deformity —the foot is dorsiflexed and everted. During manipulation sufficient pressure is maintained for 5 seconds at a time.
  2. Manipulation and strapping or corrective plaster— When the child is about 1 month old the foot is

manipulated under sedation—the adduction is corrected first followed by inversion and then equinus deformity. If this sequence is not followed, rocker-bottom foot may result (the heel remains equinus and there is midfoot breach).

3. Following reduction a below-knee plaster cast is given which is changed every 2 weeks and continued till the deformities are over-corrected. It usually needs 6 to 8 casts.

- Operative treatment:

The indications for operative treatment are—severe deformity which does not respond to nonoperative treatment, if the deformity has recurred and late or neglected clubfoot.

Usually posterior, medial and plantar soft tissue release and tendon lengthening is required. The procedure is followed by an above knee plaster that is changed after 2 weeks. The soft tissue release operations may be sufficient in children below 3 years of age. Bony operations may be required for older children.

1. Postero-medial soft tissue release (PMSTR): In this procedure the following structures are released: Posteriorly the tendo-Achilles is lengthened by a Z-plasty (Fig. 56). The posterior capsules of ankle and subtalar joints are released and posterior tibio-fibular and calcaneo-fibular ligaments are also released.

Medially 3 tendons: Tibialis posterior, flexor digitorum longus and flexor hallucis longus are lengthened, and their contracted and thickened sheaths are excised. Also, 3 ligaments: talo-navicular, superficial part of deltoid and spring ligaments are released. In severe cases interosseous talo-calcaneal ligament and capsules of naviculo-cuneiform and cuneiform-first metatarsal joints may have to be released.

Inferiorly release of plantar fascia, and short flexors of the toes (flexor digitorum brevis) and abductor hallucis from their origin on the calcaneum is required.

2. Limited soft tissue release: It is indicated when one of the components of deformity (adduction, equinus, varus or cavus) escapes correction by nonoperative treatment. For equinus, a posterior release for adduction a medial release and for cavus a planter release is required.

3. Tendon transfer: It is done in children more than 5-years of age. To balance the weak peronei (evertors) the tibialis anterior is transferred to the outer side of the foot as there are 2 strong invertor tendons – tibialis anterior and tibialis posterior.

4. Dwyer's osteotomy: It is an open wedge osteotomy of calcaneum done in children more than 3 years of age to correct varus of the heal (Fig. 56). Before 3 years of age the calcaneum is cartilaginous.

5. Dilwyn-Evan's operation: It is done in children 4 to 8 years of age. Here, the postero-medial soft tissue release (PMSTR) is combined with calcaneo-cuboid fusion to reduce the growth of the lateral side of the foot.

6. Wedge tarsectomy: It is indicated in neglected disease of the age of 8–11 years. It consists of removing a wedge of bone from the midtarsal area with its base on the dorso-lateral side. It brings the foot in normal (plantigrade) position.

7. Triple arthrodesis: It is done after the age 12 years and consists of fusion of subtalar, calcaneo-cuboid and talo-navicular joints after removing appropriate wedges to correct the deformity (Fig. 57).

8. Ilizarov's technique: It is indicated in neglected club foot and in recurrent cases. The different components of the deformity are corrected by gradual stretching using an external fixator followed by plastering.

BB Joshi from Mumbai used a simpler method known as JESS fixation.

- Methods of maintaining the correction

1. Denis-Brown splint: It holds the foot in corrected position. It is used throughout the day before the child starts walking. When walking is started, it is used at night and CTEV shoes during the day.

2. CTEV shoes: These shoes have straight inner border to prevent forefoot adduction, outer shoe raise to prevent inversion and have no heel to prevent equinus (Fig. 54).

CASE 17: ANKYLOSIS OF TEMPOROMANDIBULAR JOINT

CLINICAL DIAGNOSIS

1. The patient presents with inability to open the mouth that is of insidious onset.
2. The mouth (jaws) can be opened partially or completely.
3. In long-standing cases the chin may be receded back, and atrophic (Fig. 58 and 59).
4. There may be evidence of dental decay.

VIVA VOCE

1. **What is ankylosis?**
   Inability to open or move a joint is called ankylosis.
2. **What are the types of ankylosis?**
   The ankylosis is of two types—intra-articular and extra-articular.
3. **What are the causes of intra-articular ankylosis of temporomandibular joint?**
   It is due to lesions of the joint where the joint cavity is obliterated by bony tissue. The causes are suppurative arthritis of the temporomandibular joint. It may follow

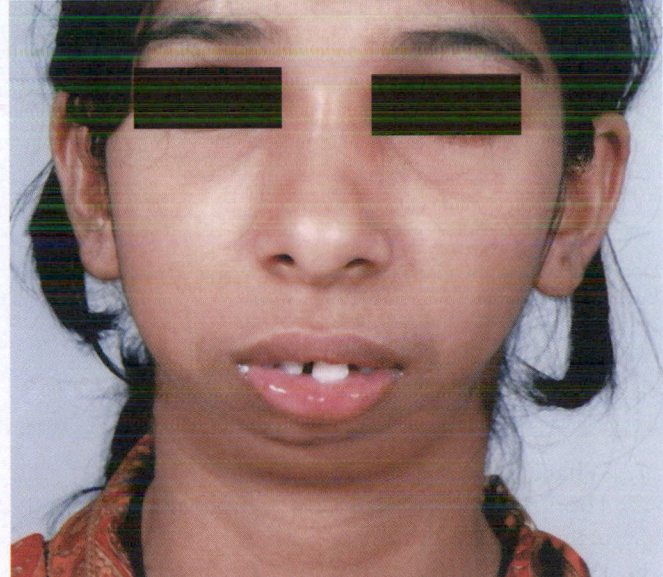

Fig. 59: Front view of an old case of ankylosis which occurred during childhood with very poor development of chin (*Courtesy:* Professor Rajiv Agarwal)

fractures of the condyle or fracture-dislocations of TMJ.

4. **What are the causes of extra-articular ankylosis?**
   It is due to lesions around the joint causing fibrosis and contracture of the soft tissues. The causes are severe periarticular infections such as cancrum oris, gun-shot injury, operations inside the mouth, destruction of the mucosa of fauces or cheek by operative or radiation injury, osteomyelitis of the mandible spreading into muscles of mastication and submucous fibrosis of the cheek.
5. **What are the effects on the health?**
   - The nutrition of the patient does not suffer as the patient continues to take liquid foods that enter the oral cavity through the spaces between the teeth and the retromolar space
   - There occurs early tooth decay as the hygiene of the oral cavity cannot be maintained
   - If the ankylosis occurs in the early childhood, the mandible fails to develop leading to receding chin directed towards the affected side. The chin does not develop and the receded and atrophic chin gives the face a bird-like facial profile (Fig. 58).

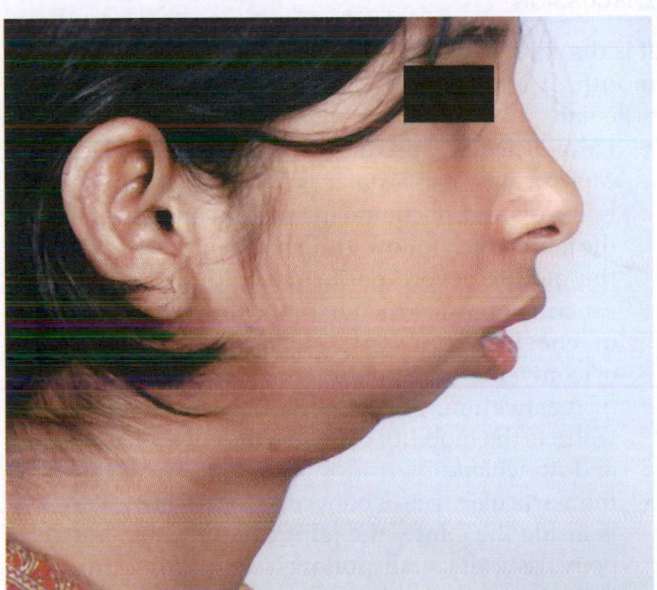

Fig. 58: Shrew-mouse appearance in a case of TMJ ankylosis (*Courtesy:* Professor Rajiv Agarwal)

6. What are the differences between extra-articular and intra-articular ankylosis of TMJ?

Feature	Extra-articular ankylosis	Intra-articular ankylosis
Site of lesion	Around the joint	Inside the joint
Causes	• Cancrum oris • Gun-shot injuries of parotid region • Radiation injury • Operations on cheek • Submucous fibrosis of cheek	• Suppurative arthritis of TMJ • Fracture dislocation of TMJ
Opening of the mouth	Some opening or movement is possible	No movement at all
X-ray	Joint space is normal	Joint space obliterated by bony tissue (Fig. 61)
Treatment	Osteotomy of mandible near the angle	TMJ arthroplasty

7. What are the investigations?

The joint is visualized by radiography (Fig. 60), orthopantomography or CT scan.

8. What are the indications of CT scan?

It is indicated when the finer details of the lesion, joint and around the joint are required to be seen.

9. How do you treat this problem?

The treatment depends upon the type of ankylosis.

10. How do you treat extra-articular ankylosis?

- It is treated by removal of the cause, e.g. repair of cancrum oris defects with flaps, excision of submucous fibrous tissue and grafting, release of fibrous contractures
- If the cause cannot be removed, the mouth may be opened by extra-articular arthroplasty of Esmarch.

11. What do you do in Esmarch arthroplasty?

A wedge of bone from the mandible just in front of angle, 2 cm broad at lower margin and tapering to a point behind the last molar is excised.

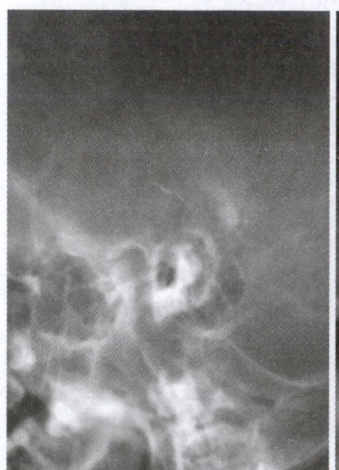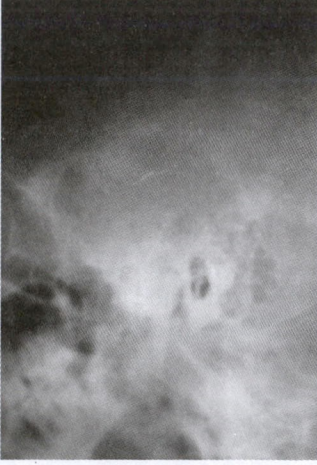

Fig. 60: Radiography of TMJ with normal right joint and ankylosed left joint

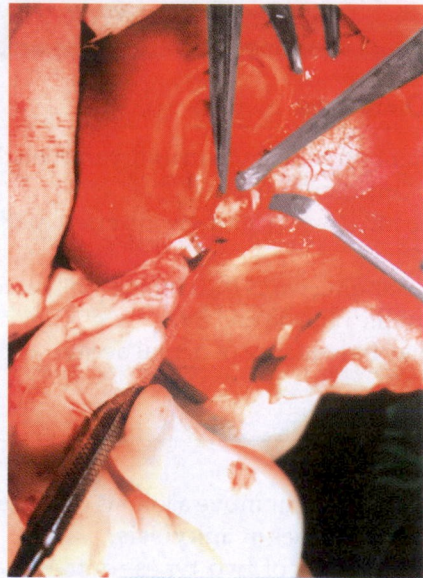

Fig. 61: Arthroplasty of TMJ for ankylosis
(*Courtesy:* Professor Divya Mehrotra)

12. How do you treat intra-articular ankylosis?

It is treated by arthroplasty in which the abnormal intra-articular bone including the condyle of the mandible is removed and a costochondral graft is kept in the joint cavity (Fig. 61).

DISCUSSION

It is the chronic limitation or inability to open the jaw or mouth. It is of two types—extra-articular and intra-articular.

- Extra-articular, false or fibrous ankylosis—Here, the cause of ankylosis is not in, but around the joint. There is fibrosis and, or contracture of the soft tissues around the joint which follow gun-shot injury, operations on the mouth, severe periarticular infections such as cancrum oris; destruction of the mucosa of the fauces or cheek by operative or radiation injury, and osteomyelitis of mandible spreading into the muscles of mastication. Submucous fibrosis of cheek also restricts the mobility of jaw as the cheek is not elastic and stretchable.

- Intra-articular, true or bony ankylosis—Here, the cause is inside the joint – the joint cavity is obliterated by bony tissue. It usually follows suppurative arthritis of the temporo-mandibular joint (TMJ). It may follow fractures of the condyle or fracture-dislocation of TMJ.

Clinical Features

Ankylosis of TMJ can occur at any age but most of the patients are children and young adults who complain of difficulty in opening the mouth. It is associated with oral sepsis, dental decay and deformity of lower face. The nutrition does not suffer as the patient continues to take liquid food without any difficulty.

The extra-articular ankylosis permits slight movement which is completely absent in intra-articular type. When the ankylosis develops in early childhood, the affected side of the mandible fails to develop fully leading to a receding chin directed towards the affected side. In bilateral ankylosis the receded and atrophic chin gives the face a bird-like or shrew-mouse appearance (Fig. 58). The gap between the upper and lower teeth is measured if the mouth can be opened.

Investigations

- Radiology: In extra-articular disease, the TMJ is normal. In intra-articular, type the joint space is occupied by bony tissue (Fig. 60).
- Orthopantomography: It shows the full mandible straightened out and both the joints.
- CT scan shows the full details of the joint and the abnormality in the joint.

Treatment

- Extra-articular ankylosis:
  1. Regular, intermittent and gradual stretching of the contracted soft tissues is done with the help of a wedge or screw or dilators. It may cause damage to front teeth.
  2. Treatment or removal of the cause, e.g. intralesional corticosteroid injection in submucous fibrosis.
  3. Extra-articular arthroplasty of Esmarch: A wedge of bone from the mandible just in front of angle, 2 cm broad at lower margin and tapering to a point behind the last molar tooth is excised (osteotomy) and jaw movements are started as early as possible.
- Intra-articular ankylosis: It is treated by arthroplasty in which the mandibular condyle including the abnormal osseous tissue is excised (Fig. 61). In the gap a costochondral graft is inserted. Postoperatively, opening of the mouth and the jaw movements are started as early as possible.
- Other measures:
  - The decaying teeth are treated by a dental colleague.
  - The receded and atrophic chin requires the attention of a plastic surgeon.

CASE 18: TORTICOLLIS (WRY-NECK)

CLINICAL DIAGNOSIS

1. The patient is a child who keeps his/her neck bent and twisted to one side (Fig. 62).
2. It may be present at birth or may be noted after second to sixth weeks of life.
3. There is hard, nontender, fibrotic mass in the sternocleidomastoid muscle (Fig. 63).
4. The muscle is shortened and appears as a protuberant band.

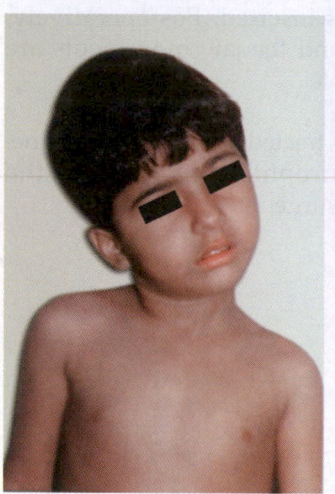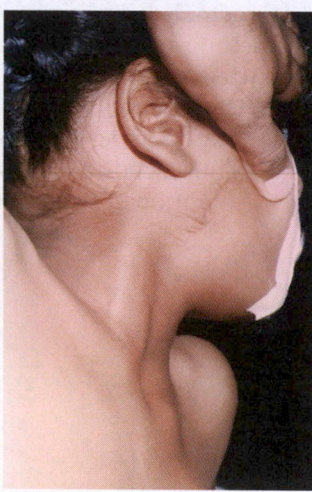

Fig. 62: Congenital torticollis
(*Courtesy:* Professor Ashish Wakhlu)

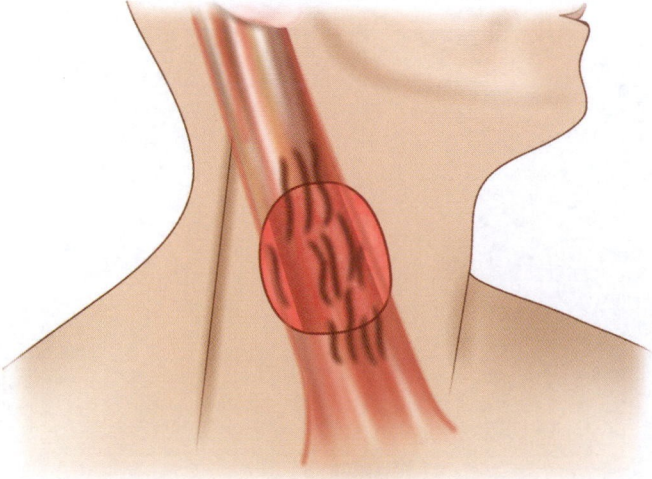

Fig. 63: Sternocleidomastoid tumor of right muscle

VIVA VOCE

1. **What is torticollis?**
   It is bending and twisting of the neck due to contracture of one of the sternocleidomastoid muscle.
2. **What is the cause of torticollis?**
   It is due to shortening of one of the sternocleidomastoid muscle where the mastoid process on the involved side is pulled down towards the clavicle and manubrium.
3. **What is the cause of shortening of sternocleidomastoid?**
   It is due to fibrosis caused by a sternocleidomastoid tumor (Fig. 63).
4. **What is a sternocleidomastoid tumor?**
   It is a tumor-like swelling in the lower part of sternocleidomastoid muscle seen in infants (Fig. 63).
5. **What is the cause of this tumor?**
   It is an organizing hematoma of sternocleidomastoid muscle due to birth trauma.
6. **What are the features of a sternocleidomastoid tumor?**
   * There is a small swelling, the size of a hazel nut, present in the lower part of sternocleidomastoid muscle.
   * It is ovoid or fusiform with its long axis in the length of muscle.
   * It is smooth, hard, nontender and well-defined.
7. **What are the consequences of torticollis?**
   If the torticollis is not treated, it may lead to a series of changes:
   * The head is drawn to the same side and rotated toward the opposite shoulder
   * The shoulder of the affected side is raised. There may be cervical and thoracic scoliosis
   * The ipsilateral face and contralateral occiput become flattened
   * Facial hemihypoplasia on the same side occurs within 6 months
   * Yellow spot (fovea) of the eye may change its position.
8. **What are the investigations?**
   No investigations are needed.
9. **How do you treat this condition?**
   * It is treated by motion exercise. The shoulders are held flat to the table and the head is tilted and rotated in a full range of motion. It is done at least four times a day for 2 to 3 months. The tumor gradually disappears and the deformity is corrected.
   * If there is no relief or the problem progresses, both the heads of sternocleidomastoid are divided just above the clavicle.

10. **Does the muscle division reverse the changes?**
    The changes that have occurred are not reversed but the further progression is prevented.

DISCUSSION

Torticollis is the twisting of the neck that is seen in newborns and probably occurs due to trauma of the muscle at the time of delivery. A history of breech delivery is present in these patients.

Initially, there is a hard, nontender, fibrotic mass in one of the sternocleidomastoid muscle which soon leads to the shortening of the muscle and torticollis and its consequences (Figs 63).

This problem occurs in both the sexes and on each side of the neck. Rarely, more than one tumor in a muscle or in both the muscles is present. Due to torticollis, if it is not treated, structural changes start occurring in the head and neck region and even the thoracic spine. The problem should be treated as early as possible by motion exercises of head (and neck) at least 4 times a day for 2 to 3 months. The tumor disappears and muscle becomes near normal. If the shortening continues or advances the shortened sternocleidomastoid is divided just above the clavicle to correct the torticollis and to prevent the progression of secondary effects.

CASE 19: CERVICAL RIB SYNDROME

CLINICAL DIAGNOSIS

1. The patient is usually a middle-aged female who presents with tingling and numbness along the medial side of the hand and forearm or with loss of power in the hand with wasting of thenar and hypothenar muscles of insidious onset.
2. There is evidence of arterial insufficiency maximally manifesting in the index finger, may be with finger tip necrosis.
3. The symptoms are relieved by elevation of the arm and aggravated by pulling it downwards.
4. If the patient takes a deep breath and turns the face to the affected side, the radial pulse in the extended arm is diminished or obliterated (Adson's test).
5. There may be a palpable swelling in the supraclavicular region.
   - It may be pulsatile and tender and on pressing it the symptoms in the upper limb are aggravated (subclavian artery elevated by abnormal rib).
   - It may be mushroom-like finely bosselated, fixed and hard (expanded free end of abnormal rib).

VIVA VOCE

1. **What is cervical rib syndrome?**
   It is a symptom-sign complex consisting of pain, paresthesia and muscular wasting in the upper limb due to neurovascular phenomenon at the thoracic outlet commonly due to cervical rib.
2. **What is the cause?**
   The neurovascular bundle of upper arm consisting of subclavian artery and first thoracic nerve may be distorted, stretched, angulated or irritated by one of the following lesions:
   1. Cervical rib.
   2. Abnormalities of scalene muscle.
   3. Post-fixed brachial plexus.
3. **What are the grades of cervical rib?**
   The grades of cervical rib are:
   - A complete rib articulating with manubrium sterni or first rib, may be with scaleni muscles attached (Fig. 64).
   - An incomplete rib with free end expanding into a large bony boss.
   - An incomplete rib ending in a tapering point attached to the scalene tubercle of first rib by a fibrous band.

- An extra rib represented by a fibrous band extending from seventh cervical transverse process to either first rib or scalenus medius muscle.
4. **What are the abnormalities of scalene muscles responsible for this syndrome?**
   The abnormalities are:
   - An additional scalene muscle.
   - Close approximation of insertions of scalenus anticus and scalenus medius.
5. **What is the nature of these abnormalities and do they always produce symptoms?**
   All these abnormalities are congenital and may remain asymptomatic throughout life.
6. **How do these abnormalities produce symptoms?**
   With the decline of youth, there is a gradual sagging of shoulder girdle due to decreased muscle tone and some atrophy of regional musculature, resulting in stretching or angulation of neurovascular bundle.
7. **How do these abnormalities affect the subclavian artery?**
   The subclavian artery is affected in the following manner:
   - Angulation of the artery over the rib.
   - Constriction or narrowing of lumen due to angulation.
   - Post-stenotic dilatation distal to constriction.
   - Thrombosis in post-stenotic dilatation and, or possibly at the site of constriction.

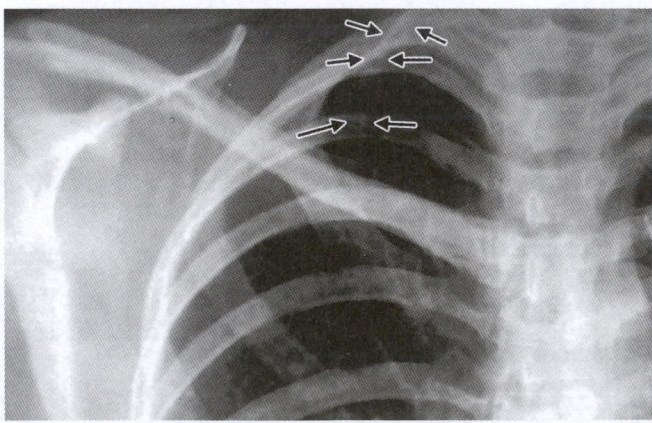

Fig. 64: Cervical rib, right side

- Distal embolization, often repeated from the thrombus in post-stenotic dilatation and its lodgement in digital arteries

8. How do they affect the local nerves?

The nerves are affected in the following manners:

1. Friction neuritis of first thoracic nerve (lowest trunk of brachial plexus due to stretch or angulation.
2. Irritation of periarterial sympathetic fibers or paralysis of sympathetic fibers contained in lower trunk.
3. Stretching of heads of median nerve by angulated artery.

9. What are the investigations?

The investigations are:

1. Radiography of cervico-thoracic junction to see for the cervical rib or any disease of cervical spine (spondylosis, disc disease) (Fig. 64).
2. Doppler probe study of subclavian artery to see for stenosis, dilatation.
3. CT scan of cervicothoracic region.

10. How do you treat this problem?

The essentials of treatment are:

1. Exercises of muscles of shoulder gridle and neck.
2. Analgesics for relief of pain.
3. Scalenotomy or excision of rib if symptoms are severe and not relieved by conservative measures.

11. What one should ensure before doing these operations?

One should make sure that upper limb symptoms are due to cervical rib and not due to some other cause as cervical ribs are found in 0.46 percent of normal people of which only 10 percent are symptomatic.

12. What are the indications of surgery?

The indications of surgery are:

- Failure of nonoperative measures.
- Severe pain.
- Wasting of muscles of hand.
- Vasomotor symptoms.

13. What is the surgical treatment of this problem?

This syndrome is treated by any or combination of the following operations:

- Scalenotomy.
- Excision of cervical rib.
- Cervicodorsal sympathectomy.

14. Do these measures always relieve the symptoms?

No.

15. What precautions will you take when you excise the rib?

It should be removed along with its periosteum.

16. Why?

A new rib may regenerate if periosteum is retained.

17. What is the indication for cervicodorsal sympathecotmy?

This operation is indicated if vasomotor symptoms are present.

18. What are the complications of these operations?

The complications are:

- Injury to subclavian artery.
- Injury to phrenic nerve, brachial plexus.
- Pneumothorax.
- Hemorrhage.
- Wound infection.

DISCUSSION

Cervical rib arising from seventh cervical vertebra is one of the common developmental abnormality which occurs in 0.46 percent of persons. It may be unilateral or bilateral, slightly more common on the right side. Majority of these ribs are asymptomatic. It is interesting to note that many times when a radiograph of cervical region is taken on account of nerve pressure symptoms no such rib is detected.

Types of cervical rib - The cervical rib is of four varieties (Fig. 65) –

- A complete rib articulating with manubrium sterni or first rib at a false joint, may be with scaleni muscles attached to it.
- An incomplete rib with free end expanding into a large bony mass.
- An incomplete rib ending in a tapering point attached to the scalene tubercle of first rib by a fibrous band.
- A fibrous band extending from seventh cervical transverse process to either first rib or scalenus medius muscle (not demonstrable in X-ray).

Pathology

At the exit from the neck the brachial plexus and subclavian artery pass through the narrow space between the first rib (base) and clavicle. If the base of this costoclavicular space is raised by the height of one vertebra by the interposition of a cervical rib, the subclavian artery and first dorsal nerve are elevated, may be angulated and not necessarily compressed. The artery is constricted at the site of angulation resulting in fusiform dilatation (poststenotic dilatation) of 2 to 4 cm of artery distal to constriction. In the dilatation and may be at constriction thrombosis occurs. The thrombus thus produced may cause distal embolism which may be repeated. Proximal propagation of thrombosis may involve the vertebral artery, and may cause cerebrovascular embolism.

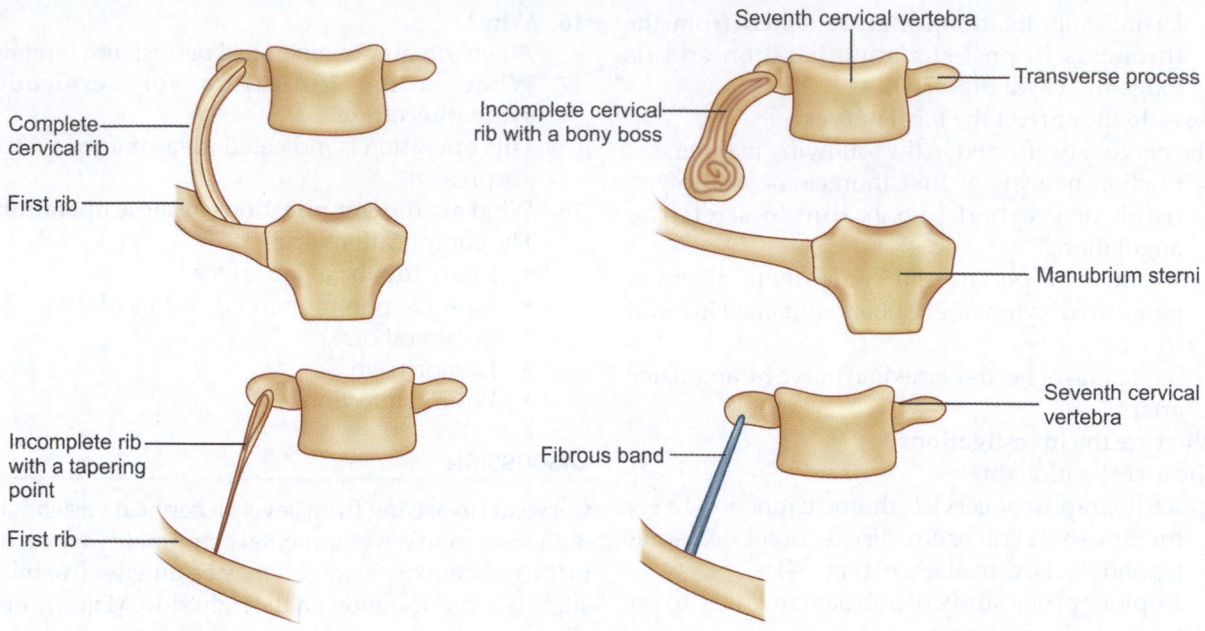

Fig. 65: Types of cervical rib

Clinical Features

Cervical rib may be entirely asymptomatic. A symptomatic rib produces three types of clinical manifestations:

a. Locally symptomatic – The patient may present with a lump in the supraclavicular fossa which is bony hard and totally fixed. The second type of rib presents with these signs.

b. Associated with vascular symptoms – They occur only in a complete cervical rib.

   The patient presents with pain in forearm which may radiate to the upper arm and brought on by the use of arm. If the arm is raised the onset of pain is aggravated. It is the pain of muscle ischemia.

   The hand on the affected side tends to be colder than the other one, becomes pale when elevated and becomes blue on making it dependent for sometime. The radial pulse may be normal, absent or feeble. There may be systolic bruit on distal subclavian artery.

   The fingers may be numb, ulcerated or gangrenous rarely.

c. Associated with nerve pressure symptoms – The so called nerve pressure symptoms may not be due to angulation of first dorsal nerve but may be due to some other cause i.e. cervical spondylosis or carpal tunnel syndrome. The patient may have tingling and numbness and there may be wasting of thenar and hypothenar muscles.

Differential diagnosis—The following conditions must be considered—lateral protrusion of intervertebral disc, carpal tunnel syndrome, angulation of ulnar nerve behind the elbow, motor neuron disease and syringomyelia.

Treatment

1. Associated with vascular symptoms—Extraperiosteal excision of the cervical rib together with any bony prominence of the first rib is the treatment of choice. It should be combined with cervicodorsal sympathectomy.

2. Associated with nerve pressure symptoms—If the symptoms are mild, the patient is advised to use a sling and exercise to strengthen the muscles of shoulder girdle.

   In severe cases, if the rib is not recognized division of scalenus anterior (scalenotomy) is recommended. It relieves symptoms in majority of cases. If rib or a band is present it should be excised. The rib is removed with its periosteum or it will regenerate. Care must be taken to prevent injury to brachial plexus and phrenic nerves.

CASE 20: RAYNAUD'S DISEASE

CLINICAL DIAGNOSIS

1. The patient is usually a young woman of 18 to 30 years who presents with Raynaud's phenomenon in the hand, i.e. developing a series of color changes when exposed to cold – white, blue (Fig. 66) and red (or WBC – white, blue and crimson).
2. The patient may have chilblains, troublesome sweating and signs of arterial insufficiency in the digits.
3. The tips of the fingers are affected maximally. The fingers waste and the pulp becomes thin and pointed.
4. The radial pulse is normal.

VIVA VOCE

1. **What is Raynaud's disease?**
   It is a vasospastic disorder of digital vessels of unknown etiology usually affecting the upper limb and occurring in young women.
2. **What is the cause of this disease?**
   The cause of this disease is not known. The arterioles are abnormally sensitive to cold:
   1. It may be the hyperactivity of sympathetic nervous system.
   2. It may be because of abnormal adrenergic receptors which are abnormally sensitive to cold exposure.
3. **What is Raynaud's phenomenon?**
   It is the clinical manifestation of Raynaud's disease consisting of sequential pallor, cyanosis and rubor following exposure of hand to cold.
4. **Where does the Raynaud's phenomenon occur?**
   Usually, it occurs in the hands. It may occur in the feet (Fig. 67), ears, nose and lips.

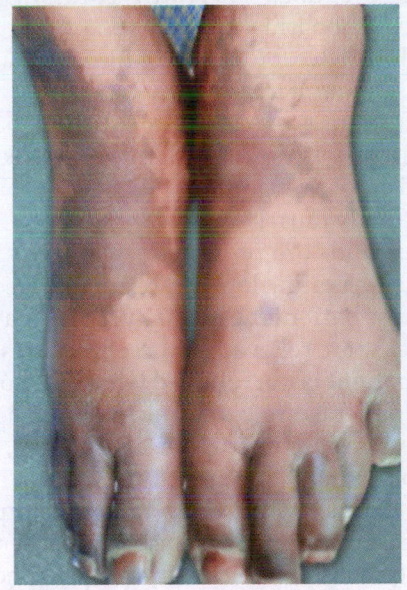

Fig. 67: Raynaud's Phenomenon in lower limbs (*Courtesy:* Professor Sandeep Tewari)

5. **What is the difference between Raynaud's disease and Raynaud's phenomenon?**
   Raynaud's disease is one of the cause of Raynaud's phenomenon. There are many causes of Raynaud's phenomenon other than Raynaud's disease (Table 1).
6. **What are the causes of Raynaud's phenomenon?**
   - Immunologic and connective tissue disorders, e.g. scleroderma, systemic lupus erythematosus, polymyositis, Sjogren's syndrome, vasculitis
   - Neurovascular compression and occupational disease—Carpal tunnel syndrome, thoracic outlet obstruction, vibration injury, cold injury
   - Drugs—Serotonin agonists, sympathomimetic drugs, ergotamine

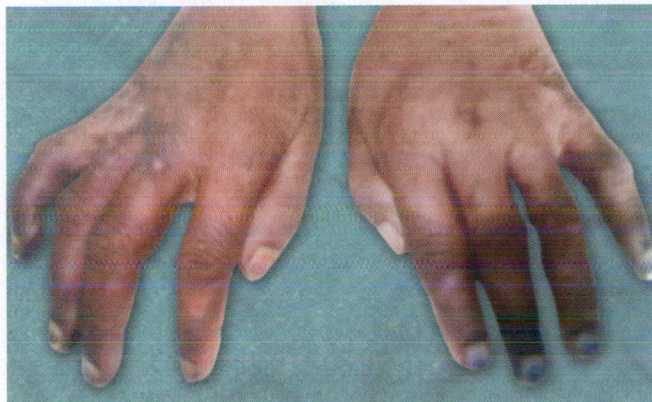

Fig. 66: Raynaud's Phenomenon—The blue fingers following exposure to cold. (*Courtesy:* Professor Sandeep Tewari)

Table 1: **Differences between Raynaud's disease and RP**

Features	Raynaud's disease	Raynaud's phenomenon (RP)
Age	15-30 years	Variable
Sex	Almost always in females	Variable
Side	Usually bilateral	May be unilateral
Extent	Fingers and distal palm	May be limited to one digit
Secondary changes	Uncommon	Pitting, ulceration and gangrene are common
Nailfold capillary abnormality	Not present	Present
Etiology	Not known	Signs of the cause present
Nature	Relatively benign	More virulent
Treatment	Conservative measures	Treatment of cause

- Hematologic disorders, e.g. cryoglobulinemia, polycythemia, cold agglutinins
- Other causes—Hypothyroidism, repeated microembolism

7. How do you treat Raynaud's disease?

The essentials of treatment are:

- Avoidance of cold exposure, tobacco, oral contraceptives, beta-adrenergic blocking agents and ergot preparations
- The body must be kept warm.
- The hands are protected from injury. Softening and lubricating lotions are applied frequently. Many patients, especially those having mild disease are relieved by these measures.

8. If the patient is not relieved what will you do?

These patients are given calcium channel blockers like slow release nifedipine, amlodipine, felodipine or nisoldipine.

Other drugs, which may relieve symptoms are angiotensin converting enzyme inhibitors, sympatholytic drugs (prazosin), topical nitrates, phosphodiesterase inhibitors (e.g. sildenafil, tadalafil and vardenafil), selective serotonin reuptake inhibitors (fluoxetine) and endothelin receptor inhibitors (e.g. bosentan).

Transdermal prostaglandins, ketanserin and cilostazol may relieve symptoms in some patients. Cervicodorsal sympathectomy may be done in severe disease.

9. What is the indication for cervicodorsal sympathectomy?

It is indicated in a severe case who fails to respond to conservative measures.

10. What do you do in this operation?

In this operation 1 to 3 thoracic sympathetic ganglia are removed preserving the cervical portion of stellate ganglion.

11. What will happen if the stellate ganglion is removed completely?

It will result in Horner's syndrome.

12. What are the approaches of this procedure?

This operation can be done through a cervical approach, and axillary approach or by a dorsal incision.

13. What are the results of this operation?

The immediate results are good but there is a gradual recurrence of symptoms in a large number of patients.

14. What are the causes of recurrence following operation?

The causes of recurrence are:

- Incomplete excision of sympathetic cord.
- Regeneration and relinking of the sympathetic fibers.

- Increased sensitivity of denervated limb to circulating catecholamines.
- The patient had Raynaud's phenomenon and not disease and the cause is not treated, e.g. untreated scleroderma.

15. What are the complications of cervicodorsal sympathectomy?

The complications are:

- Perforation of pleura leading to pneumothorax.
- Hemorrhage, hemothorax or retropleural hematoma.
- Lymph fistula following damage to thoracic duct in left-sided operation.
- Horner's syndrome.

RAYNAUD'S PHENOMENON

Raynaud's phenomenon (RP) is a syndrome consisting of sequential pallor, cyanosis and redness of fingers (or toes) following exposure to cold. It is an exaggerated response of digital arteries to cold or emotional stress.

Etiology

Etiologically RP is of two types—idiopathic or primary where the cause is not known which is same as Raynaud's disease, and secondary where it is a symptom of some disease. The causes of secondary Raynaud's phenomenon are:

- Immunologic and connective tissue diseases, e.g. scleroderma, systemic lupus erythematosus, polymyositis, Sjogren's syndrome and vasculitis
- Neurovascular compression and occupational diseases, e.g. carpal tunnel syndrome, thoracic outlet obstruction, vibration injury, cold injury
- Drugs: Serotonin agonists, sympathomimetic drugs, ergotamine
- Hematologic diseases, e.g. cryoglobulinemia, polycythemia, cold agglutinins
- Other causes—hypothyroidism, repeated microembolism.

The Raynaud's disease is a benign lesion, while the Raynaud's phenomenon (RP) is a more virulent entity.

Pathology

The pallor of the RP is due to excessive vasoconstriction and the redness (rubor) is caused by the vasodilatation of the recovery phase.

The arterial system is normal in Raynaud's disease.

In secondary RP the pathologic changes in the body depend upon the causative disease.

Clinical Features

Raynaud's disease occurs in 2 to 6 percent of adults, and is common in young females between 15 to 30 years of age.

In early phase of disease only one or two fingertips may be affected. As the disease advances all fingers upto the distal palm may be involved. The thumbs are rarely involved. Both the hands are symmetrically affected.

Following dipping the hand in cold water (exposure to cold), the hand becomes pale (pallor), cold and numb and a little later somewhat bluish (cyanosis). When the attack passes off (after removing the hand from cold water spontaneously or dipping in warm water) there may be intense rubor (redness), throbbing, paresthesia, pain and slight swelling. Stiffness, diminished sensation and aching pain may be present. There are no symptoms and signs between attacks. The peripheral pulses are normal.

The primary Raynaud's phenomenon is bilateral and involves all the fingers and distal palm, while the secondary RP may be unilateral and may involve only one or two fingers. Skin tightening, loss of extremity pulse, rash, swollen joint, digital pitting or ulceration are usually seen in secondary RP.

Nailfold capillary abnormalities – A drop of grade B immersion oil is put at the cuticle and seen with an ophthalmoscope set to 20 to 40 diopters. In secondary RP (most commonly due to scleroderma) dilatation or drop out of the capillary loops is seen.

Investigations

- Raynaud's disease—Investigations are normal.
- In secondary RP investigations are done depending upon the clinical suspicion of the cause of symptoms.

Treatment

The primary RP is treated according to the severity of the disease. The secondary problem is treated by removing its cause if possible. Digital sympthectomy may improve its symptoms.

1. **Mild Raynaud's disease:**
   - Avoidance of cold exposure, smoking, oral contraceptives, beta-adrenergic blocking agents and ergotamine preparations
   - The body is kept warm
   - The hands are protected from injury. Softening and lubricating agents are frequently applied.
   Many patients are relieved by these measures.

2. **Severe Raynaud's disease:**
   - Calcium channel blockers—Drugs like slow release nifedipine 30 to 180 mg per day or amlodipine (5-20 mg per day), felodipine or nisoldipine are better than verapamil and diltiazem. These drugs are more effective in primary than in secondary RP.
   - Other drugs which are sometimes effective are angiotensin converting enzyme inhibitors, sympatholytic drugs (e.g. prazosin), topical nitrates, phosphodiesterase inhibitors (e.g. sildenafil, tadalafil and vardenafil), selective serotonin reuptake inhibitors (fluoxetine), and endothelin receptor inhibitors (e.g. bosentan).
   - Transdermal prostaglandins, ketanserin and cilostazol may relieve symptoms in some patients.
   - Cervicothoracic sympthectomy (excision of T1, T2 and T3 ganglia) may be helpful in Raynaud's disease when the medical treatment fails. It is not helpful in secondary RP.
   - Raynaud's phenomenon is more common than the Raynaud's disease. It is recognized by history and physical signs of the causative lesion. To confirm the diagnosis the following investigations are done – Blood counts, ESR, urea, electrolytes, antinuclear factor, rheumatoid factor, cryoproteins, immunoglobulins, cold agglutinins, chest radiography, skin biopsy.

Prognosis

- Raynaud's disease is more of a nuisance than risk
- In secondary RP, the prognosis depends upon the causative disease.

CASE 21: DUPUYTREN'S CONTRACTURE (OR DISEASE)

CLINICAL DIAGNOSIS

1. The patient is usually a middle-aged or elderly person commonly a male who presents with a flexion deformity of the ring or little finger or both.
2. The finger may be so much flexed that its nail may dig into the palm of the hand.
3. The metacarpophalangeal (MP) and the proximal interphalangeal (PIP) joints are flexed and the distal interphalangeal joint is extended (Fig. 68).
4. The flexion deformity is not lessened by flexion of the wrist joint.
5. The palmar fascia is thickened and one or two nodules may be present in the palm, near the base of the ring finger.
6. Each nodule is spherical, irregular, 1 to 2 mm in diameter firm, and ill-defined.

VIVA VOCE

1. **What is Dupuytren's contracture?**
   It is a localized thickening of the palmar fascia (rarely plantar fascia) with contracture of unknown etiology resulting in flexion deformity of affected fingers.
2. **What is the cause of this condition?**
   - It is an autosomal dominant trait which is associated with Anglo-saxon lineage
   - It is associated with smoking, use of vibrating tools, pulmonary tuberculosis, idiopathic epilepsy, antiepileptic drugs, AIDS, alcoholic cirrhosis and diabetes
   - It is not work-related as it may occur in people who do not work.
3. **Where does this disease start?**
   This disease starts most commonly near the base of little finger and soon draws the finger into the palm of the hand.
4. **What is the course of this disease?**
   After involving the little finger, it affects the ring finger and, less often the middle and then the index fingers in the same manner (Fig. 68).
5. **What are the long-term effects of this lesion?**
   In long-standing disease permanent changes occur in the metacarpophalangeal and proximal interphalangeal joints which make any attempt to straighten the fingers futile subsequently.
6. **How do you treat this condition?**
   The treatment is outlined below:
   - *Early case*—Night splintage, gentle stretching by the patient and fasciotomy

- *Advanced disease*—Excision or partial fasciectomy and repair by Z-plasty.
- *Very advanced disease*—If above measures fail, the affected finger is amputated (ray amputation). Sometimes arthrodesis of the proximal interphalangeal joint may be done in semiextended position.

7. **What are the complications of operative treatment?**
   They are digital infarction, flap necrosis, hematoma, scarring, stiffness, digital nerve injury and reflex sympathetic dystrophy (causalgia).
8. **What is reflex sympathetic dystrophy?**
   It is severe burning pain affecting the entire hand which becomes cold, cyanotic and moist.
9. **What are the results of treatment?**
   The disease can recur. The chances of success are higher for MP joint than PIP joint.

DISCUSSION

Dupuytren's contracture is a disease (palmar fasciitis) of unknown etiology characterized by tightness of the palmar fascia resulting in flexion deformity of ring and little fingers at the metacarpophalangeal joint (coachman's hand) (Fig. 68).

Etiology

It is an autosomal dominant trait which is associated with Anglo-saxon lineage, smoking, use of vibrating tools, pulmonary tuberculosis, idiopathic epilepsy (may be to antiepileptic drugs), AIDS, alcoholic cirrhosis and diabetes.

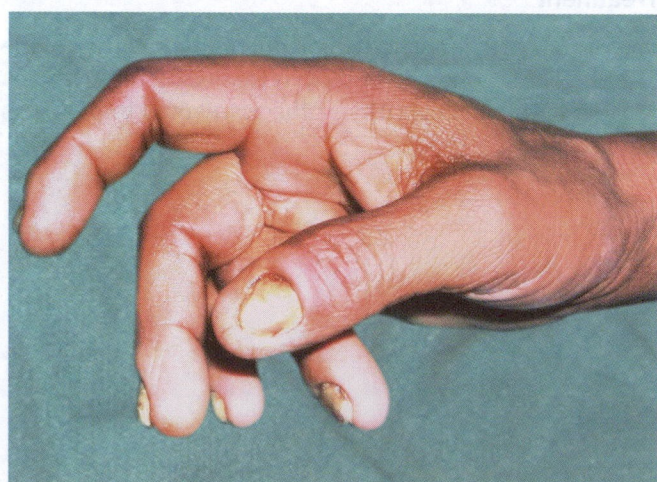

Fig. 68: Dupuytren's contracture of hand. This patient has diseased nails. (*Courtesy:* Professor Rajiv Agarwal)

It may occur in people who do not work, and in the hand of the labourers that does the least work. Hence, it is not work-related.

Pathology

The cellular and biochemical changes in the palmar fascia are the same as seen in healing wounds.

Clinical Features

It is mostly seen in males over 50 who are of sedentary habits. It is bilateral in about 50 percent of patients. It may be acute, subacute or chronic.

The patient presents with flexion deformity of the ring or little finger or both of insidious onset. The ring finger may be so much flexed that its nail may dig into the palm of hand. It may involve any finger or web space.

The metacarpophalangeal and the proximal interphalangeal joints are flexed and the distal inter-phalangeal joints are extended. The flexion deformity is not reduced by flexing the wrist (opposite to Volkmann's contracture).

The findings include thickening of the palmar fascia with one or two nodules near the base of ring finger, skin puckering, cords of the palm and digits, flexion contracture of fingers and thickened skin on the dorsum of proximal interphalangeal joint (Garrod's knuckle pads).

This disease may occur in the plantar fascia of instep (Ledderhose disease), and sometimes in penis (Peyronie's disease).

Treatment

- There is no drug which can help in this disease.
- *Surgery*—Fasciectomy is indicated when there is 30^0 flexion at MP joint or any flexion contracture of PIP joint. It is done by longitudinal incisions which are sutured by Z-plasties. Zig-zag incisions are also effective. Depending upon the extent of skin shrinkage skin grafting may be required.
- Fasciotomy is indicated in cases where the skin is normal and moves freely over the contracted fascial band.

  Active movements are started 3 to 5 days after surgery. Dynamic splints and steroid injection into the joints in the vicinity are helpful.

  The complications of operation are—digital infarction, flap necrosis, hematoma, fibrosis, stiffness, digital nerve injury and reflex sympathetic dystrophy.
- An acute tender nodule may be treated by local triamcinolone injection
- If the little finger is grossly contracted amputation may be a better option.

Prognosis

- Recurrence can occur
- The chances of success are higher for MP joint than PIP joint.

Non-clinical Practical Examination

Apart from the examination on the clinical cases the candidate has to appear in the nonclinical practical examination. It consists of the following -
- Examiner I — 1. Surgical pathology
- 2. Clinical radiology and other imaging methods
- Examiner II— 1. Surgical instruments and equipment
- 2. Operative surgery including surgical anatomy

SURGICAL PATHOLOGY

In clinical practice the diseases are diagnosed by symptoms and signs. Apart from this a surgeon has to recognize the abnormal or diseased organs and tissues during the operation. Hence a candidate is examined on the preserved specimens of excised lesions and diseased organs. Usually a candidate is examined on 3 specimens of different systems. Examples of some of the specimens kept in the examination (KG's Medical University) are:
- Gastric ulcer, perforated peptic ulcer, bleeding peptic ulcer (an artery in the floor of the ulcer with a hole), carcinoma of stomach, hour-glass stomach, trichobezoar, stricture of bowel, tuberculous ulcer, typhoid ulcer, Meckel's diverticulum, intussusception, carcinoma of colon, ulcerative colitis, rectal adenoma.
- Gall stones, chronic cholecystitis, mucocele of gall bladder, carcinoma of gall bladder, gall stones.
- Amebic abscess of liver, hydatid cyst, metastases, hemangioma, melanoma, cyst.
- Renal cell carcinoma, horse-shoe kidney, polycystic kidney, renal tuberculosis, hydronephrosis, pyonephrosis, Wilms' tumor, carcinoma-bladder, enlarged prostate, carcinoma-penis, testicular tumor, infarcted testis of torsion.

- Tuberculous nodes, Hodgkin lymphoma, carcinoma of breast, osteoclastoma, osteosarcoma, fibrosarcoma, dermoid cyst, ameloblastoma of mandible, multinodular goiter, aortic aneurysm, bronchiectasis, lung abscess, bronchogenic carcinoma, pulmonary tuberculosis.

What is to be done by the examinee?

- *First step*—The candidate should examine or see the specimen from all sides and angles so as not to miss any finding, as the diagnosis depends upon the gross appearance of the specimen. The specimen must not be damaged during examination.
- *Second step*—The examinee tells about the specimen under the following headings – organ or part, findings and diagnosis.

Questioning

Three questions are usually asked after the candidate identifies the specimen and makes a diagnosis:
- What are the reasons for making this diagnosis?
- What is this disease?
- How will you manage it?

Further questioning depends upon the response of the candidate and the time available.

One must remember that the examiner is a surgeon, not a pathologist. Hence, he is unlikely to ask you the details of the pathology. The questioning starts in pathology and ends in surgery.

AN EXAMPLE OF VIVA ON A PATHOLOGICAL SPECIMEN

Examiner: See this specimen and tell me the findings and diagnosis.

Candidate

- It appears to be an enlarged lymph node which is markedly enlarged, nearly round in shape, pinkish gray in color and has an uneven surface (Fig. 1).
- The cut surface is pinkish grey and uneven. There is no evidence of necrosis or liquefaction (Fig. 2). The diagnosis is lymphoma.

VIVA VOCE

1. **Why is it not an enlarged tuberculous lymph node?**
   It is not a tuberculous lymph node as it is not having any area of caseous necrosis (yellowish area) and liquefaction.
2. **How will you confirm the diagnosis?**
   By histopathological examination of excised lymph node.

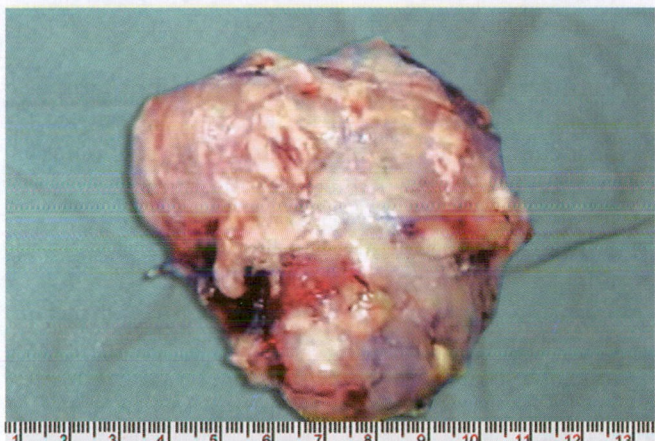

Fig. 1: Excised markedly enlarged inguinal lymph node

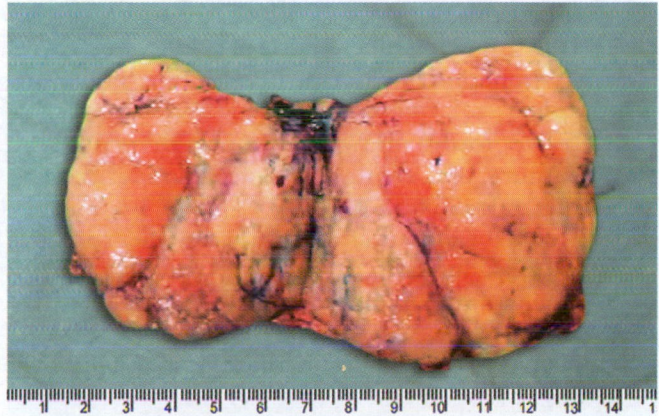

Fig. 2: The cut surface of the lymph node

3. **What are the types of lymphomas?**
   The lymphomas are of two types:
   1. Hodgkin lymphoma.
   2. Non-Hodgkin lymphoma.
4. **What is the microscopic picture of a Hodgkin lymphoma?**
   It is characterized by Reed-Sternberg cells surrounded by an inflammatory infiltrate consisting of lymphocytes, plasma cells, eosinophils and histiocytes.
5. **What are Reed-Sternberg cells?**
   They are the malignant cells which are relatively large cells with abundant basophilic or amphophilic cytoplasm and two or more vesicular nuclei (mirror-image nuclei). Each nucleus has a thick nuclear membrane and a single prominent acidophilic or amphophilic nucleolus surrounded by a clear halo (owl-eye cells).
6. **What is cell of origin of Reed-Sternberg cells?**
   The Reed-Sternberg cell is derived from B lymphocytes of germinal cell origin.
7. **What is the clinical presentation of Hodgkin's lymphoma?**
   - The patient is usually in 20s or over 50 years of age
   - There is a painless mass (enlarged node), commonly in the neck (A stage)
   - Constitutional symptoms – Fever, weight loss, drenching night sweats or generalized pruritus may be present (B stage)
   - There may be pain in the enlarged lymph node following alcohol ingestion.
8. **What are the stages of this disease?**
   The stage are (Ann Arbor):
   - Stage I—Single lymphatic site involved.
   - Stage II—Two or more lymphatic sites involved on one side of diaphragm.
   - Stage III—Lymph node sites involved on both sides of diaphragm.
   - Stage IV—Disseminated disease with bone marrow or liver involvement.
   - Each stage is divided in 2 stages:
     - A – Constitutional symptoms absent
     - B – Constitutional symptoms present
9. **What are the types of Hodgkin lymphoma?**
   It is of four subtypes:
   - Lymphocyte predominance
   - Nodular sclerosis
   - Mixed cellularity
   - Lymphocyte depletion.

10. **How do you treat Hodgkin lymphoma?**
    - IA and II A – Radiotherapy (may be combined with limited chemotherapy)
    - Others – Combination chemotherapy consisting of doxorubicin (Adriamycin), bleomycin, vincristine and dacarbazine (ABVD)

11. **What is non-Hodgkin lymphoma?**
    Non-Hodgkin lymphomas are a heterogeneous group of malignant tumors of lymphocytes.

12. **What is the clinical presentation?**
    - Apart from painless lymphadenopathy (retroperitoneum, mesentery or pelvis), there may be extra-nodal sites of disease, e.g., skin, gastrointestinal tract.
    - There is no pain following alcohol ingestion.

13. **How do you treat nonhodgkin lymphoma?**
    - Limited disease (very few patients)– Radiotherapy
    - Indolent lymphoma, if asymptomatic and not bulky (most patients) – Keep under observation
    - Low grade lymphoma – Anti-CD 20 antibody rituximab, or rituximab+ chemotherapy (R-CVP or R-CHOP)
    - Aggressive lymphoma - Allogenic transplantation
    - High risk lymphoma - Autologous stem cell transplantation.

14. **What is the prognosis?**
    - Hodgkin lymphoma—Good as 70 percent patients are cured
    - Non-Hodgkin lymphoma—Poor as the median survival of patients with indolent lymphomas has been 6 to 8 years.

CLINICAL RADIOLOGY AND OTHER IMAGING METHODS

The internal organs, structures and tissues of the body can be seen or picturized by radiography (plain and contrast), ultrasonography, CT scan, MRI and radio-isotope studies. These methods or techniques of imaging have a great value in confirming the diagnosis. Hence, a clinician should know how to examine or read them and then interpret them. Therefore, a candidate is examined on these pictures in the nonclinical part of practical examination.

Usually 3 pictures are given to the candidate who sees them carefully and systematically so as not to miss any finding. Then the candidate describes each picture one by one under the following headings:
- Part – skull, neck, chest, abdomen, limbs
- Nature of imaging – Radiography, US, CT or MRI
- Plain/contrast
- View – AP/ lateral, oblique, sagittal, transverse, others
- Findings
- Diagnosis.

Questioning

- Some simple questions may be asked about that imaging method, e.g.
  1. What is the nature of energy used in this diagnostic method – X-rays in radiography and CT scan, sound waves in ultrasonography and magnetic waves in MRI.
  2. What are the advantages and disadvantages or limitations of this method?
- Some questions about the disease you have diagnosed by seeing the pictures given to you – what is this disease, how does it present, what is its cause and how do you treat it?

The imaging pictures commonly kept or likely to be kept in the practical examination are given below:
- Plain radiography:
  Radiographs of abdomen showing radio-opaque shadows (stones, calcifications, foreign bodies), soft tissue shadows, gas shadows and fluid levels, volvulus of sigmoid.
  Radiographs of the chest showing lung abscess, hydatid cyst, fracture of ribs, hemothorax, bronchogenic carcinoma, pulmonary tuberculosis, subphrenic abscess, enlargement of mediastinum or mediastinal shadows, gas under diaphragm.
  Bones—Fractures, tumors and osteomyelitis
  Joints—Dislocations, tuberculosis.
  Tumors—Osteosarcoma, Ewing's sarcoma, osteoclastoma, metastases, chondrosarcoma, exostosis, ameloblastoma, Colles' fracture, supracondylar fracture of humerus, skull fracture, fracture of neck of femur.
- Contrast
  1. Achalasia cardia, carcinoma of esophagus, stomach and colon, peptic ulcer; ileo-cecal tuberculosis, stricture, intussusception, hiatus hernia, colonic diverticulosis.
  2. IVU's showing tuberculosis of urinary tract, RCC, hydronephrosis, horse-shoe kidney, polycystic kidney.
  3. Cystography showing tumors, diverticulum, rupture, and small contracted bladder, vesico-ureteral reflux.
  4. Urethrography showing stricture, rupture, diverticulum.
  5. Aneurysm, atheroma, vascular malformations.
  6. ERCP.
- Ultrasound—Gall stones, hydatid cyst of liver, liver abscess, cysts, others
- CT scan/MRI—Tumors and diseases of deep seated organs (e.g. pancreas adrenal), skull, mediastinum, vertebral column

- Others—Bone scan showing skeletal metastases, RAI scan showing cold nodule in thyroid, hyperthyroidism and metastases of follicular carcinoma.

AN EXAMPLE OF VIVA ON A DIAGNOSTIC IMAGING PICTURE

Examiner – See this picture (Fig. 3), describe the findings and give diagnosis.

Candidate

- Part—Biliary tract
- Nature—MRI (MRCP)
- Findings—There is fusiform dilatation of common bile duct with normal gall bladder and normal intrahepatic biliary ductal system (Fig. 3)
- Diagnosis—Choledochal cyst.

VIVA VOCE

1. **What is a choledochal cyst?**
   It is a congenital dilatation or dilatations of extra-hepatic or, and intra-hepatic biliary ductal system.
2. **What is the cause of this condition?**
   The etiology is not known; it is a developmental defect.
3. **What are the types of choledochal cyst?**
   The types of choledochal cyst are:
   Type I—Diffuse cystic.
   Type II—Diverticulum of common bile duct.
   Type III—Dilatation of pancreatic part of common bile duct.
   Type IV—Apart from bile duct, there is intra-hepatic involvement.
   Type V—Cystic dilatation of intrahepatic ducts
4. **Which is the type?**
   It is diffuse cystic type (type I).
5. **Which is the commonest type?**
   Type I is the most common and accounts for 75 percent of patients.
6. **How does it present clinically?**
   The patient presents with obstructive jaundice, fever, abdominal pain and swelling in right upper abdomen which is cystic and ill-defined.
7. **How do you confirm the diagnosis?**
   - Ultrasonography shows the dilatation of the ductal system
   - MRI (MRCP) reveals the details of its anatomy, especially the relationship of lower end of the bile duct with the pancreatic duct.
   - CT scan may be done, especially to see the intra-hepatic ductal system.

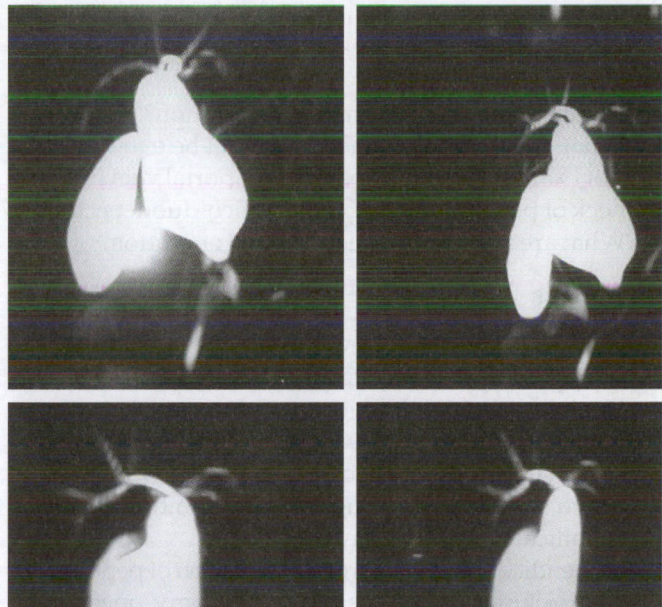

Fig. 3: MRI (MRCP) showing fusiform dilatation of common bile duct with normal gall bladder and normal intrahepatic biliary channels—Type I choledochal cyst
(*Courtesy:* Dr PR Gupta)

8. **How do you treat this condition?**
   It is treated by complete excision of cystic dilatation with reconstruction of bile duct using a Rouxen-Y loop of jejunum (hepaticojejunostomy).
9. **Why don't you treat it by anastomosing the cyst with the small bowel to relieve obstructive jaundice?**
   The anastomosis is not done because of two reasons:
   1. The complete excision of the cyst is done as a cholangiocarcinoma is more likely to develop in the abnormal ductal tissue.
   2. The other complications of anastomosis are stricture formation and cholangitis.

OPERATIVE SURGERY

In this part of oral examination, questions are asked about some common operations. One operation is allotted to each candidate by lottery.

Sometimes the examiner may ask about the operation which the candidate has done himself during residentship, or which he knows the best. The senior author was asked to select the operation in this way and he selected cholecystectomy.

Questioning

The questions which may be asked are:
- What is done in this operation?
- What are the indications?

- What is the nature of anesthesia?
- What is the position of the patient on operating table?
- Describe the incision.
- What are the essential steps of operation?
- What are the points when one must be extra careful? (for example during separation of portal vein from the neck of pancreas during pancreatico-duodenectomy).
- What are the complications of this operation?

Operations

- Lymph node biopsy, vasectomy, eversion of sac, suprapubic cystostomy, circumcision, exposure of kidney.
- Excision of sebaceous cyst, subcutaneous neurofibroma, lipoma.
- Inguinal herniotomy in children, Should ice operation, Mayo's double breasting for a paraumbilical hernia, umbilical herniorrhaphy.
- Appendicectomy, closure of perforation of peptic ulcer, gastrojejunostomy, ileostomy, colostomy, opening the abdomen by a right paramedian incision or McBurney's incision.
- Tracheostomy, cholecystectomy, hemorrhoidectomy, internal sphincterotomy for anal fissure, fistulotomy, excision of a rectal polyp.
- Cystoscopy, gastroscopy and laparoscopy.

An Example of Viva on Operative Surgery

Suprapubic cystostomy is the operation allotted to the candidate by lottery.

Viva Voce

1. **What do you do in this operation?**
   In this operation, the urinary bladder is opened and kept opened for some time by keeping a suprapubic catheter.
2. **What is cystotomy?**
   It is the opening the bladder, doing the job inside the bladder (e.g. removing a stone, or foreign body) and closing it afterwards.

3. **What are the indications?**
   Suprapubic cystostomy is indicated:
   - For removing bladder stones which cannot be removed by litholapaxy or percutaneous method
   - For relieving acute retention of urine when a catheter cannot be passed per urethra
   - For removing a very large prostate which cannot be resected transurethrally
   - For removing a bladder diverticulum and foreign bodies in the bladder.
4. **What is the anesthesia used?**
   This operation can be done in general, spinal or local anesthesia.
5. **What is the incision used?**
   - It is usually done by a vertical midline suprapubic incision (Fig. 4)
   - It can be done by a transverse incision.
6. **Describe the steps of operation.**
   - The patient lies supine with a pillow behind the sacrum
   - If the bladder is not full, it is filled by a urethral catheter with sterile fluid or saline
   - The incision divides skin, subcutaneous tissue and rectus sheath. The rectus and pyramidalis muscles are retracted laterally on each side
   - The distended bladder and the peritoneum covering its upper part are recognized
   - The peritoneum is stripped by blunt dissection and retracted upwards
   - The bladder is held steady by two stay sutures on either side of midline and then opened by a stab taking care not to puncture its posterior wall. The leaking urine or fluid is sucked
   - The bladder incision is extended by a pair of scissors as required
   - The interior of the bladder is examined including the internal urinary meatus
   - The procedure inside the bladder is done, e.g. stones are removed or enlarged prostate is enucleated

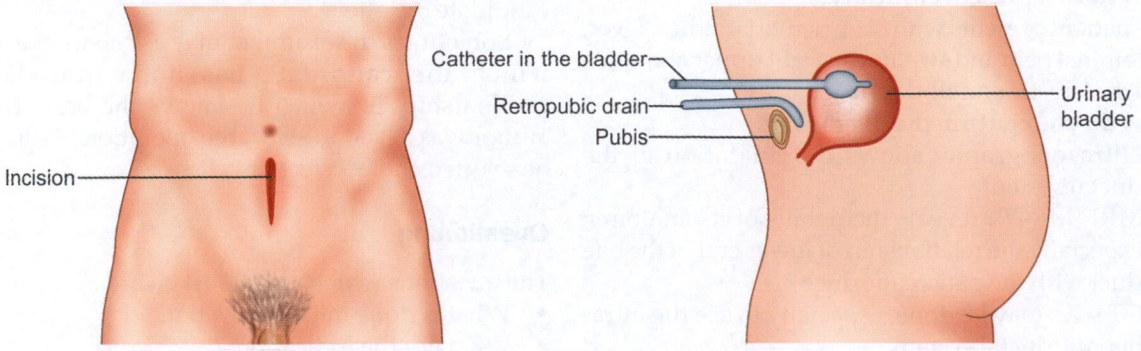

Fig. 4: Suprapubic cystostomy

- The bleeding is controlled and the bladder is washed clean
- A suprapubic self-retaining catheter is put in the bladder and the bladder is closed in 2 layers by continuous absorbable sutures around the catheter.
- A drain is left in the retropubic space of Retzius, and the parietal wound is closed in 3 layers—rectus sheath, subcutaneous tissue and skin.
- The catheter is connected to urine collecting bag.

7. **How do you recognize the bladder?**
The bladder is recognized by its globular feel, longitudinal muscle fibers and large veins of its surface.

8. **How will you confirm the presence of urinary bladder?**
It can be confirmed by needle aspiration when the urine or distending fluid comes out in the syringe.

9. **How will you know that the peritoneum is opened?**
It is recognized by omentum or small bowel peeping through the wound.

10. **What will you do if the peritoneum is opened?**
It is closed by suturing before proceeding further with the operation.

11. **What are the complications of this operation?**
The complications are—bleeding, bowel injury, vesico-cutaneous fistula and low fixation of bladder. When the steps are described, they are described in the third person, passive voice, e.g. an upper abdominal midline incision is given and the abdomen is opened.

SURGICAL INSTRUMENTS

During surgical procedures a large number of instruments are used. Some commonly used instruments are kept in the examination. Usually three instruments are given to each candidate and the following questions are asked:
- What is the name of this instrument?
- What are the important structural features?
- What are its uses?
- How will you sterilize it?
With the last question, many questions may be asked on sterilization.

Viva on a Straight Hemostat

1. **What is the name of this instrument?**
Straight hemostat (Fig. 5)

2. **What are the main structural features?**
- It has two limbs joined together by a joint where the limbs cross each other

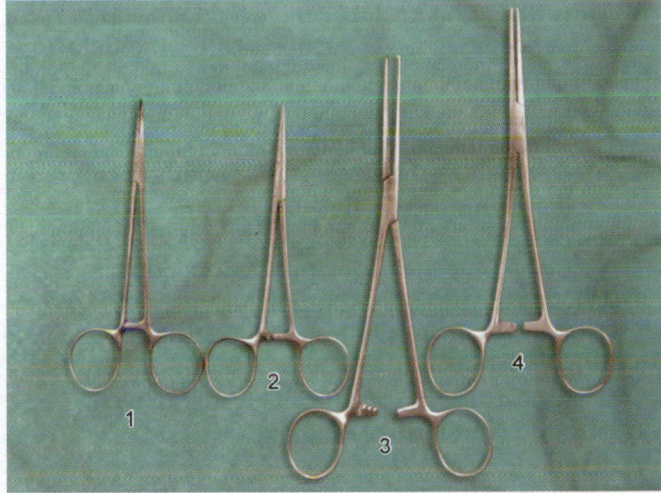

1. Needle holder (for comparison)
2. Straight hemostat
3. Kocher's hemostat
4. Large straight hemostat

Fig. 5: Needle holder and some straight hemostats

- The part proximal to the joint (handles) have a ratchet for locking the instrument in closed position
- The part distal to the joint have two jaws or blades having serrations for slipless grip.

3. **What are its uses?**
The uses are:
- For catching bleeding points or vessels
- For catching a vessel before it is divided and ligated
- For holding cut edges of fascia, sheaths, stay sutures and small round swabs (peanuts) for dissection
- As a substitute for other instruments for example needle holder, dressing forceps
- For clamping various tubes and catheters.

4. **How do you differentiate if from a needle holder?**
A needle holder is a heavier and stronger instrument with small jaws having grooves and serrations for a firm grip on a stitching needle.

5. **How do you differentiate it from a sinus forceps?**
A sinus forceps has olivary tipped jaws with a few serrations and no ratchet at the handle.

6. **Why is it called a hemostat?**
It is called hemostat as most commonly it is used for controlling bleeding (hemostasis) by catching divided vessels or for preventing bleeding by catching a vessel before division.

7. **What is an artery forceps?**
A hemostat is also called artery forceps as it is used to catch divided arteries or arterial bleeding points.

8. **How does a hemostat achieve hemostasis?**
   A hemostat achieves hemostasis by the following mechanisms:
   - Compression of bleeding point or vessel in the jaws of the instrument
   - By crushing the vessel wall resulting in curling of the intima to plug the lumen
   - By helping in electrocoagulation of small bleeders'
   - By helping in ligation of bleeding points.

9. **What is the purpose of serrations inside the jaws?**
   They are there for slipless grip of the bleeding point.

10. **What are the disadvantages of serrations?**
    They obstruct the cleaning of the instrument.

11. **How do you sterilize it?**
    It is done by autoclaving.

12. **How do you autoclave the instruments?**
    They are put in an autoclave in a drum and treated by steam at 15 pounds pressure at 120°C for half an hour.

13. **Why do you not sterilize it by boiling?**
    - The boiling does not kill the spores of bacteria.
    - It leads to deposition of salt dissolved in water on the surface of instruments.

SURGICAL ANATOMY

- Bones are kept for asking some simple questions, marking common fractures, some important attachments are relations.
- Skull—foramina and what passes through them, signs of fracture of various cranial fossae
- Questions about the surgical anatomy of the operative procedure allotted, for example boundaries of Callot's triangle if cholecystectomy is allotted, branches of facial nerve if parotidectomy is being discussed.

  It is not viva on pure anatomy, but on SURGICAL ANATOMY. Only simple questions are asked. Hence, the candidate need not be nervous.

Index